Fundamentals of

Assessment and Care Planning for Nurses

Fundamentals of

Assessment and Care Planning for Nurses

IAN PEATE, OBE, FRCN

Head of School, School of Health Studies
Visiting Professor of Nursing, St George's University of London,
Kingston University London
Editor in Chief, British Journal of Nursing
Visiting Senior Clinical Fellow, University of Hertfordshire
University of Gibraltar

WILEY Blackwell

Registered Office(s)
John Wiley & Sons, Inc., 111 River Street, Hoboken, NJ 07030, USA
John Wiley & Sons Ltd, The Atrium, Southern Gate, Chichester, West Sussex, PO19 8SQ, UK

Editorial Office
9600 Garsington Road, Oxford, OX4 2DQ, UK

For details of our global editorial offices, customer services, and more information about Wiley products visit us at www.wiley.com.

Wiley also publishes its books in a variety of electronic formats and by print-on-demand. Some content that appears in standard print versions of this book may not be available in other formats.

Library of Congress Cataloging-in-Publication Data

Names: Peate, Ian, author.
Title: Fundamentals of assessment and care planning for nurses / Ian Peate.
Description: Hoboken, NJ : John Wiley & Sons, Inc., 2020. | Includes
    bibliographical references and index. |
Identifiers: LCCN 2019019196 (print) | LCCN 2019021655 (ebook) | ISBN
    9781119491767 (Adobe PDF) | ISBN 9781119491743 (ePub) | ISBN 9781119491750
    (pbk.)
Subjects: | MESH: Nursing Assessment | Patient Care Planning
Classification: LCC RT48 (ebook) | LCC RT48 (print) | NLM WY 100.4 | DDC
    616.07/5–dc23
LC record available at https://lccn.loc.gov/2019019196

Cover Design: Wiley
Cover Images: © T VECTOR ICONS/Shutterstock, © matsabe/ Shutterstock, © Ben Davis/Shutterstock, © Toko Icon/Shutterstock, © Crispyicon/iStockphoto, © dem10/Getty Images

Set in 9/11pt Myriad by SPi Global, Pondicherry, India
Printed and bound in Singapore by Markono Print Media Pte Ltd

10 9 8 7 6 5 4 3 2 1

Contents

Contents

vi

Preface

The *Fundamentals of Assessment and Care Planning for Nurses* has been written to help develop the assessment and care planning skills of the nurse. In order to assess needs effectively in a patient-centred way the nurse is required to have a detailed understanding of the nursing process and the skills needed to plan care that is individual and holistic. Assessment and care planning are set against a backdrop of a dynamic and changing nursing profession as well as how contemporary care is being provided (Chapters 1 and 2).

The initial nursing assessment, the first step in the five steps of the nursing process, demands the systematic and continuous collection of data. Chapter 4 provides details concerning the systematic, cyclical nature of the nursing process. The nurse is required to systematically organise and analyse the data that has been gathered. Once primary and secondary data have been gathered there is a need to document and communicate findings in a care plan (Chapter 5) so that care can be delivered in response to an individual's unique sociocultural and physical needs, incorporating evidence-based practice.

Using the nursing process effectively demands the application of critical thinking skills that have been applied during the various phases of the nursing process. Critical thinking skills and the decision-making process feature in Chapter 3. The nursing process is a decision-making framework that helps the nurse work with the patient where appropriate. The use of a nursing model (Chapter 6) can help develop and steer the plan of care.

During nursing assessment information is gathered regarding the patient's individual physiological, psychological, sociological, and spiritual needs. This phase is the first phase required for the successful evaluation of care interventions. Working in partnership with the patient, the nurse collects subjective and objective data throughout the nursing process, the skills needed to do this are outlined in Chapter 7.

The *Fundamentals of Assessment and Care Planning for Nurses* discusses the general and focussed assessment of needs in relation to the body systems. There are a variety of assessment tools that are available to help the nurse in the assessment phase (see Chapter 8).

The first eight chapters of *Fundamentals of Assessment and Care Planning for Nurses* provide the foundations needed to be able to assess, make a diagnosis, plan care, implement that care, and devise strategies to evaluate outcomes. The nature of nursing offers insight into contemporary health and social care provision. Emphasis is placed on how care provision is dynamic and the voice of the service user is the key driver in how nurses and care providers respond to needs.

Key to understanding the primary and secondary source data that has been collected when assessing needs is the application of critical thinking and clinical decision making in order to formulate a plan of care. The skills and attributes of a critical thinker are outlined as the nurse applies the five phases of the nursing process and the planning of individual care plans using a model of nursing to steer and guide data collection.

The initial nursing assessment is a key component of nursing practice, it begins the nursing process. The use of assessment tools can, when appropriate and when utilised correctly, yield objective data, this is then used to implement care and evaluate impact. There are many assessment tools available and their content varies, they aim to help the nurse provide safe and evidence-based care. Assessment tools are described in Chapter 8.

The Nursing and Midwifery Council's (NMC) (2018a) Code is clear when it states that the nurse must ensure that people's physical, social, and psychological needs are assessed and responded to. In order to demonstrate compliance with this clause the nurse must undertake a comprehensive and systematic nursing assessment, plan nursing care in partnership with the patient and respond in an effective way to changing needs and changing situations.

There are 12 chapters of *Fundamentals of Assessment and Care Planning for Nurses* dedicated to the assessment of body systems. Each of these chapters begin with a discussion of the anatomy and physiology of the body system. Within these chapters the reader is provided with information and understanding associated with the gathering of subjective and objective data as the nurse conducts a health history interview and performs a physical examination. A practical approach is adopted, urging the nurse to learn the art and science associated with assessment to develop and hone their skills.

This text is timely as the NMC introduces its new Standards of Proficiency for Nurses (NMC 2018b). The proficiencies specify the knowledge and skills that registered nurses must demonstrate when caring for people, these are the proficiencies that the nurse must have met prior to being allowed entry on to the professional register as they gain their licence to practise. Within these new standards, platforms three and four focus on assessing needs and planning care; and providing and evaluating care (respectively).

Those who provide nurse education are required to develop and deliver programmes that give nurses the skills, knowledge and behaviours they need. The NMC's new Standards for Pre-registration Nursing set out how they must do this (NMC 2018c). The *Fundamentals of Assessment and Care Planning for Nurses* echo many of the requirements around assessing needs and planning care, providing and evaluating care.

There have been further developments in the profession as the NMC have also produced standards that outline the proficiencies for Nursing Associates (NMC 2018d) along with the Standards for Pre-registration Nursing Associate Programmes (NMC 2018e). The nursing associate is required to provide compassionate care and contribute to on-going assessment, recognising when needed to refer to others for reassessment.

Each chapter begins with an aim and learning outcomes, enabling the reader to contextualise and focus on the chapter content and the NMC proficiencies. The *Fundamentals of Assessment and Care Planning for Nurses* adopts a practical approach in order to facilitate learning, apply theory to practice, and encourage a person-centred approach, and to aid recall, a number of features and activities have been incorporated to assist with this. The book is fully illustrated throughout with clear artwork. There are a number of interactive learning features, encouraging the reader to review their learning, take note of key issues, and engage with the various elements associated with the 6Cs. Where appropriate the reader is drawn to cultural considerations where there are specific issues that have to be given due consideration. A fictitious family, the Samudas, is introduced to help link further the assessment of needs, focusing on the individual needs of a family member and the family unit. The chapters have several summary sections interspaced, enabling the reader to digest the bite-sized theory.

There are a number of mnemonics used throughout the book. Their inclusion is to assist and promote comprehensive history taking and a systematic, focused physical assessment. The mnemonics, however, should not be viewed simply as tick boxes, but rather as a way of triggering the nurse during history taking and examination addressing areas of importance.

I have very much enjoyed writing *Fundamentals of Assessment and Care Planning for Nurses*, it comes at an interesting time for nurses, the nursing profession, and those who work with us, as we are experiencing much change within and without the profession. My intention has been to help you understand, to apply what it is you are reading as you offer care to people (often the most vulnerable in society), to whet your appetite and inspire you to delve deeper and to stimulate curiosity, but most of all to ensure that the patient is truly at the heart of all you do.

References

Nursing and Midwifery Council (2018a). The Code. Professional standards of practice and behaviour for nurses, midwives and nursing associates. www.nmc.org.uk/globalassets/sitedocuments/nmc-publications/nmc-code.pdf last accessed October 2018.

Nursing and Midwifery Council (2018b). Standards of proficiency for registered nurses. www.nmc.org.uk/globalassets/sitedocuments/education-standards/future-nurse-proficiencies.pdf last accessed October 2018.

Nursing and Midwifery Council (2018c). Standards of pre-registration nursing programmes. www.nmc.org.uk/globalassets/sitedocuments/education-standards/programme-standards-nursing.pdf last accessed October 2018.

Nursing and Midwifery Council (2018d). Standards of proficiency for nursing associates. www.nmc.org.uk/globalassets/sitedocuments/education-standards/nursing-associates-proficiency-standards.pdf Last accessed October 2018.

Nursing and Midwifery Council (2018e). Standards for pre-registration nursing associate programmes. www.nmc.org.uk/globalassets/sitedocuments/education-standards/nursing-associates-programme-standards.pdf Last accessed October 2018.

Acknowledgements

I would like to thank my partner Jussi Lahtinen, who continues to encourage and support me. I acknowledge my gratitude to my friend Mrs Frances Cohen. I owe thanks to my brother Anthony Peate, who helped with the illustrations. Thank you to the library staff at Gibraltar Health Authority and the Royal College of Nursing. Special thanks to Magenta Styles at Wiley – your enthusiasm is palpable.

Meet the family

One of the features used in *Fundamentals of Assessment and Care Planning for Nurses* centres around a fictitious family, the Samudas (all names and details are fictional in accordance with the Nursing and Midwifery Council's (2018) Code). Inclusion of the family helps to provide context to the chapters that focus on assessment of the body systems. In each of these chapters a family member is discussed and the reader is encouraged to consider that individual family member's needs as well as how their condition may impact on the family unit.

The Samuda family live in a small town on the South West coast, all within walking distance of each other apart from Howard, who lives in Norwich. The Samudas live in a housing complex in Welltown south of the river. They own a four-bedroomed semi-detached house.

You will meet various members of the Samuda family in several chapters of the book. There are nine members of the Samuda family, take some time to get to know them (see the genogram in Figure 1).

Ruby Coleman 70 years old (grandmother). Ruby lives in the same street as the Samuda family and offers her daughter support with the family when she can. Ruby is a member of the local bridge club and enjoys watching the soaps. She enjoys baking.

Bob Coleman, 74 years old (grandfather). Bob lives in the same street as the Samuda family. Bob meets up with his mates, with whom he worked on the railway. He finds getting around a little more difficult now as he has been getting 'caught short' once too often lately.

Shahine Samuda Mother: 39 years old, part-time ward clerk. Shahine spends most her time when not working looking after the family. She likes to swim. Shahine and her best friend Marie also like to dance, they are learning to salsa.

Maurice Samuda Father: 44 years old, is a full-time civil servant. Maurice spends most his free time fixing up old motor bikes in his shed, he gets little physical exercise. He is overweight, smokes 60 cigarettes a week. Maurice drinks alcohol to excess.

Howard Samuda Son: 23 years old, works full time in a law firm. Howard lives in Norwich, left home six years ago after a disagreement with his father. He keeps in touch with the family via Kam. Howard is an avid traveller and is studying part-time for a Master's degree in Law.

Kamina (Kam) Samuda Daughter: 17 years old, student at Goodenough School and is about to undergo her A levels. Kam has found being at home recently a little overwhelming at times; she tends to spend her time at her boyfriend's house, where she says it is much a calmer. Kam wants to go to university and study electrical engineering; she is studying hard at school.

Oswald (Ossie) Samuda Son: 13 years old with special needs, student also attending Goodenough School. Ossie is the youngest child. He uses a wheelchair for mobility and he has a special education needs teacher who supports him at school. Shahine is Ossie's main carer. Ossie enjoys swimming and playing on his PlayStation.

Judith Higgins (Daughter of Ruby and Bob): 45 years old (Aunty Judy). Judith lives in close proximity to the Samudas and the Colemans. Judy has not worked for the last five years. Judy and her husband Winston are close to the family. They have no children. However, her niece, Shahine, has expressed concerns about Judith's cognitive state.

Winston Higgins (Son in law of Ruby and Bob): 43 years (Uncle Winston). Winston lives in close proximity to the Samudas and the Colemans. He enjoys cycling and hiking in the highlands whenever he can get a chance, he is a postman. Winston lives with Judith. He is becoming more and more a key carer of Judith, who he says has become very short-tempered and even more forgetful.

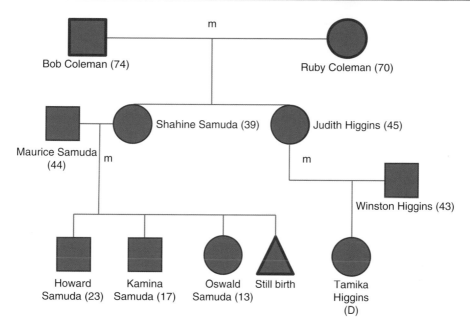

Figure 1 Genogram.

Reference

Nursing and Midwifery Council (2018) The Code. Professional standards of practice for nurses, midwives and nursing associates. www.nmc.org.uk/globalassets/sitedocuments/nmc-publications/nmc-code.pdf last accessed October 2018.

Chapter 1

The nature of nursing

Aim

The aim of this chapter is to introduce the reader to the nature of nursing and offer an overview of how care is offered.

Learning outcomes

By the end of the chapter the reader will be able to:

1. Provide a timeline outlining key points in the development of contemporary nursing practice
2. Identify how care provision over the years has impacted on contemporary practice
3. Discuss how the NHS was formed and its current role in the provision of health and social care
4. Consider local, national, and international care perspectives

Introduction

The past is where lessons have been learnt and the future is where those lessons learnt are applied. However, living in the past can hinder progress. In an unidentified source, 'you cannot tell where you are going unless you know where you have been' is the key theme of this chapter. Much is to be learnt from the past in order to help us in the future, to learn from our mistakes and to help us and the services we provide to develop in an appropriate and patient-centred manner.

Before the mid-nineteenth century, nurses, whether employed in hospitals or in private homes, were very often uneducated and usually had no formal training. In Britain in the 1840s nursing sisterhoods were founded to improve standards of nursing, these mimicked the Catholic nursing orders in other European countries. St John's House, an Anglican Nursing Sisterhood founded in 1848, was one example of these. As a thank-you to Florence Nightingale for her accomplishments during the 1854–1856 Crimean War, a fund was raised by public donations to allow her to establish a training school for nurses in London, the Nightingale School set up at St Thomas' Hospital in 1860. Other hospitals, both voluntary hospitals and workhouse infirmaries, formed their own training schools, and many of these were run by superintendents who had trained at the Nightingale School. Nightingale based her curriculum on the following beliefs:

- Nutrition is an important part of nursing care.
- Fresh, clean air is beneficial to the sick.
- Sick people require occupational and recreational therapy.
- Nurses should help identify and meet patients' personal needs and these include the provision of emotional support.

Fundamentals of Assessment and Care Planning for Nurses, First Edition. Ian Peate.
© 2020 John Wiley & Sons Ltd. Published 2020 by John Wiley & Sons Ltd.

- Nursing should be directed towards two conditions: health and illness.
- Nursing is separate and distinct from the practice of medicine and as such should be taught by nurses.
- Nurses need continuing education.

Review

Think about the list of Nightingale's beliefs (those that were a part of her nursing curriculum) and reflect on the course or programme of study you are enlisted on and determine if these beliefs are still the foundation of nursing education today.

Provision was also provided to train district nurses to care for the sick and poor in their own homes, and in 1887 the Queen's Institute of District Nursing was founded.

The 1919 Nurses Registration Act set up the General Nursing Council, which was charged with maintaining a register of nurses to ensure that in future all nurses were appropriately trained. As a result of a shortage of nurses, the Nurses Act established in 1943 provided a roll of assistant nurses.

In 1930 county councils took over the workhouse infirmaries from the Boards of Guardians and the London County Council also acquired all the hospitals that had been previously managed by the Metropolitan Asylums Board. Most hospitals and mental institutions in 1948 passed to the National Health Service (NHS), with the majority of them becoming the responsibility of the regional hospital boards. Four boards assumed responsibility in London and the South East, as well as the North East, North West, South East, and South West Metropolitan Hospital Boards. In each hospital region an Area Nurse Training Committee was established, with the aims of financing, advising and improving all nurse training institutions in the region.

County councils became responsible for district nursing as well as for other personal health services in 1948. All health services were transferred to the newly formed regional and area health authorities in 1974, replacing the regional hospital boards, and in 1982 area health authorities were abolished. There have been numerous other reorganisations that have followed.

The National Health Service

The NHS is over 70 years old, and the NHS and those people it offers a service to today are very different now than in 1948 when it was born. This difference between then and now must be taken into account in any discussion that includes contemporary service provision. Today Britain has become a wealthier society, it is more socially and morally liberal and as a result of this, public expectations have changed considerably. However, the impact that social and economic changes have had on society have been uneven, and there are inequalities.

The NHS was created out of the notion that good healthcare should be available to all, irrespective of wealth. When the NHS was launched on 5 July 1948, it was based on three core principles, that it:

1. Meets the needs of everyone
2. Be free at the point of delivery
3. Be based on clinical need, not ability to pay

(the National Health Service Act – see figure 1.1).

These three principles are still very apparent today, they continue to guide the development of the NHS and remain at its centre. The NHS is the largest employer in the UK, there are roughly 1.5 million people employed by the NHS across the UK. By country:

- In England 1.2 million
- In Scotland 162 000
- In Wales 89 000
- In Northern Ireland (NI) 64 000

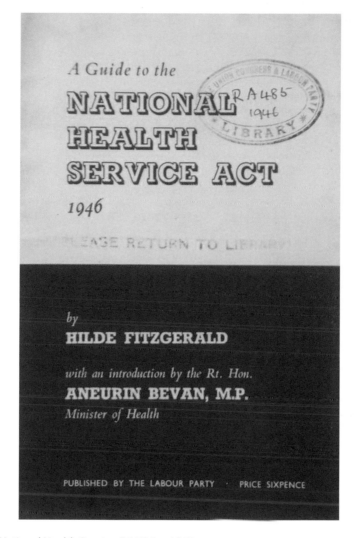

Figure 1.1   The National Health Service (NHS) Act 1946.

This data does not include everyone working in the health sector. They leave out some people, for example temporary staff, GPs, dentists, optometrists, and other staff in the independent sector or private hospitals (Full Fact 2017).

In England, around 824 000 clinical staff (those directly involved in patient care) work in the NHS, including 141 000 doctors and 329 000 nurses, midwives and health visitors (National Audit Office 2016).

So far

The NHS was launched in 1948. It was born out of a long-held ideal that good healthcare should be available to all, regardless of wealth. The NHS provides healthcare for all UK citizens based on their need for healthcare as opposed to their ability to pay for it. It is funded by taxes.

The NHS is the largest employer in the UK – there are around 1.5 million people employed by the NHS across the UK.

Department of Health and Social Care

The purpose of the Department of Health (DH) is to help people live better for longer, the DH shapes and funds health and care in England, ensuring that people have the support, care and treatment they require, with the compassion, respect and dignity that they deserve. The dynamic and changing health and care organisations work together with the DH to achieve this common purpose. In 2018 the Department of Health became the Department of Health and Social Care (DHSC).

The DH facilitates health and social care bodies to deliver services according to national priorities, working with other parts of government to achieve this and setting objectives and budgets and holding the system to account on behalf of the Secretary of State for Health. Ultimate responsibility for ensuring that the whole system works together to meet the needs of patients and the public sits with the Secretary of State for Health. Figure 1.2 provides a visual overview of the DH.

NHS England

NHS England assists NHS services nationally ensuring that money spent on NHS services provides the best possible care for patients. It funds local clinical commissioning groups (CCGs) to commission services for their communities and ensures that they do this effectively. NHS England brings together expertise to ensure that national standards are consistently in place across the country. Throughout its work it promotes the NHS Constitution and the Constitution's values and commitments.

Clinical commissioning groups

These are clinically led statutory NHS bodies responsible for the planning and commissioning of healthcare services for their local area. Membership of CCGs includes nurses and other clinicians, such as GPs and consultants. They are responsible for approximately 60% of the NHS budget and commission the majority of secondary care services as well as playing a part in the commissioning of GP services.

Health and wellbeing boards

Health and wellbeing boards (HWBs) were established by local authorities to act as a forum for local commissioners across the NHS, social care, public health, and other services. The aims of the HWBs are to increase democratic input into strategic decisions about health and wellbeing services and strengthen working relationships between health and social care.

Public Health England

Public Health England (PHE) provides national leadership and expert services to support public health and works with local government and the NHS to respond to emergencies.

Vanguards

These were introduced in 2015. Fifty chosen vanguards are required to develop new care models and potentially redesign the health and care system. It is intended that this could lead to better patient care and service access, and a more simplified system.

Regulation and safeguarding people's interests

Responsibility for regulating particular aspects of care is shared across a number of different bodies, for example:

- The Care Quality Commission (CQC)
- NHS Improvement is an umbrella organisation bringing together a number of other organisations
- Individual professional regulatory bodies, that include the Nursing and Midwifery Council (NMC), the General Medical Council, the General Dental Council and the Health Care Professions Council

The health & care system from April 2013

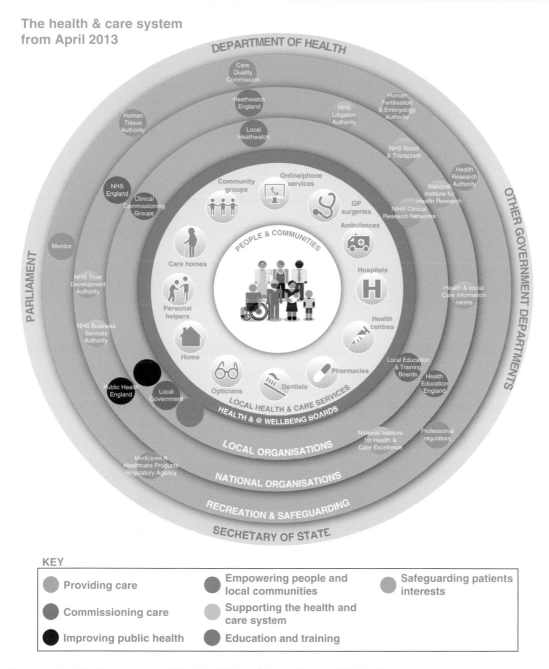

KEY

- ● Providing care
- ● Commissioning care
- ● Improving public health
- ● Empowering people and local communities
- ● Supporting the health and care system
- ● Education and training
- ● Safeguarding patients interests

Figure 1.2   The Department of Health (DH) explained. Source: DH (2013) (permission open government licence: www.nationalarchives.gov.uk/doc/open-government-licence/version/3).

The health care system in Scotland

Scotland's NHS operates under separate management, administration and political authority since devolution in 1999. Budgets for each branch of government spending, including the NHS, are determined not by Westminster but by the Scottish government, which decides how to split its block grant between public services.

The responsibility for delivering health services is mainly devolved to the health boards. There are 14 territorial health boards, which arrange services for their local population, and there are seven special health boards which provide a specific service for the whole of Scotland. Since the 1st April

2016, territorial health boards and local authorities have integrated certain health and social care services with the creation of 31 integration authorities.

Health boards are accountable to Scottish Ministers and ultimately to the Scottish Parliament. They are held to account through a number of measures such as Local Delivery Plan standards and annual accountability reviews.

The health care system in Wales

NHS Wales is the publicly funded national healthcare service of Wales, providing healthcare to around three million people who live in the country.

The NHS Wales provides services through seven Health Boards and three NHS Trusts in Wales. Primary care services are provided by GPs, nurses, and other health care professionals in health centres and surgeries across Wales. Secondary care is delivered through hospital and ambulance services and tertiary care is provided by hospitals, treating people with particular types of illness such as cancer. Community care services are usually provided in partnership with local social services and delivered to patients in their own homes.

The health care system in Northern Ireland

The DH sets the policy and legislative context for health and social care in NI. An annual Commissioning Plan Direction sets out ministerial priorities, key outcomes and objectives, and related performance indicators.

The Health and Social Care Board (HSCB), in conjunction with the Public Health Agency (PHA), then produces a Commissioning Plan.

Commissioning is about securing and monitoring health and social care services for the population of NI. The variety and complexity of the services provided is huge, with some local services being designed and secured for a population of a few thousand and for rare disorders, services need to be considered regionally or even nationally. NI's approach to integrated governance for health and social care sets it apart from other UK jurisdictions.

So far

Since devolution in 1998, the UK has had four increasingly distinct health systems, in England, Northern Ireland, Scotland, and Wales. The key tenets of the NHS, free at the point of need, still feature in all four countries.

Review

Consider health and social care provision in the country where you are working. Analyse the pros and cons of a devolved health and social care provision for the people you offer care and support to and yourself.

The NHS Constitution

The NHS Constitution (DH 2015) establishes the principles and values of the NHS in England, setting out rights to which patients, public, and staff are entitled and pledges which the NHS is committed to achieve, along with responsibilities, which the public, patients, and staff owe to one another, ensuring that the NHS operates fairly and effectively. The Secretary of State for Health, all NHS bodies, private and voluntary sector providers supplying the NHS with services, and local authorities in the exercise of their public health functions have to by law take account of the Constitution in their decisions and actions.

Box 1.1 The seven key principles

1. The NHS provides a comprehensive service, available to all.
2. Access to NHS services is based on clinical need, not an individual's ability to pay.
3. The NHS aspires to the highest standards of excellence and professionalism.
4. The patient will be at the heart of everything the NHS does.
5. The NHS works across organisational boundaries.
6. The NHS is committed to providing best value for taxpayers' money.
7. The NHS is accountable to the public, communities and patients that it serves.

Source: DH (2015).

Box 1.2 The six values

1. Working together for patients
2. Respect and dignity
3. Commitment to quality of care
4. Compassion
5. Improving lives
6. Everyone counts

Source: DH (2015).

The seven key principles guide the NHS in all it does. They are underpinned by core NHS values, derived from extensive discussions with staff, patients, and the public (see Box 1.1).

The key principles are underpinned by six values (see Box 1.2). The NHS values provide common ground for cooperation to achieve shared aspirations, at all levels of the NHS.

For the first time in the history of the NHS, the NHS Constitution brings together details of what staff, patients and the public can expect from our NHS. The Constitution also explains what patients can do to help support the NHS, help it work effectively and help in ensuring that resources are used responsibly.

Review

The Code (NMC 2018) requires you to keep to the laws of the country in which you are practising. What does this mean and how can you ensure that you adhere to this clause?

Nursing

What is nursing? This is a complex question. It is also difficult to answer because nursing is dynamic, it is evolving and is a comparatively new profession. It is not easy to define nursing because the concept is as complex as its numerous activities. According to Nightingale (1859):

> Nature alone cures… And what nursing has to do…is to put the patient in the best condition for nature to act upon him.

This is a classic definition of nursing with an emphasis on the promotion of health and healing as opposed to a cure of illness, the definition has a focus on the interconnected triumvirate (see Figure 1.3).

All three of Nightingale's features are still central to modern definitions of nursing.

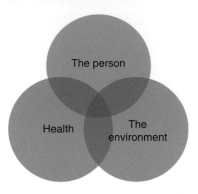

Figure 1.3   The triad.

Review

How would you define nursing? Write down your definition. Ask some others about their definition of nursing: do their definitions match yours? What are the similarities, if any?

There are a number of definitions of nursing available. Virginia Henderson (1960), for example, stated that the purpose of nursing is:

To assist the individual, sick or well, in the performance of those activities contributing to health or its recovery (or to a peaceful death) that he would perform unaided if he had the necessary strength, will, or knowledge and to do this in such a way as to help him gain independence as rapidly as possible.

The Royal College of Nursing (RCN 2014) defines nursing as:

The use of clinical judgement in the provision of care to enable people to improve, maintain, or recover health, to cope with health problems, and to achieve the best possible quality of life, whatever their disease or disability, until death.

The RCN's definition is supported by six defining characteristics (see Table 1.1 and Figure 1.4).
Wild (2018) notes that the RCNs definition draws on what are seen as the purposes of nursing, they are:

- To promote and sustain health
- To care for those whose health has been compromised
- To aid in the recovery process
- To facilitate independence
- To meet needs
- To improve/maintain wellbeing/quality of life.

Review

Compare your earlier definition of nursing with Henderson's 1960 definition and the RCN's 2014 definition. In your own description of nursing, can you identify what Wild (2018) refers to as the purposes of nursing?

So far

The ability to define nursing and what nurses do is elusive, and this may be a good thing as what it is nurses do will (or should) be determined by the unique needs of the person receiving care. There are a number of definitions of nursing available; some may be of use and others may not.

The 6Cs of nursing

The 6Cs of nursing represent the professional commitment to always deliver exceptional care. Each value is equal, no one is more important than the other. Each of them focuses on putting the person who is being cared for at the heart of the care that they are given. See Table 1.2 for an overview of the 6Cs.

The code

Nurses are required to adhere to the principles of a Code of Conduct. The Code (NMC 2018) presents the professional standards that all nurses, midwives and nursing associates have to uphold if they wish to be registered to practise in the UK.

Table 1.1　The RCN's six defining characteristics.

Defining characteristic	Definition
One	A particular purpose: the purpose of nursing is to promote health, healing, growth and development and to prevent disease, illness, injury, and disability. The purpose of nursing when people become ill or disabled is to minimise distress and suffering and to enable people to understand and cope with their disease or disability, its treatment, and its consequences. In death, the purpose of nursing is to maintain the best possible quality of life until its end.
Two	A particular mode of intervention: nursing interventions are concerned with empowering people, helping them to achieve, maintain, or recover their independence. Nursing is an intellectual, physical, emotional, and moral process which includes the identification of nursing needs; therapeutic interventions and personal care; information, education, advice, and advocacy; and physical, emotional, and spiritual support. In addition to direct patient care, nursing practice includes management, teaching, and the development of knowledge and policy.
Three	A particular domain: the specific domain of nursing is people's unique responses to and experience of health, illness, frailty, disability, and health-related life events in whatever environment or circumstances they find themselves. Responses may be physiological, psychological, social, cultural, or spiritual, and often they are a combination of all of these. This includes people of all ages, families, and communities, throughout the life span.
Four	A particular focus: the emphasis of nursing is the whole person and the human response as opposed to a particular aspect of the person or a particular pathological condition.
Five	A particular value base: nursing is based on ethical values; these respect the dignity, autonomy and uniqueness of human beings, the privileged nurse–patient relationship and the acceptance of personal accountability for any actions and omissions.
Six	A commitment to partnership: nurses work in partnership with patients, their relatives, and other carers, and in collaboration with others as members of a multidisciplinary team. Where appropriate they will lead the team, prescribing, delegating, and supervising the work of others; at other times they will participate under the leadership of others. At all times, however, they remain personally and professionally accountable for their own decisions and actions.

Source: Adapted RCN (2014).

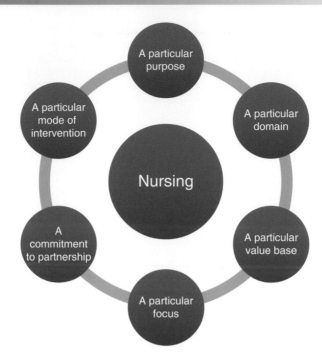

Figure 1.4 The six defining characteristics and the how they inform and support the definition of nursing. Source: RCN (2014).

Table 1.2 The 6 Cs.

Care	Care is our core business and that of our organisations, and the care we deliver helps the individual person and improves the health of the whole community. Caring defines us and our work. People receiving care expect it to be right for them, consistently, throughout every stage of their life.
Compassion	Compassion is how care is given through relationships based on empathy, respect and dignity – it can also be described as intelligent kindness, and is central to how people perceive their care.
Competence	Competence means all those in caring roles must have the ability to understand an individual's health and social needs and the expertise, clinical, and technical knowledge to deliver effective care and treatments based on research and evidence.
Communication	Communication is central to successful caring relationships and to effective team working. Listening is as important as what we say and do and essential for 'no decision about me without me'. Communication is the key to a good workplace with benefits for those in our care and staff alike.
Courage	Courage enables us to do the right thing for the people we care for, to speak up when we have concerns and to have the personal strength and vision to innovate and to embrace new ways of working.
Commitment	A commitment to our patients and populations is a cornerstone of what we do. We need to build on our commitment to improve the care and experience of our patients, to take action to make this vision and strategy a reality for all and meet the health, care and support challenges ahead.

Source: DH (2012).

If a nurse fails to comply with the Code, this could bring their fitness to practise into question. Within the Code are the professional standards that nurses must uphold. Whether the nurse is providing direct care to individuals, groups, or communities or bringing their professional knowledge to bear on nursing and midwifery practice in other roles, such as leadership, education, or research,

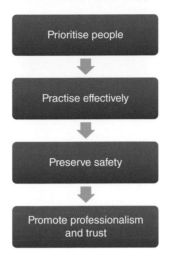

Figure 1.5   The four themes underpinning good nursing practice. Source: NMC (2018).

they must, at all times, act in line with the Code. The values and principles set out in the Code can be interpreted in a number of ways and in a range of practice settings. Regardless of this, the principles are not negotiable or discretionary.

There are four themes within the Code. When used together they signify good nursing practice (see Figure 1.5).

The Code provides a focuses on:

- Compassionate care – kindness, respect, and compassion
- Teamwork – working in cooperative way
- Record keeping – keep clear and accurate records
- Delegation and accountability – delegate responsibly, be accountable
- Raising concerns – reporting concerns immediately
- Cooperating with investigations and audits – includes those against individuals or organisations and acting as a witness at hearings

Take note

Delegation

- Only delegate tasks and duties that are within the other person's scope of competence, making sure that they fully understand your instructions.
- Make sure that everyone you delegate tasks to is adequately supervised and supported so they can provide safe and compassionate care.
- Confirm that the outcome of any task you have delegated to someone else meets the required standard.

Source: NMC (2018).

The term 'registered nurse' is a protected title. To become a registered nurse entails three years of education, as well as registration with the NMC, the regulatory body that can call to account and ultimately strike off those not adhering to the Code.

So far

The Code (NMC 2018) details the professional, ethical and moral standards nurses are required to uphold. Whilst the Code is not law, much of it derived from legislation. Nurses may be called to account for their actions or omissions and will be judged against the standards detailed in the Code. The nurse is first and foremost accountable to the patient, they must act in the patient's best interests at all times.

The role of the nurse

The role of the nurse has been expanded and extended in many ways over the years. As health care becomes more complex, so too must the ways in which care is delivered in order to meet the multi-faceted needs of those we offer care and support to. The contribution of nurses is key in ensuring that we meet twenty-first-century health care challenges. Regardless of the many advances that have been made in disease prevention and health promotion, there is still a need to offer people education and advice about healthy lifestyles and provide care for and assist people if and when they do become ill, disabled, or unable to care for themselves.

As health care systems become more complex, the economic, technical, and social factors that shape the nature of any health care experience will shape the nurses' role and function. Nurses are required to collaborate on the organisation of care with other members of the health care team (the multidisciplinary team) across systems and contexts of care and across the life span. They are seen as the pivot, the conductor conducting the orchestra, or the glue that holds an organisation together. See Figure 1.6 for some of the partnerships associated with the role of the nurse.

The fundamental role of the nurse is to provide services that promote health and wellbeing, encourage self-care and deliver personalised health outcomes which can be in a hospital, in the person's own home, in a local general practice, or in the community. These services have to be appropriately combined with social care and properly signposted so that, whether for urgent or more planned treatments, a full range of coordinated, high-quality, accessible, and well-understood services are in place for people to use and to use effectively.

As the role of the nurse expands (beyond the realms of the hospital and the NHS), there is an even greater need for a thorough knowledge of the nursing process and problem solving. The nursing process is a multi-step tool and process that uses assessment, diagnosis, planning, implementation, and evaluation to teach, learn, think, and reason about nursing care wherever this occurs. The nurse takes on the role of caregiver, educator, collaborator, advocate, leader, and manager.

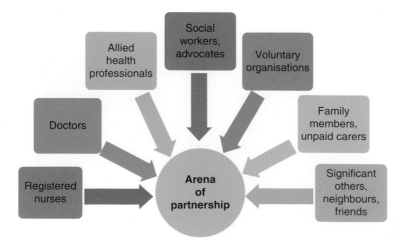

Figure 1.6   Partnerships.

Review

Write notes about the role of the nurse in relation to:

1. Caregiver
2. Educator
3. Collaborator
4. Advocate
5. Leader
6. Manager

Professionalism

The provision of safe and effective health care is very complex. Nurses make up the largest group of health care professionals, playing an especially important role within health and care delivery. Health care delivery represents a number of elements that when gathered together offer a description of the spirit of professional nursing practice.

The many roles that nurses play within health care delivery as well as the features required of professional nurses include the behaviours that nurses integrate into all patient care encounters, making every contact count. These include:

- Professionalism
- Clinical judgement
- Leadership
- Ethics
- Patient education
- Health promotion

Competence is another important consideration that is associated with professionalism, this refers to being competent or well-qualified to undertake and complete a skill or task. In order for the nurse to perform in a competent manner they must possess the appropriate knowledge, skills, and attributes that are essential for the provision of safe and effective care.

Nurses deliver health care in a variety of contexts using various approaches and models. The chosen model has to reflect the context of care, the client group, the healthcare infrastructure, and various philosophies.

So far

The role and function of the nurse is diverse and changes as the needs of the people they offer care to change. Nursing encompasses autonomous and collaborative care of people of all ages, families, groups, and communities, be they sick or well and in all settings. Nurses promote health, aim to prevent illness, and provide care and support to those who are ill and those who are dying. Nurses work in a number of large specialties, sometimes working independently and as part of a team to assess, diagnose, plan, implement, and evaluate care. At all times the patient is at the centre of all that the nurse does.

Technology and nursing

In our own lives we have become more and more digitally literate, using smart phones, utilising TV and news media, booking our holidays online or using home delivery supermarket services. When motivated to learn, we do. Many of the skills we use in our personal life can be easily transferred to our work lives, where we can use them in supporting the best outcomes for those people we offer care to.

Take note

Social media

If used correctly and appropriately, social networking sites may provide a number of benefits for nurses, midwives, and students. However, registration with the NMC may be jeopardised if a nurse acts in any way that is unprofessional or unlawful on social media, including (but not limited to):

- Sharing confidential information inappropriately
- Posting pictures of patients and people receiving care without their consent
- Posting inappropriate comments about patients
- Bullying, intimidating or exploiting people
- Building or pursuing relationships with patients or service users
- Stealing personal information or using someone else's identity
- Encouraging violence or self-harm
- Inciting hatred or discrimination

Source: NMC (2017).

The Royal College of Nursing (2017) defines eHealth (sometimes known as digital health) as concerned with promoting, empowering, and facilitating health and wellbeing with individuals, families, and communities and the enhancement of professional practice through the use of information management and information and communication technology (ICT). There is more to eHealth than just technology. It is about finding, using, recording, managing, and communicating information to support health care provision, in particular when decisions need to be made about patient care. Computers (and other ICT devices) are only the technology that enables this to occur.

The technological revolution and digitalisation are developing at tremendous speed. It will continue to impact on a number of aspects of people's lives, it also has the potential to change how nursing care is delivered creating opportunities for the population as well as those who provide. It can stimulate innovation and enable the nurse to work in different ways.

Review

Analyse the characteristics of the organisation where you work with respect to the technology used there.

Strengths	Weaknesses
Opportunities	Threats

In order for the nurse to get the most out of current and future digital and technological advances, they must be prepared to lead and to deliver this change, working together with patients and with other members of the multi-professional team. With the rapid pace of change in technologies that have been developed to support and improve individual care and outcomes, this means that everyone has to be ready to support and lead on change and innovation (Health Education England [HEE] n.d.).

Digitally-enabled, individual-centric care already occurs through the digital recording of high-quality data, improved information management, communication, and collaboration on care plans and real-time monitoring of a patient's journey. These digital innovations have led to less duplication of activity, a reduction in miscommunication, and enhanced patient safety.

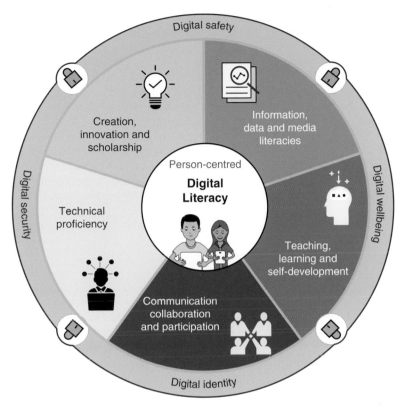

Figure 1.7   Digital literacy. Source: Health Education England (n.d.)).

Becoming or developing further as a digitally literate nurse involves developing a range of skills, as well as attitudes, values, and behaviours that can be categorised under the following domains (HEE n.d.) (see Figure 1.7):

- Digital identity, wellbeing, safety, and security
- Communication, collaboration, and participation
- Teaching, learning, and personal/professional development
- Technical proficiency
- Information, data, and media literacies
- Creation, innovation, and scholarship

Nurses will be coordinating care and supporting people navigating complex care environments. They ensure that services are patient-centred through collaboration with people about their preferences, alerting people to new options such as accessing social networks within their community.

Improving digital literacy throughout health and social care needs to be entrenched in organisations as well as individual nurses. The use of technology is not intended to be an additional responsibility or burden for the nurse, it should be seen as an enabler and supporter to providing improved individual care, reducing the administrative burden, helping people to have more control over their own health and wellbeing, and using the potential of technologies to close gaps in funding and efficiency as well as care provision, care quality, and safety.

Conclusion

The health and organisational challenges that the NHS is facing are not unlike those that are being faced by many national healthcare systems globally. Life expectancy has been increasing across the world and this has brought with it increases in chronic diseases and long-term conditions such as cancer and neurological disorders. Negative environment and lifestyle influences have generated a pandemic in obesity and associated conditions, for example diabetes and cardiovascular disease. Health inequalities still exist across the UK and are disturbingly increasing, with minority and ethnic groups experiencing most serious illnesses, premature death, and disability.

The focus, practice, and provision of healthcare services are being and will continue to be transformed from having traditionally offered treatment and supportive or palliative care to increasingly dealing with the management of long-term and chronic disease and rehabilitation regimens and providing disease prevention and health promotion interventions.

The use of technology is growing and will continue to grow. Nurses are the largest users and generators of information in clinical practice. Safe and effective patient care and nursing practice have always relied on the effective management of information. Nurses are increasingly relying on appropriate health information technology systems in order to ensure that communication is effective for meaningful collaboration, for monitoring and making decisions where the patient is at the centre of all that is done.

References

Department of Health (DH) (2012). Compassion in practice: Nursing, midwifery and care staff. Our vision and strategy. www.england.nhs.uk/wp-content/uploads/2012/12/compassion-in-practice.pdf (accessed December 2017)

Department of Health (DH) (2013). The health and care system explained. www.gov.uk/government/publications/the-health-and-care-system-explained/the-health-and-care-system-explained

Department of Health (DH) (2015). The NHS Constitution. The NHS belongs to us all. www.gov.uk/government/publications/the-nhs-constitution-for-england/the-nhs-constitution-for-england (accessed December 2017)

Full Fact (2017). How many NHS employees are there https://fullfact.org/health/how-many-nhs-employees-are-there (accessed December 2017)

Health Education England (HEE) (n.d.) Improving digital literacy. www.hee.nhs.uk/sites/default/files/documents/3146%20-HEE%20RCN%20Report%2016%20pages%20FINAL.pdf (accessed December 2017)

Henderson, V. (1960). *Basic Principles of Nursing Care*. London: International Council of Nurses.

National Audit Office (2016). Managing the supply of NHS clinical staff in England. www.nao.org.uk/wp-content/uploads/2016/02/Managing-the-supply-of-NHS-clinical-staff-in-England.pdf (accessed December 2017)

Nightingale, F. (1859). *Notes on Nursing: What it is and What it is Not*. London: Harrison.

Nursing and Midwifery Council (2018). The Code. Professional Standards of Practice and Behaviour for Nurses, Midwives and Nursing Associates. https://www.nmc.org.uk/globalassets/sitedocuments/nmc-publications/nmc-code.pdf last accessed 8 May 2019

Nursing and Midwifery Council (NMC) (2017). Guide on using social media responsibility. www.nmc.org.uk/globalassets/sitedocuments/nmc-publications/social-media-guidance.pdf (accessed December 2017)

Royal College of Nursing (RCN) (2014). Defining nursing. www.rcn.org.uk/professional-development/publications/pub-004768 (accessed December 2017)

Royal College of Nursing (RCN) (2017). What is eHealth. www.rcn.org.uk/clinical-topics/ehealth (accessed December 2017)

Wild, K. (2018). The professional nurse and contemporary health care. In: *Nursing Theory and Practice*, 2e (ed. I. Peate and K. Wild), 24–49. Oxford: Wiley.

Chapter 2

The provision of care

Aim

This chapter aims to introduce the reader to four key underpinning concepts concerning the provision of care: accountability, confidentiality, autonomy, and advocacy.

Learning outcomes

By the end of the chapter the reader will be able to:

1. Understand why those who provide and prescribe care are professionally and legally accountable for their actions and omissions
2. Discuss why confidentiality is seen as the cornerstone of care provision
3. Discuss the importance of encouraging autonomy when offering care and support to people
4. Consider ways in which the nurse can act as an advocate

Introduction

The provision of safe and effective care is based on a number of factors, with an overarching aim of doing the patient no harm. Nursing is a profession that is focused on collaborative relationships that promote the best possible outcomes for patients. The relationships may be interprofessional, involving a variety of health care professionals who are working together to deliver quality care within and across settings, or it can be intraprofessional, where nurses work with multiple members of the same profession as they deliver quality care within and across settings.

Nurses recognise and work within the bounds of their competence (or their scope of practice), and they are responsible for their actions. The nurse acts in the best interests of people, ensuring that they put them first. They provide nursing care that is safe and compassionate and use their knowledge and experience to make evidence-based decisions and solve problems.

The four key concepts of care – accountability, confidentiality, autonomy, and advocacy – are evident when assessing needs and planning care. An awareness of these four elements is essential when care that is provided is patient-centred, appropriate, and delivered in a timely manner. Nurses hold a position of responsibility, patients and other people rely on them for a number of things.

Across health care in the UK there are a number of different kinds of care plan in use, and despite their differences, they all share three aims:

1. To ensure that the patient receives the same care irrespective of which staff are on duty
2. To ensure that the care offered and delivered is recorded
3. To support the patient as they identify, manage, and, if appropriate, solve their problems.

Fundamentals of Assessment and Care Planning for Nurses, First Edition. Ian Peate.
© 2020 John Wiley & Sons Ltd. Published 2020 by John Wiley & Sons Ltd.

The care plan, which can be electronic or paper-based, is amended constantly throughout the day and defines the areas that the care plan will address. There are a number of ways of doing this. Some adopt a simple approach focusing on the essentials of care, for example:

- Nutrition
- Mobility
- Sleeping
- Positioning
- Oral hygiene care
- Personal hygiene

Others, however, can be detailed and may address issues related to:

- Falls prevention
- Psychological needs
- Recording of clinical signs
- Communication and information
- Sexuality

An individual care plan has to be prepared for each patient. Where possible, it should be put together 'with' the patient, as opposed to 'for' the patient; remember that the patient is at the centre of all that is done.

Reading and using care plans will help guide practice with individual patients. Understanding what care plans contain and the information within them in the care area where you work is essential. You should also determine who in the care area has responsibility for keeping the care plans up to date – this will vary from area to area.

Review

Find out from the care plan where you are working who has responsibility for keeping care plans up to date. This responsibility will differ from area of care to area of care.

Duty of care

The 'duty of care' concerns the obligations that are placed on people to act towards others in a particular way and in alignment with certain standards (Royal College of Nursing 2018a). Sometimes the term is used to address legal and also professional duties that a nurse and other health care professionals may have towards others. However, there are distinctions between the two. The law imposes a duty of care on a nurse in conditions where it is 'reasonably foreseeable' that the nurse might cause harm to patients through what it is that they do or do not do (their actions or omissions). This is the case irrespective of whether this is a nurse, nursing associate, midwife, health care assistant, or assistant practitioner. The duty exists when the nurse has assumed some sort of responsibility for the patient's care. This can be fundamental personal care such as washing a patient, providing catheter care or a complex procedure, for example the administration of medications. In essence, duty of care relates to the nurse's requirement to perform to a certain standard of conduct for the protection of another against an unreasonable risk of harm.

The legal standard of care

To fulfil the legal duty of care, the nurse (or any other health care practitioner) has to act in accordance with the relevant standard of care. Generally, this is assessed as the standard to be expected of an 'ordinarily competent practitioner' or an ordinary competent registered nurse carrying out that particular task or role. The standards that are expected are not normally affected by any personal attributes, for example the level of experience. The legal standard of care to generally be expected of a newly-qualified nurse is the same as that expected of a more experienced nurse who would be performing the same task.

Professional duty of care

The NMC's standards for education, conduct, training, and ultimately performance are those set out in the Code (NMC 2018). Those standards can be used to inform the legal standard described above. NMC guidance (in its many forms) is useful when considering best practice.

So far

The 'duty of care' refers to the duties placed on people to act towards others in a particular way, in accordance with specific standards. The term is sometimes used to address *legal* and *professional* duties that nurses and health care practitioners may have towards others.

Professionalism

The NMC (2017) suggest that professionalism is characterised by the autonomous evidence-based decision making by members of an occupation who share the same values and education. In nursing, professionalism is achieved through relationships that are purposeful and supported by environments that enable the nurse to practise professionally. Nurses demonstrate and accept accountability for their actions whenever they offer care to people. They are also answerable for the times when they make any decisions related to the omission of care.

The ultimate purpose of professionalism in nursing is to ensure that there is consistent provision of safe, effective, person-centred outcomes that support people as well as their families and carers, in order to achieve the level of health and wellbeing. Practising nurses receive educational input that has prepared them with the behaviours, knowledge, and skills needed to provide safe, effective, person-centred care and services. Nurses have been professionally socialised to practise in compassionate, interprofessional, and collaborative ways. They are required to demonstrate that they have continuing registered nurse status with the NMC. Practice and behaviour are underpinned by the Code (NMC 2018) and are demonstrated through a number of characteristics or fundamentals of nursing practice, namely:

- Being accountable (Practising effectively)
- Being a leader (Promoting professionalism and trust)
- Being an advocate (Prioritising people)
- Being competent (Preserving safety)

The Code. Professional standards of practice and behaviour for nurses, midwives, and nursing associates

The Code (NMC 2018) is the NMC's principal publication that sets out the standards that are expected of all nurses, midwives, and nursing associates. It is clear within the Code that all nurses keep to the laws of the country in which they are practising.

The Code symbolises the key principles and values of the profession and as such underpins practice. There are four principles on which the Code has been established (see Figure 2.1). The overriding aim is public protection.

Review

Go to this NMC link and retrieve the documents 'Concerns, Complaints and Referrals': www.nmc.org.uk/concerns-nurses-midwives/concerns-complaints-and-referrals/
Have look at the documents and consider the various ways that referrals are made to the NMC.
Access the NMC website and determine the Standard of Proof used by the NMC. What does this mean?

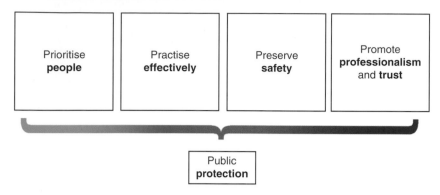

Figure 2.1   The four guiding principles underpinning the Code (NMC 2018).

Generally, the four key principles (rules that govern the provision of care: accountability, confidentiality, autonomy, and advocacy) apply to all nursing activities, regardless of patient group or the environment in which is being care is delivered.

So far

Professionalism can mean something different to everyone who works as a nurse. It can be acting as an inspiring role model working in the best interests of people, regardless of what position the nurse holds and where they deliver care, professionalism is what brings practice and behaviour together in harmony.

The Code presents the professional standards that nurses are required to uphold in order to be registered to practise in the UK.

Accountability

The term 'accountability' is sometimes an elusive and ambiguous term. Nevertheless, it has implications for professional practice. The importance of accountability along with responsibility are recurrent themes in contemporary nursing. It is essential that the nurse has an understanding of the various terms so that the care provided is safe and the public are protected. Often the terms 'accountability' and 'responsibility' are used synonymously. Accountability is doing the right thing consistently, day in and day out, in the tasks and duties being performed and in relationships we have with others.

Accountability stands for professionalism and is a higher standard than responsibility, including being able to accept accountability for one's actions and being able to provide justification for one's actions; this equates to knowing when to do something and when not to do something (Cornock 2011). When a nurse fails to meet a required standard, then they could be sanctioned by their regulatory body (the NMC) or a court of law. Accountability is the term that is used in law to impose standards and boundaries on professional practice.

It is clearly stated in the NMC's various Standards that their function is first and foremost to protect patients, enhance confidence in nurses and to be at the forefront of healthcare regulation. The NMC has a key role in regulating and registering qualified nurses, setting standards of practice and conduct, assuring the quality of nurse education and ensuring that those whose name is entered on the NMC register keep up to date with the overall aim of strengthening patient protection.

According to Williams (2018), in agreement with Cornock (2011), accountability means to take responsibility for one's actions. Professional accountability she continues is a nurse's responsibility

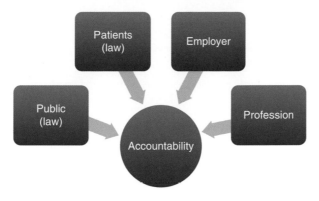

Figure 2.2   Spheres of accountability.

to meet the patient's health care needs in a safe, effective, and caring way. Accountability also involves behaviours, for example seeking assistance when unsure, carrying out nursing activities in a safe manner, reporting and documenting assessments undertaken and interventions carried out, and evaluating the care that was given and the response that the patient makes to this. Accountability also includes a commitment to continuing education in order to stay current and knowledgeable. Nurses are accountable for their decisions and actions and the outcomes of those actions; they are not accountable for the decisions or actions of other health and social care professionals.

There are some common concepts that are associated with accountability. There is an obligation, and this brings with it a duty that usually comes with consequences, there is a willingness that is accepted by choice or without reluctance or coercion, and there is intent, and this is the purpose that accompanies the care plan. The nurse has ownership, having power or control over what it is they are doing, and, finally, they are committed. All these concepts are key to ensuring accountability (see Figure 2.2).

Spheres of accountability

When a nurse harms a patient or there is loss of property or damage to property, the nurse may be liable and can be called to account. Dimond (2015) refers to the spheres of accountability as the arenas of accountability, and divides them up as follows:

Public:	Criminal law
	Criminal courts
Public:	Civil law
	Civil courts
Profession:	Code of conduct
	Committees of the NMC
Employer:	Contract of employment
	Employment tribunal

A nurse may be required to give reasons for any decisions that they make in their professional practice and they should be able to justify the decisions made in the context of legislation (the law), professional standards and guidelines, evidence-based practice, and professional and ethical conduct. The nurse is accountable legally and professionally for their practice, for the decisions that they make and the consequences that follow as a result of those decisions.

Take note

Are you willing to make the necessary changes in yourself to provide the highest quality of care? Can you commit to each of these statements?

- I take full responsibility for myself, my decisions, and everything I do when providing care.
- I am willing to take responsibility for any mistakes that I make and learn from helpful feedback.
- I am accountable for my actions and omissions
- I commit to actively supporting the people I work with and helping them remember what their commitments are. I am aware that this means that I may have to challenge them in a courteous way.

So far

Accountability is a complex concept. Each registered nurse is accountable for the care they provide, they answer for their own judgements and actions. They carry out these actions in a way that is agreed with patients and the families and carers of their patients, doing this in such a way that they meet the requirements of the NMC, their employer, and the law.

Confidentiality

The cornerstone of an effective therapeutic nurse–patient relationship centres on trust and being able to ensure that confidentiality forms part of that trust. Confidentiality and being able to maintain it is essential in all areas of care provision.

Preserving confidentiality demonstrates that the nurse is protecting a person's right to privacy, it is a key element of a nurse's work, it respects a person's human rights. Article 8 of the European Convention of Human Rights refers to confidentiality, the right to respect for private and family life. In the course of their duty the nurse obtains private and personal information from those who use services, their relatives, or from other health care professionals as part of their role. Nurses have a duty to keep any personal information about those who use services safe and only share this information with others who have a right to know or when a person has given their permission to disclose information about them. People expect that the information given to a health or care worker will only be used for the purpose for which it was given, and that disclosure will only occur with their permission.

When considering privacy, one element of privacy is that people have the right to control access to their own health information. It is not acceptable for nurses and/or other health care professionals to discuss matters related to the people in your care outside the work area, and you must not discuss a person with colleagues when you are in public and where there is a possibility that you may be overheard, or leave records unattended where they may be read by unauthorised people.

If those nurses who offer care fear giving information to health care professionals because they feel that they cannot trust them with that information, then this may have the potential to prevent the patient from seeking healthcare or providing the nurse with other information that may be required in order to offer the patient and the wider community high-quality care. Failing to provide a confidential health and social service as a result of non-adherence to confidentiality regulations and policies can impact negatively on the therapeutic nurse–patient relationship.

The nurse has a professional duty to the patient to maintain confidentiality as well as a legal duty. The Code (NMC 2018) makes it clear that confidentiality is a professional requirement clause 5:

> As a nurse, midwife or nursing associate, you owe a duty of confidentiality to all those who are receiving care. This includes making sure that they are informed about their care and that information about them is shared appropriately.

Nurses are also obliged through their contract of employment to maintain confidentiality, and they are correspondingly required to uphold organisational policy and procedures that their employer may have in place. It has to be remembered that any discussion regarding the issue of confidentiality will have general but also specific aspects associated with it. Any guidance that is issued will not be able to deal with every facet of confidentiality, in every situation, in every care setting. Guidance is just that: guidance. The context of care must be given full consideration. Legally there are a number of elements of legislation that must be respected and upheld as a part of any health care professional's duty. In some areas expert legal advice may need to be sought.

Review

You meet an ex-patient who you nursed on a surgical ward a week ago. He was being cared for in a six-patient bay. One of the other patients in the bay was a gentleman who was receiving palliative care for carcinoma of the head of the pancreas.

Your ex-patient notices you as you are doing your shopping in the local supermarket and asks: 'How is old Mac doing, nurse? The old man with cancer, he wasn't well at all.'

What would be the most appropriate response to this question?

Duty of confidentiality

Dimond (2015) points out that every healthcare employee (including those providing clinical services to patients, administrative staff, and those staff who support the provision of care delivery) has a duty to ensure confidentiality of information. This duty of confidentially will even continue after a patient has died (British Medical Association [BMA] 2016). The nurse has duties imposed on them by their contract of employment; they must keep information obtained from work confidential as well as acting within the realms of the law through statutory duties, such as the Data Protection Act 1998.

A duty of confidence occurs when a patient divulges information to another in situations where it is reasonable to assume that the information will be held in confidence. The duty to respect and protect the confidence of patients is a professional and legal requirement. All members of staff who receive personal information about patients in order to provide or support care are required by a legal duty of confidence to protect confidentiality; this includes nurses and those in nurse education.

Confidentiality is key to the development of trust between nurses, doctors, other health care professionals, and patients. Patients must be able to expect that information about their health is kept confidential unless there is a persuasive reason that it should not. There is a strong public interest in confidentiality as those who need treatment will be encouraged to seek treatment and to disclose information that is relevant to it.

A nurse owes a duty of confidentiality to all those who are receiving care. This includes ensuring that they are informed about their care and that any information about them is shared appropriately. In order to do this the NMC (2018) note that you must:

- Respect a person's right to privacy in all aspects of their care
- Make sure that people are informed about how and why information is used and shared by those who will be providing care
- Respect that a person's right to privacy and confidentiality continues after they have died
- Share necessary information with other healthcare professionals and agencies only when the interests of patient safety and public protection override the need for confidentiality
- Share with people, their families and their carers, as far as the law allows, the information they want or need to know about their health, care and ongoing treatment sensitively and in a way that they can understand.

The Human Rights Act 1998 protects and enforces the patient's right to confidentiality. Article 8 – covering the right to respect for private and family life – ensures that the nurse uses information provided to them only for the purposes for which it was given, it is also expected that this information will not be disclosed without permission. It is also important to remember that patients have the right to control information that belongs to them. This means that the nurse has to obtain permission from the patient prior to sharing that information with other people.

Policies and procedures will be in place in the areas where you work. There will be a confidentiality policy, which will include the appropriate (and legal) ways in which the sharing of confidential information can occur. The issue of confidentiality is also covered in your contract of employment and you could also be required to sign a confidentiality agreement.

A person's notes, care plans, or other details must be stored in a locked cupboard and not left where unauthorised people can see them. When using computers or mobile devices these have to be protected by a password and firewall. Where possible (and this may not always be possible), people should provide their consent when information is being transferred.

Confidential information

Confidential information, which is seen as identifiable patient information, be this written, computerised, visually or audio recorded, or simply held in the memory of the nurse, is subject to the duty of confidentiality. It includes:

- Any clinical information about a person's diagnosis or their treatment
- A picture, photograph, video, audiotape, or other image of the person
- Who the person's primary health care provider is (i.e. clinical nurse specialist, doctor) and what clinics that person has attended
- Anything else that could directly or indirectly lead to identifying of the person

Disclosure of confidential information

The duty of confidentiality is not absolute and there are instances where confidential information can be disclosed:

- The patient has the capacity to consent and consents to the disclosure (the patient gives their permission)
- It is required by statute (law), for example in relation to certain communicable diseases
- It is required by a court order
- It is seen to be justified in the public interest

Confidential information may be disclosed without consent where the public interest in the disclosure is necessarily strong. These can include disclosures that are necessary to prevent a serious and imminent threat to public health, national security, the life of the individual or a third party or to prevent or detect a serious crime. Any disclosure must be both necessary – the goal cannot be achieved without it – and also proportional – this means only as much information as is necessary to achieve the goal should be disclosed.

Disclosure to the police without consent is a complex situation and the nurse should seek advice before doing this. As is the case with all other requests for information, the presumption is that confidential information will only be disclosed to the police where the patient has provided explicit consent. There are exceptions to this, for example where there is a court order requiring disclosure, where the public interest in preventing or prosecuting a serious crime outweighs the person's right to confidentiality, or where there is someone at risk of death or serious harm.

Any health information about identifiable patients is confidential and as such the nurse must ensure that they take great care that they do not disclose such information to friends or colleagues unless, in the case of colleagues, they are directly involved in the provision of care to the patient.

Those nurses who choose to disclose confidential information during informal conversations in public places, for example on a bus, in a lift, or on a train, will be subject to strong condemnation by the NMC for breaches of confidentiality. The Health and Care Professions Council (HCPC) (2017) has provided registrants with guidance concerning confidentiality and what they consider to be best practice.

Identifiable information may include:

- The patient's personal details, such as names and addresses
- Information about a patient's health, treatment, or care that could identify them
- Photographs, videos, or other images
- Other information that a patient, family member, or carer shares with the nurse or healthcare professional that is not strictly related to the care, treatment, or other services provided

Anonymised information is information about a patient that has had all identifiable information removed from it and where there is little or no risk of a patient being identified from the information available. In some circumstances the nurse may be able to share anonymised information more openly. However, the nurse should always consider carefully what it is that they are sharing and who it is they are sharing the information with (HCPC 2017).

The 1998 Data Protection Act

The 1998 Data Protection Act aims to control the way information is handled and to give legal rights to those who have information stored about them. This aspect of legislation protects personal data that is stored on computers or in an organised paper filing system.

Everyone responsible for using data has to adhere to the 'data protection principles'. Nurses must ensure that the information is:

- Used fairly and lawfully
- Used for limited, specifically stated purposes
- Used in a way that is adequate, relevant and not excessive
- Accurate
- Kept for no longer than is absolutely necessary
- Handled according to people's data protection rights
- Kept safe and secure
- Not transferred outside the European Economic Area without adequate protection

The health and social care sectors handle some of the most sensitive personal data, and patients have the right to expect that information will be looked after. The Data Protection Act identifies what it calls 'sensitive information'. Because information about those matters could be used in a discriminatory way and is likely to be of a private nature, it is assumed that this data needs to be treated with greater care than other personal data. Sensitive personal data refers to personal data that consists of information noted in Box 2.1.

Caldicott Guardian

A Caldicott Guardian is a senior person in an NHS organisation who is responsible for protecting the confidentiality of patient and service-user information and enabling appropriate information sharing. Each NHS organisation is required to have a Caldicott Guardian, and this covers all organisations that have access to patient records.

The Guardian has a key role to play in ensuring that NHS, Councils with Social Services Responsibilities and partner organisations satisfy the highest practical standards for handling patient identifiable information. The Caldicott Guardian acts as the 'conscience' of the organisation, enabling information sharing where it is appropriate to share as well as advising on options for lawful and ethical processing of information. The Caldicott Principles can be found in Box 2.2.

Box 2.1 Sensitive data

a. the racial or ethnic origin of the data subject
b. his political opinions
c. his religious beliefs or other beliefs of a similar nature
d. whether he is a member of a trade union (within the meaning of the Trade Union and Labour Relations (Consolidation) Act 1992)
e. his physical or mental health or condition
f. his sexual life
g. the commission or alleged commission by him of any offence
h. any proceedings for any offence committed or alleged to have been committed by him, the disposal of such proceedings or the sentence of any court in such proceedings

Source: Information Commissioners Office (2018).

Box 2.2 The Caldicott principles

Principle	Discussion
Justify the purpose(s):	Every proposed use or transfer of personal confidential data within or from an organisation should be clearly defined, scrutinised and documented, with continuing uses regularly reviewed, by an appropriate guardian.
Do not use personal confidential data unless it is absolutely necessary:	Personal confidential data items must not be included unless this is essential for the specified purpose(s) of that flow. The need for patients to be identified should be considered at each stage of satisfying the purpose(s).
Use the minimum necessary personal confidential data:	Where use of personal confidential data is considered to be essential, the inclusion of each individual item of data should be considered and justified so that the minimum amount of personal confidential data is transferred or accessible as is necessary for a given function to be carried out.
Access to personal confidential data should be on a strict need-to-know basis:	Only those individuals who need access to personal confidential data should have access to it, and they should only have access to the data items that they need to see. This may mean introducing access controls or splitting data flows where one data flow is used for several purposes.
Everyone with access to personal confidential data should be aware of their responsibilities:	Action should be taken to ensure that those handling personal confidential data – both clinical and non-clinical staff – are made fully aware of their responsibilities and obligations to respect patient confidentiality.
Comply with the law:	Every use of personal confidential data must be lawful. Someone in each organisation handling personal confidential data should be responsible for ensuring that the organisation complies with legal requirements.
The duty to share information can be as important as the duty to protect patient confidentiality:	Health and social care professionals should have the confidence to share information in the best interests of their patients within the framework set out by these principles. They should be supported by the policies of their employers, regulators, and professional bodies.

Source: UK Caldicott Guardian Council (2017).

Review

Who is the Caldicott Guardian where you are working?

Confidentiality: NHS Code of Practice

The NHS Code of Practice (Department of Health 2003) underpins much information governance work that is undertaken in healthcare organisations today. The NHS Code of Practice is often a key point of reference with regard to information management systems.

The Code sets out what health and care organisations must do to meet their responsibilities concerning confidentiality and patients' consent to use their health records. It is based on legal requirements and best practice.

Autonomy

Autonomy is regarded as an essential element of professional status. It is not possible for accountability to be realised unless the nurse has the ability to practise and provide care autonomously. Varjus et al. (2011), in their review of the literature, suggest that autonomy refers to a nurse's ability to 'make some decisions within their own profession and their right and responsibility to act according to the shared standards of that profession'. Professional autonomy arises from the ability to use a number of kinds of knowledge in an analytical way that will offer safe, high-quality health care to people. The levels of autonomy vary depending on some key factors, for example legislation, the organisation, and individual factors.

Review

What do you understand by the phrase 'scope of practice'?

A key element to practising safely as an autonomous practitioner is associated with decision making. Being able and willing to make decisions and be accountable for them is an essential quality of a professional nurse. What is also an important part of this equation is the nurse's ability to accept the consequences of one's own actions. Making any decision is not without risk, and nurses have to realise this and accept this in order to practise in an autonomous and accountable way.

The features of autonomous nursing practice include the ability to observe, conceptualise, diagnose, and analyse complex issues that are related to health, possess a knowledge of a wide range of theory that is relevant to understanding health problems, and have an ability to select and justify the application of theory deemed to be the most useful in understanding those problems and in determining a wide range of treatment options. As the nurse's skills develop and they become more competent and confident, the degree of autonomy will increase.

Advocacy

An advocate is a person who pleads the cause for another. Regardless of the many changes to the role and function of the nurse, it is the case that nurses are and will remain the care giver acting, when needed, as the patient's advocate. Often the nurse acts as advocate to the most vulnerable in our society.

As an advocate, one aspect of this duty is to speak up for others when they are unable to do this for themselves. Speaking up for others, acting in their best interest, means that you are dedicated to those you offer care to and you raise concerns and speak up when things are not right. Those who

Box 2.3 The goals of the nurse when acting as advocate

Assess the need for advocacy
Develop a plan of action
Communicate with other healthcare team members
Provide individual and family teaching
Assist and support individual decision making
Serve as a change agent in the healthcare system
Participate in health policy formulation
Achieve the best outcomes for patients

Source: Adapted Tomajan (2012).

may be in vulnerable situations require an advocate, and the advocate may be required to uphold that person's human rights. In order to be able to act as advocate the nurse must ensure that they are up to date with current legislation, local policy, and procedure. If the nurse witnesses any activity that they feel puts the people they are offering care to at risk or they have any concerns about safeguarding, there is a duty to challenge this. The NMC (2018) make clear that the nurse must act as an advocate for the vulnerable, challenging poor practice and discriminatory attitudes and behaviour relating to their care. The goals of the nurse practising as an advocate are outlined in Box 2.3.

The College of Nursing Ontario (2015) points out that one of the nurse's roles is to advocate for client-centred care plans, advocating for patients' choices. Care provided must address the patient's wishes or needs, and the nurse needs to be aware when these wishes are not being met, and in so doing put themselves in a position to advocate for the patient's wishes. One aspect of advocating is assessing that the patient has all the information required to make informed choices. Advocating means talking about the patient's wishes with the right people, with the purpose of respecting those wishes. Advocacy must involve communicating in a way that supports the best care possible for the patient, whilst helping the health care team understand what their need and wishes are.

So far

Those who are receiving care may be unable or unprepared to make independent decisions. The nurse as an advocate will actively promote the person's rights to autonomy and freedom of choice (even if the nurse disagrees with what the person chooses). Speaking up for the person, facilitates communication between the person and others, as well as protecting the individual's right to self-determination or autonomy. Advocacy, empowerment, patient-centred care, and patient involvement in their care are key principles underpinning nursing practice.

Take note

Nurses out of all health care providers spend the most time with patients, and because of this they also experience first-hand the health care system's limitations. This puts nurses in the best position to speak up about their patients' needs and any safety concerns.

Delegation

Delegation can be defined as directing another to carry out work or perform a duty, it focuses on allowing another person to act on behalf of another. The National Leadership and Innovation Agency for Healthcare (2010) summarise delegation of duties as follows:

> Delegation is the process by which you (the delegator) allocate clinical or non-clinical treatment or care to a competent person (the delegate). You will remain responsible for the overall management of the service user and be accountable for your decision to delegate. You will not be accountable for the decisions and actions of the delegate.

Registered nurses have a duty of care and a legal liability with regard to the patient. If the registered nurse has delegated an activity to a health care assistant, for example, then they have to ensure that it has been appropriately delegated (RCN 2017).

The NMC Code (NMC 2018) notes that nurses must be accountable for their decisions to delegate tasks and duties to other people, and they must:

- only delegate tasks and duties that are within the other person's competence
- make sure that everyone they delegate tasks to is adequately supervised and supported
- confirm that the outcome of any task they have delegated to someone else meets the required standard.

Take note

Delegation must be safe and aim to improve the care of all patients within any given setting.

Responsibility also falls on employers. They have to ensure that their staff are trained and supervised properly until they have been deemed competent (RCN 2018b). An employer accepts vicarious liability for their employees. This means if their employees are working within their sphere of competence and in association with their employment, then the employer is also accountable for their actions. Principles of delegation have been highlighted by the RCN (2018b) (see Box 2.4).

Box 2.4 The principles of delegation

- Delegation has to be, at all times, in the best interest of the patient and not performed in order to save time or money.
- The person being delegated to (the support worker) must have been suitably trained to undertake the intervention.
- Full records of training given, including dates, should be kept.
- Evidence that support workers' competence has been assessed should be recorded, preferably against recognised standards such as National Occupational Standards.
- There should be clear guidelines and protocols in place so that the support worker is not required to undertake a standalone clinical judgement.
- The role should be within the support worker's job description.
- The team and any support staff need to be informed that the activity has been delegated.
- The person delegating the activity (the registered nurse) must ensure that an appropriate level of supervision is available and that the support worker has the opportunity for mentorship. The level of supervision and feedback required depends on the recorded knowledge and competence of the support worker, the needs of the patient, the service setting, and the activities allocated.
- Support workers must have ongoing development to ensure that their competency is maintained.
- The whole process must be assessed to identify any risks.

Source: Adapted RCN (2018b).

The 6Cs

Competence is one of the 6Cs and means all those in caring roles must have the ability to understand an individual's health and social needs and the expertise, clinical and technical knowledge to deliver effective care and treatments based on research and evidence.

How do you know if you are competent in what you are doing?

Conclusion

Underpinning all we do are four key themes: accountability, confidentiality, autonomy, and advocacy. The concepts of accountability, confidentiality, autonomy, and advocacy are inherently linked in determining how we practise. Nurses hold positions of responsibility, and they are therefore required to be accountable for their practice. Responsibility and accountability are the foundations of professional nursing practice and are epitomised as key principles in our Code.

References

British Medical Association (BMA) (2016). Confidentiality and Health Records Tool Kit. www.bma.org.uk/advice/employment/ethics/confidentiality-and-health-records/confidentiality-and-health-records-tool-kit (accessed January 2018)

College of Nursing Ontario (2015). Advocating for your client. www.cno.org/en/learn-about-standards-guidelines/magazines-newsletters/the-standard/january-2016/advocacy (accessed February 2018)

Cornock, M. (2011). Legal definitions of responsibility, accountability and liability. *Nursing Children and Young People* 23 (3): 25–26.

Department of Health (2003). Confidentiality: NHS Code of Practice. www.gov.uk/government/uploads/system/uploads/attachment_data/file/200146/Confidentiality_-_NHS_Code_of_Practice.pdf (accessed February 2018)

Dimond, B. (2015). *Legal Aspects of Nursing*, 7e. Harlow: Pearson.

Health and Care Professions Council (HCPC) (2017). Confidentiality: Guidance for registrants. www.hpc-uk.org/assets/documents/100023F1GuidanceonconfidentialityFINAL.pdf (accessed January 2018)

Information Commissioners Office (2018). Key definitions of the Data Protection Act. https://ico.org.uk/for-organisations/guide-to-data-protection/key-definitions (accessed February 2018).

National Leadership and Innovations Agency for Healthcare (2010). All Wales guidelines for delegation. www.wales.nhs.uk/sitesplus/documents/829/All%20Wales%20Guidelines%20for%20Delegation.pdf (accessed February 2018)

Nursing and Midwifery Council (2018). The Code. Professional Standards of Practice and Behaviour for Nurses, Midwives and Nursing Associates. https://www.nmc.org.uk/globalassets/sitedocuments/nmc-publications/nmc-code.pdf last accessed 8 May 2019

Nursing and Midwifery Council (NMC) (2017). Enabling professionalism. www.nmc.org.uk/standards/professionalism (accessed February 2018)

Royal College of Nursing (RCN) (2017). Accountability and delegation: A guide for the nursing team. www.rcn.org.uk/professional-development/publications/pub-006465 (accessed February 2018)

Royal College of Nursing (RCN) (2018a). Duty of care. www.rcn.org.uk/get-help/rcn-advice/duty-of-care (accessed January 2018)

Royal College of Nursing (RCN) (2018b). Accountability and delegation. www.rcn.org.uk/professional-development/accountability-and-delegation (accessed February 2018)

Tomajan, K. (2012). Advocating for nurses and nursing. *The Online Journal of Issues in Nursing* 17 (1).

UK Caldicott Guardian Council (2017). A manual for Caldicott Guardians. www.gov.uk/government/uploads/system/uploads/attachment_data/file/581213/cgmanual.pdf (accessed February 2018)

Varjus, S.L., Leino-Kilpi, H., and Suominen, T. (2011). Professional autonomy of nurses in hospital settings: A review of the literature. *Scandinavian Journal of Caring Sciences* 25 (1): 201–207. https://doi.org/10.1111/j.1471-6712.2010.00819.x.

Williams, P. (2018). *deWit's Fundamental Concepts and Skills for Nursing*, 5e. St Louis: Elsevier.

Chapter 3

Critical thinking and clinical decision making

Aim

This chapter provides the reader with insight into critical thinking and the components associated with this essential activity in order to make safe and effective clinical decisions.

Learning outcomes

By the end of the chapter the reader will be able to:

1. Describe the various components that are required to think in a critical manner
2. Discuss the importance of thinking critically when offering people safe and effective care
3. Demonstrate an understanding of the assessment, judgement and decision-making processes required to improve practice
4. Consider implications for patient care

Introduction

Often the terms clinical reasoning, clinical judgement, problem solving, decision making, and critical thinking are used interchangeably. This chapter focuses on critical thinking and clinical decision making, both of which require clinical judgement and problem solving. Clinical reasoning describes the process by which nurses gather cues, process the information, come to an understanding of the issue, plan and implement interventions, evaluate outcomes, and then reflect on and learn from the process (see Figure 3.1).

The critical reasoning process is not a linear process, it is a dynamic cyclical process. In a cyclical process, the system starts in a particular state and returns to that state after undergoing a number of different processes. The cycle runs clockwise, beginning at 12 o'clock with the issue.

Take note

Clinical reasoning is an essential component to 'thinking like a nurse', the same goes for critical, creative, scientific, and formal criterial reasoning.

Fundamentals of Assessment and Care Planning for Nurses, First Edition. Ian Peate.
© 2020 John Wiley & Sons Ltd. Published 2020 by John Wiley & Sons Ltd.

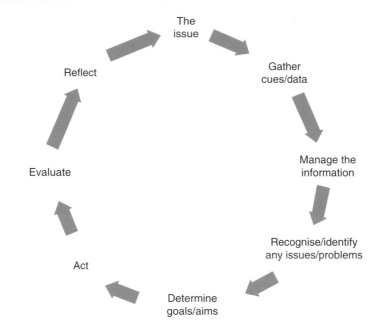

Figure 3.1   The critical reasoning process.

Nursing practice requires practitioners to display sound judgement and decision-making skills as critical thinking and clinical decision making are crucial elements of nursing practice. The nurse's ability to recognise and respond to signs of patient deterioration in a timely manner plays a central role in patient outcomes (Purling and King 2012). Tomlinson (2015) notes that errors in clinical judgement and decision making account for more than half of adverse clinical events.

So far

Clinical reasoning can be challenging and requires a different approach to that used when learning other routine nursing procedures. When the nurse learns to reason effectively this does not happen by chance; it requires determination as well as deliberate active engagement in practice for continued learning. It also requires the nurse to reflect, particularly on those activities that are meant to improve performance.

Critical thinking

The NMC (2018) defines critical thinking as the practice of analysing and considering all aspects of a situation and evidence about what works best, when making decisions or taking action. Critical means to require careful judgement and in this context thinking means to reason.

Clinical reasoning requires the nurse to make reliable observations concerning a person's health and wellbeing and to then draw sound conclusions from the data that has been obtained from the patient and from other sources. Together critical thinking and clinical reasoning are required to creatively problem solve and produce new ideas and solutions. The underpinning of good clinical decision making is clinical reasoning and the development of clinical judgement. The outcome of clinical reasoning is clinical judgement which is the conclusion or decision (a nursing diagnosis maybe) that you arrive at by using your clinical reasoning skills. The ability of the nurse to think critically, apply their knowledge and skills and provide expert hands-on nursing care lies at the centre of all nursing practice.

Critical thinking, clinical reasoning and clinical judgement are central to the nursing process. Critical thinking is applied by nurses as they work with patients in order to solve problems. It is a key component of the decision-making process. It is an essential process for safe, effective, and skilful nursing interventions. Critical thinking involves a variety of skills it is the mental active process and subtle perception, analysis, synthesis, and evaluation of information that has been collected or the result of observation, experience, reflection, reasoning, or the communication leading to a need to take action, it also requires the nurse to listen attentively (De Wit et al. 2017).

Review

When you are at handover, listening to a report for a patient or a group of patients, think about how you actually listen. What is attentive listening? How did using critical thinking enable you to gather the data needed to help you care safely and effectively for a patient(s).

When the nurse employs attentive listening they are consciously focusing on the topic of discussion, it also takes much practice to develop the skills of attentive listening. You have to pay attention to each word as well as the meaning the speaker is trying to convey.

Review

Practice attentive listening.

Work with a partner. Ask your partner to tell you about something of interest. When they have finished, repeat back the main ideas of what was stated. Confirm with your partner that you heard correctly.

Take note

As we live our busy lives, often we tend to rush ahead to form an answer or ask a question as opposed to waiting until the speaker has finished or the information has been imparted.

Identifying a problem, working out the best solution and choosing the most effective method to solve the problem are all elements of the critical thinking process. After undertaking the plan, a critical thinker will reflect on the situation to determine if the intervention (s) was effective and if it could have been done better.

Take note

Critical thinking is a transferable skill that can be and is used in several facets of your life. Personal and professional. Almost everything a human does involves decisions.

Clinical judgement a concept critical to nursing can be complex, as nurses are required to use the skills of observation, identify information that is relevant, to identify the relationships amongst given components through reasoning and judgement. Clinical reasoning is a process by which nurses observe the patient's condition, take the information and process it, the nurse then comes to an understanding of the patient's problem, planning care and implementing appropriate interventions and evaluating outcomes. This process is best done with reflection and learning from the activity (Levett-Jones et al. 2010). Nurses are responsible at all times for their actions and they are accountable for nursing judgement and action or inaction (NMC 2018).

Review

What does the Nursing and Midwifery Council say in the Code about accountability?

The skills and attributes of a critical thinker are detailed in Box 3.1.

Review

Think about the activities listed in Box 3.1. What activities do you do frequently in your personal life where you use the attributes of a critical thinker when you want to accomplish things?

The ability to think critically, apply knowledge and use evidence and experience to solve problems and make informed decisions are transferrable skills and very often, without even being aware of it, nurses critically think their way through each day, not only as they interact with patients and other healthcare professionals but as they carry on their day-to-day lives. However, as nursing decisions can very often impact profoundly on patients' lives, it is important that the thinking process that guides nursing practice has to be:

- Organised
- Purposeful
- Disciplined

Box 3.1 Some skills and attributes of a critical thinker

A critical thinker has the ability to:

- Keep an open mind and a questioning outlook.
- Be confident, competent, flexible, creative and aware.
- Recognise one's own limitations and prejudices.
- Be tenacious in their resolve to seek solutions.
- Separate relevant information from irrelevant information.
- Recognise inconsistencies in gathered data.
- Identify any missing information.
- Consider all possibilities with curiosity.
- Anticipate any potential problems.
- Employ an organised and systematic approach to problems.
- Confirm accuracy and reliability of data.
- Prior to making a decision consider all possible solutions.
- Acknowledge what you do not know.
- Reason logically and reflect on experience.
- Strive for excellence and improvement.
- Draw valid conclusions from the evidence or data.
- Set priorities and make carefully well-thought-out decisions.
- Be empathic, modest, honest and realistic.

Critical thinking is used in a number of spheres of practice, it is not limited to problem solving or decision making. Nurses use critical thinking to make observations, draw conclusions and evaluate and in particular when they evaluate the impact of care interventions.

Take note

Using critical thinking and the nursing process can help you develop good clinical reasoning skills that result in solid clinical judgement.

So far

Critical thinking and clinical reasoning are key components that are needed to problem solve in a creative way and to bring about new ideas and solutions. Good clinical decision making is underpinned by clinical reasoning and the development of clinical judgement. The outcome of clinical reasoning is clinical judgement which is seen as the conclusion or decision that the nurse has arrived at by using their clinical reasoning skills.

Clinical decision making

Clinical decisions are concerned with the needs of the patient as well as the most appropriate interventions that are required to meet those needs as well as the goals and outcomes that have been agreed upon. Clinical decisions help nurses to describe how they give meaning to problems that are being faced by patients, with the ultimate aim of eliminating or alleviating the problem.

Nurses are active clinical decision makers. In being active clinical decision makers nurses are required to access, review and incorporate research evidence into their professional judgement and clinical decision making (NMC 2018). The number and types of decisions that nurses face are related to the work environment, how they see their clinical role, the amount of autonomy required to perform their job, and the degree to which they themselves are seen as active and influential decision makers. Nurses working on a busy surgical ward with multiple patients to care for with multiple dependency levels will face a different set of decision challenges compared to those nurses who are working in a residential care home.

Review

How might the clinical decisions, the ways in which these decisions are made, and the urgency of these decisions made by nurses in a critical care unit and a residential care home for older people differ?

Banning (2008) provides a definition of clinical decision making suggesting it is about choosing between alternatives, it is a skill that improves as a nurse gains experience, both as a nurse and also within a specific specialty. To reiterate, clinical decision making requires good-quality judgement and this includes critical thinking (Thompson and Stapley 2011).

When working in the care setting, nurses are constantly faced with demands to make decisions related to care. The process of coming to a choice is at the heart of decision making, and this can be a complex process.

So far

Nurses use their clinical judgement and decision-making skills in number of clinical environments. Nurses are regarded as key decision makers within the health and social care team, they are also required to use the best available evidence in their judgements and decisions. There are a number of technological and educational interventions available to assist nurses with judgement and decision-making skills.

There are many different ways to think about decisions, decision-making theory differs. There are specific and non-specific (general) theories associated with decision making.

Review

These are examples of some decisions and of the theoretical problems that they may pose.
Will I need sunglasses today? – The decision is dependent on something that is unknown, such as whether the sun will shine, requiring the wearing of sunglasses.
I am looking for a bicycle to buy. Shall I purchase this one? – This bicycle looks fine, but perhaps there will be a better bicycle for the same price if I continue searching. When will I stop the search procedure?
Am I going to have another alcoholic drink? – One single alcoholic drink may be no problem, but if I make the same decision on many occasions then there is potential that I may cause harm.
Now think of the theoretical problems these decisions may pose:

- I am looking to buy a house.
- I am searching for a restaurant to eat in.
- Am I going to have cake?

Decision making can be defined in very general terms as a process or set of processes that result in the selection of one item from a number of potential alternatives. Within this general definition, the processes might be natural and conscious, for example a deliberate choice between alternatives, but they may also be unconscious. Decisions can be about what to do (action) and also about what to believe (opinion). There are usually two or more options, including making a decision or not, and they require a deliberate mental choice based on indications, hints, signals, or evidence.

Decisions can be made with or without a framework. Options can be considered, followed by a list of factors that are important will enable us to make a choice or a decision, and, finally, we opt for what we think is going to be the correct decision. Some decisions are hurried and there are others that require time, when we may need to deliberate or take our time. It is more likely that the right decision will be made if all options have been thoroughly explored and thought through.

Review

Think of a time in your personal or professional life when you have had to make:

- A decision that was required in a hurry
- A decision that needed more time (contemplation)

What factors led to the hurried decision and what factors led to the decision that required more time?

Table 3.1 Some of the factors that need to be taken into consideration with regard to decision making.

- What is the decision that needs to be made? This needs to be defined – the *definition*.
- What is it that you need to know in order to make the decision? This is the *aim*.
- What needs to be kept in mind? These are the *criteria*.
- Work out what the *options* might be.
- Consider if there are there any decision-making *tools* that might need to be used.
- Review the decision

The decision being made can be either an individual or group decision. The outcome of the decision can be almost instantaneous, or it could take a little longer or a lot longer. In Table 3.1 some of the factors that may be involved when making a decision have been listed.

When a healthcare provider makes a clinical decision, it is different to making a decision generally; the consequences of the decision being made have to be given much thought. It is essential, therefore, that the nurse strives to make the correct clinical decision. Almost every aspect of health care is associated with uncertainty and this is also true when making decisions that are health care related. Nurses have to be mindful of this and address this uncertainty in their decision making. The construction and implementation of evidence-based policies and practice will impact on how this is done and also on the quality of decision making.

Review

The decisions nurses make can range from consulting with a speech and language therapist regarding a patient's ability to swallow following a stroke to deciding what dose of an analgesic a patient requires when they are in pain.

It would be very difficult, if not impossible, to list all of the clinical decisions that a nurse makes in clinical practice. In trying to put together such a list you would have to take into account the many activities and the various contexts of care in which the nurse practises. Nurses are continually making decisions; it could be suggested that sometimes the nurse may not be aware that he/she is making these decisions.

Try to make a list of some clinical decisions that you see nurses make.

Which care environment is the decision being made in?

Are they decisions that the nurse makes alone or do the decisions require others to have an input?

What were the consequences on patient care?

So far

Clinical decision making is about choosing between alternatives. This is a skill that improves as the nurse gains experience and is exposed to various situations and environments. In order to make safe and effective clinical decisions, good-quality judgement which also includes critical thinking skills is required.

It should always be remembered that whenever any decision is made, there are consequences. These consequences can be positive or negative and can impact on a patient's health and wellbeing. The nurse is accountable for their actions or omissions.

Normative, prescriptive, and descriptive models

The decision-making process (particularly in complex dynamic care environments) occurs in environments of uncertainty, which is an inescapable fact of decision making in modern health care. There are several models that nurses choose from (either consciously or unconsciously) when making care decisions.

MacNeela et al. (2017) describe three models that are associated with judgement and the decision-making process:

1. Normative
2. Prescriptive
3. Descriptive

Normative models

These models are associated with rational, logical, scientific, evidence-based decisions informed by statistical analysis of large-scale experimental and survey research (representative of a target population to who the findings will be applied). Rationality is the key to this model, with the assumption that when people make decisions, they wish to be logical in their approach. Normative models are evaluated against their theoretical adequacy in enabling decision makers to make predictions and explain the outcomes of decisions. Clinical trials that test the usefulness of new medicines and treatments can be cited as examples of this approach.

Prescriptive models

Prescriptive models acknowledge that when we use information this is rarely optimal. However, the approach recognises that there are ways to make improvements. Prescriptive models according to Thompson and Dowding (2009) describe underlying cognitive processes that support and influence decision making and judgement, for example attitudes, biases, and schemas, and they suggest better ways of making better use of the information that is available. Prescriptive models often apply principles and findings of previous scientific research (those associated with normative models), for example in the development of tools used in assessment and the production of clinical guidelines, the focus is on the accuracy of the decision being made. Prescriptive models can be supported by strategies such as:

- Decision analysis techniques and decision trees
- Critical incident analyses to learn from near misses and previously ineffective actions
- Organisational preparedness for managing critical events
- Training initiatives that encourage rule-based or formal models of decision making in the care environment.

Descriptive models

Descriptive models are associated with studies that observe, describe, and analyse how decisions are made by managers and professionals as they carry out their day-to-day responsibilities. They demonstrate how people actually make judgements as opposed to how they ought to. MacNeela et al. (2017) would suggest that behind descriptive models is the notion that people are not very good at using information in order to form conclusions or when making choices. Descriptive models characteristically stress our dependence on intuitions, beliefs, and feelings over objective evidence and logical analysis. For Dowding et al. (2011) this raises the question of the accuracy of any subsequent judgements. In health and social care settings, this is an important question, particularly if practitioners are relying on intuition, beliefs, and feelings as opposed to, for example, a simple statistical combination rule.

Benner (1984) described the transition from being a rule-governed novice to becoming an intuitive expert nurse by obtaining practitioners' accounts of 'reflection-on-action'. She did this in tape-recorded 'phenomenological' interviews and then applied the findings to support the model. Benner (1984) described five levels of nursing experience, coining the phrase 'from novice to expert' (see Figure 3.2).

So far

The decision-making process often acted out in complex dynamic care environments occurs in environments of uncertainty, which is an inevitable aspect of decision making in modern health care. There are a number of models that might help the nurse, either consciously or unconsciously, when making care decisions.

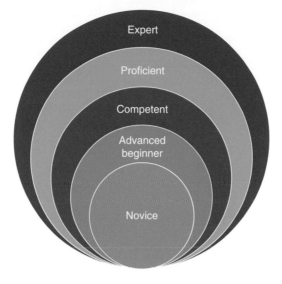

Figure 3.2   Benner's novice to expert. Source: Benner (1984).

The decision-making process

Thompson and Dowding (2009) emphasise that it is important to have an understanding of the decision-making process so as to make the most appropriate health care decisions. There are several models available outlining the decision-making process or the steps that are involved in the decision-making process. In 1993 Tschikota considered the various elements of decision making and identified six elements:

1. Cue
2. Hypothesis
3. Knowledge base
4. Nursing intervention
5. Search
6. Assumption

In Table 3.2 each element is described, defined, and an example is provided.

Review

Reflect on the care you have given to a patient and think about a decision that was required concerning that person's care. Can you identify the six elements that Tschikota (1993) identified?

So far

There are a number of important steps that compromise the active decision-making process. Nurses may use these consciously or subconsciously regardless, these steps are evident when nurses make decisions. It is important for the nurse to have an understanding of the decision-making process so as to make the most appropriate health care decisions.

Table 3.2 The decision-making process in action.

Element	Definition	Example
1. Cue	A piece of information or data	All the time patients are providing nurses with pieces of information. This might be something that they say or do, signs and symptoms, or it might be information obtained from the patient when the nurse was undertaking a nursing history. Other pieces of information might be data that the patient's vital signs reveal, e.g. his/her oxygen saturation percentage or the blood pressure measurements. Other data may include laboratory values, for example results of blood tests or the outcome of an investigatory procedure such as an exercise stress test During this aspect of the decision-making process the nurse is required to gather preliminary information. This can happen before the nurse meets the patient, e.g. the gathering of information from the patient's health and social history from the patients' records or when meeting the patient. This stage is also known as the cue acquisition stage.
2. Hypothesis	This is a proposed possibility or a projected likelihood. Often the words 'query' or 'might' are used at this stage, for example, what concerns might the patient have? Other words used are 'probably', 'if', 'could be', 'maybe' or 'perhaps'. When the hypothesis made is tentative: 'What might be the patient's problems?'	The number of hypotheses generated is generally between four and six. 'Probably urinary tract infection.' 'Could be a kidney infection.' 'May be an appendicitis.' 'If we administer prescribed analgesia this may change the patient's pain score.'
3. Knowledge base	The information that has been acquired is used to support any statements made by the patient. The information – correct or incorrect – is used as a rationale for any proposed action.	'Because the patient is pale, tachycardia and pyrexia he/she probably has anaemia.' 'Because the patient is hypotensive, tachycardic and oliguric he/she is probably hypovolaemic.' 'Because the patient is hypertensive, bradycardic and drowsy he/she may have raised intracranial pressure.'
4. Nursing intervention	Any proposed nursing activity	Nurse the patient upright. Perform all the activities of living. Encourage a high-protein diet.
5. Search	A need to search for additional or supplementary information regarding the situation	'I think we need to know what the patient's liver function tests are.' 'Do we know if the patient is allergic to anything that could have exacerbated the current condition?'
6. Assumption	A conclusion. Whereby there is insufficient information or data to make a definitive judgement. This can lead the nurse to carry on searching for more additional information regarding the situation	'With the information I have, I think the patient is experiencing hallucinations, as her behaviour suggests that she is talking to an imagined thing, and she has told me she feels she is being followed.' 'I think the patient has a urinary tract infection: his urine is concentrated, it is malodourous, and he is passing small amounts frequently. He has a tachycardia and pyrexia. He tells me it is painful when he micturates.'

Source: Adapted Thompson and Dowding (2009) and Tschikota (1993).

Factors impacting on clinical decision making

It has already been noted that decision making about individual patient care is a complex and a contextually dependent process. In a review undertaken on behalf of the NHS Confederation, Williams and Brown (2014) wished to understand what factors influence decisions, impacting on quality and costs in health care and non-health care contexts. They determined that the following factors could be seen as impacting on decision making:

- Decision characteristics, for example complexity, urgency of the need to make the decision
- Decision-maker characteristics
- Availability of information (tacit and explicit knowledge)
- Economic factors, such as the financial environment
- Politics and regulation

Several other factors influence decision making, for example past experience, cognitive biases, age and individual differences, and belief in personal relevance. These influence what choices people make. Understanding the factors that influence decision-making process is important to understanding what decisions are made (de Bruin et al. 2007; Jullisson et al. 2005; Stanovich and West 2008).

Barriers to effective clinical decision making

Thompson et al. (2013) note that there is evidence from healthcare systems around the world that suggests that judgements and decisions that are made by clinicians could be improved. Approximately 50% of all adverse events have some kind of error at their core.

If nurses are to continue to enhance patient care, one way in which this can occur is through effective decision making, in which case it is necessary to understand what the barriers may be to effective clinical decision making. There are several factors that can have a negative influence on the decision-making process. The following could be considered barriers to effective clinical decision making:

- Inadequate knowledge base
- Inadequate skills
- Emotional difficulties
- Lack of opportunity
- Dependence on others

As the nurse's skills, knowledge, competence and confidence develop and grow, the factors that can have detrimental impact on decision making may lessen and the nurse will become more proficient at making effective decisions. Becoming more involved in the decision-making process as the nurse's career progresses will enable confidence to grow. Becoming a proficient clinical decision maker comes with experience and learning. Learning takes place once the nurse has been exposed to various scenarios related to patient care. In Table 3.3 there is a list of some dos and don'ts that are associated with decision making.

Take note

Never rush your decision making; the right decision at the wrong time is equally as bad as the wrong decision made at the right time. If it is possible, suspend your decision making and avoid making those snap decisions.

So far

When decisions are made erroneously, this can have an impact on a person's health and wellbeing. It has been suggested that judgements and decisions made by clinicians could be improved, as around half of all adverse events have some kind of error at their core. Understanding the factors that impact on decision making is a key requirement of the professional nurse as this may avert errors in the future.

Table 3.3   Some dos and don'ts of decision making.

The Dos	The don'ts
Try to collect good relevant information before you make a decision.	Make snap decisions.
Use all appropriate information to the best of your ability and 'think outside the box'.	Make decisions for the sake of making them, avoid wasting your time making decisions that do not have to be made.
Take time to consider the pros and cons of the issue you are dealing with.	Feel that there is a right or wrong decision – decisions are choices amongst alternatives.
Try not to let decisions that are to be made build up and accumulate – make your decisions as you go along.	Regret making a decision.
	Rush, pre-judge and jump to a conclusion.
Delay or revise a decision as you deem necessary – trust yourself and do not be frightened to do this.	Make decisions in an attempt to defend any decision you have made earlier.
Remember that any decision that you make will have consequences.	Be forced or pressured into making a decision.
Avoid basing decisions on tradition, hearsay, and ritual: 'the way things are always done here'.	

Table 3.4   From novice to expert.

Stage	Description
Novice or beginner	The nurse at this stage has no experience in the situation which they are exposed to and are dependent on rules in order to guide their actions. They lack confidence to demonstrate safe practice and are reliant on continual verbal and physical cues.
Advanced beginner	Nurses at the advanced beginner stage demonstrate marginally acceptable performance as the nurse had prior experience in actual situations. They often need help establishing priorities and cannot reliably determine what is most important in complex situations, they need help to prioritise.
Competent	This nurse demonstrates efficiency, is coordinated and has confidence in what they do. They are able to plan and sort out which aspects of a situation are important and which can be ignored or delayed. However, this nurse does not have the speed and flexibility of a proficient practitioner, they do show an ability to cope with and manage change in practice.
Proficient	The proficient nurse is someone who addresses the situation as a whole as opposed to parts. They understand clinical situations holistically, and this results in quick and more accurate decision making. These nurses consider fewer options and are quick in homing in on accurate issues of the problem.
Expert	These nurses are no longer reliant on rules or guidelines, to rapidly understand the problem. They have an extensive background of experience that demonstrates an intuitive grip related to complex situations. They are able to focus on the accurate region of the problem without first considering ineffective options.

Source: Adapted Benner (1984).

From novice to expert

Benner's stages of clinical competence (see Table 3.4) describe how nurses might progress through skill acquisition as they develop specific levels of proficiency. The different levels can also be applied to how nursing judgements and decision making advances as does skill acquisition.

Review

Can you identify any intuitive feelings you have had (personal and/or professional)? How do you think they came about? How did you manage them?

Can you think of some other words that that are used alongside or instead of 'intuition'?

Box 3.2 Factors influencing decision making

- Knowledge (technical knowledge and tacit knowledge)
- Evidence-based practice (scientific knowledge)
- Experience (this is gained over time)
- Intuition (associated with the nurse's perception of the situation)
- Ethics (doing no harm)
- The relationship between the nurse and the patient (engaging the patient in the decision-making process)
- The professional role (being accountable)
- Constraints on time (time available, urgency of need to make a decision)
- Rules and culture (respecting norms and beliefs)

Source: Adapted Benner and Tanner (1987).

Benner is the author who is most connected with developing the intuitive model (the intuitive-humanistic decision-making model) and the distinction between theoretical knowledge and experiential knowledge in the discipline of nursing (Thompson 1999). According to Benner and Tanner (1987), decisions are influenced by a number of factors (see Box 3.2).

Conclusion

Clinical reasoning, clinical judgement, problem solving, decision making, and critical thinking are terms often used interchangeably. This chapter has concentrated on critical thinking and clinical decision making, which both require clinical judgement and problem solving. Clinical decision making is a key component of the role of the professional nurse. Those nurses who make clinical decisions are also required to accept responsibility and be prepared to be held accountable for the consequences as a result of those decisions, or the failure to make a decision. In order to do this those factors that impact on the decision-making process and decision makers have to be understood. The outcome of effective decision making results in finding solutions, offering safe and effective nursing care, and the provision of an individual, holistic approach to care. There has been an association between patient outcomes and nurses' decision making, and thus one way to enhance patient care is to improve the nurse's capacity to make effective decisions.

References

Banning, M. (2008). A review of clinical decision making: models and current research. *Journal of Clinical Nursing* 17 (2): 187–195.

Benner, P.E. (1984). *From Novice to Expert: Excellence and Power in Clinical Nursing Practice*. Menlo Park: Addison-Wesley.

Benner, P.E. and Tanner, C. (1987). Clinical judgement: how expert nurses use intuition. *American Journal of Nursing* 87 (1): 23–31.

de Bruin, W.B., Parker, A.M., and Fischhoff, B. (2007). Individual differences in adult decision-making competence. *Journal of Personality and Social Psychology*. 92 (5): 938–956.

de Wit, S.C., Stomberg, H.K., and Vreeland Dallred, C. (2017). *Medical Surgical Nursing: Concepts and Practice*, 3e. St Louis: Elsevier.

Dowding, D.W., Cheyne, H.L., and Hundley, V. (2011). Complex interventions in midwifery care: reflections on the design and evaluation of an algorithm for the diagnosis of labour. *Midwifery* 27 (5): 654–659.

Jullisson, E.A., Karlsson, N., and Garling, T. (2005). Weighing the past and the future in decision making. *European Journal of Cognitive Psychology* 17 (4): 561–575.

Levett-Jones, T., Hoffman, K., Dempsey, Y. et al. (2010). The 'five rights' of clinical reasoning: an educational model to enhance nursing students' ability to identify and manage clinically 'at risk' patients. *Nurse Education Today* 30 (6): 515–520.

MacNeela, P., Scott, A., Clinton, G. et al. (2017). Judgement and decisions making. In: *Becoming a Nurse: Fundamentals of Professional Practice for Nursing*, 2e (ed. D. Sellman and P. Snelling), 327–349. Oxford: Routledge.

Nursing and Midwifery Council (2018). The Code. Professional Standards of Practice and Behaviour for Nurses, Midwives and Nursing Associates. https://www.nmc.org.uk/globalassets/sitedocuments/nmc-publications/nmc-code.pdf last accessed 8 May 2019.

Purling, A. and King, L. (2012). A literature review: Graduate nurses' preparedness for recognising and responding to the deteriorating patient. *Journal of Clinical Nursing.* 21 (23–24): 3451–3465.

Stanovich, K.E. and West, R.F. (2008). On the relative independence of thinking biases and cognitive ability. *Journal of Personality and Social Psychology* 94 (4): 672–695.

Thompson, C. (1999). A conceptual treadmill: The need for 'middle ground' in clinical decision making theory in nursing. *Journal of Advanced Nursing* 39 (5): 1222–1229.

Thompson, C. and Dowding, D. (2009). *Essential Decision Making and Clinical Judgement for Nurses.* Edinburgh: Elsevier.

Thompson, C. and Stapley, S. (2011). Do educational interventions improve nurses' clinical decision making and judgement? A systematic review. *International Journal of Nursing Studies* 48 (7): 881–893.

Thompson, C., Aitken, L., Doran, D., and Dowding, D. (2013). An agenda for clinical decision making and judgement in nursing research and education. *International Journal of Nursing Studies* 50: 1720–1726.

Tomlinson, J. (2015). Using clinical supervision to improve the quality and safety of patient care: a response to Berwick and Francis. *BioMedical Central Medical Education* 103 (15): https://doi.org/10.1186/s12909-015-0324-3.

Tschikota, S. (1993). The clinical decision making process of student nurses. *Journal of Nursing Education* 32 (9): 389–398.

Williams, I. and Brown, H. (2014). Factors influencing decisions of value in health care: A review of the literature. www.nhsconfed.org/-/media/Confederation/Files/Publications/Documents/DOV_HSMC_Final_report_July_281.pdf (accessed March 2018).

Chapter 4

The nursing process

Aim

This chapter aims to provide the reader with an introduction to the nursing process and its five phases.

Learning outcomes

By the end of the chapter the reader will be able to:

1. List the five components of the nursing process
2. Discuss and apply the five components of the nursing process
3. Discuss the importance of ensuring that the patient is at the centre of all that is done
4. Discuss the nurse's professional duties when applying the nursing process in practice

Introduction

The nursing process was explained by Orlando (1961) (initially the process had four stages: assessing, implementing, planning, evaluating), with ongoing development of the nursing process by Yura and Walsh (1967), who suggested that it could be considered the most influential change in approaches to thinking about nursing care. It has been described as being a decision-making model that focuses on patients' needs and helps to solve problems that they may have. The nursing process supports professional nursing practice. Stonehouse (2017) aptly suggests that in contemporary practice the nursing process may be better called 'the caring process', involving all members of the multidisciplinary phase. The systematic approach to care provision can also be used for the provision of patient education as well as health education interventions. There are a number of scenarios provided in this chapter that are used to develop key concepts further.

The nursing process

The nursing process, a cyclical model, is clear and straightforward, and it comprises five concepts of nursing: assessment, diagnosis, planning, implementation, and evaluation. The key element of the nursing process is that it considers the patient first and then thinks about the care that the patient requires. This is in contrast to the nurse deciding what care he or she thinks it is that the patient needs and then thinking about the patient and how this might be implemented.

Fundamentals of Assessment and Care Planning for Nurses, First Edition. Ian Peate.
© 2020 John Wiley & Sons Ltd. Published 2020 by John Wiley & Sons Ltd.

Lappin (2018) discusses the nursing process, suggesting that it is broken down into a five-step procedure that is known as ADPIE:

Assess: observing, measuring, and communicating
Diagnosis: identifying the patient's problems
Planning: planning care and setting patient-centred goals
Implement: being able to apply the nursing actions identified in planning
Evaluation: determining if the goals set have been achieved and, if needed, reassessing

This cyclical process (see Figure 4.1) emphasises the importance of assessment as well as encouraging nurses to identify with the patient's potential and actual health needs. The patient is truly at heart of all that is done when the nurse uses the nursing process.

The nursing process can help improve the critical thinking process and provides for the formation, evaluation, and re-evaluation of various actions to be implemented and continually modified until the appropriate outcome has been achieved. This is why the process is a cyclical process and not linear. The nursing process permits nurses to assess and use an organised framework for thinking through problems as well as expanding further on their critical thinking skills. One of the advantages of this process is that it offers flexibility and is adaptable, as opposed to limiting the ways in which the nurse can use a framework in order to meet the needs of patients. It is a tool that assists in the provision of nursing care while allowing creativity as well as providing an opportunity for nurses to look at alternative ways to provide care (Yildirim and Ozkahraman 2011).

Review

Apply the nursing process to a familiar life activity, for example buying a car, buying a house, planning a holiday. As you plan your holiday, the assessment consists of a list of needs, for example are you looking for a beach holiday, a self-catering apartment or hotel, a holiday at home or abroad, and what is your budget? The process is planned; you might go online to view the proposed property or use other online tools to determine if your conditions have been met. The diagnostic phase equates to you choosing the holiday in the location, for what it is you can afford. The intervention is when you actually go on that holiday. Evaluation of the holiday is ongoing and occurs throughout the holiday; you will assess the hotel, the apartment, the weather, the beach, and you will go on assessing and reassessing – you will move to another part of the beach if you do not like one part, you may even check out of the hotel and into another if it does not meet your needs.

Now try doing the same activity with another familiar life activity.

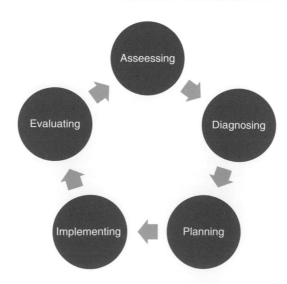

Figure 4.1   The cyclical nursing process.

Using a systemic framework or approach to care delivery can help the nurse ensure that care is truly holistic, along with the provision of quality care to the patient irrespective of the person's age, gender, diagnosis, or care setting. The various components of the nursing process will address the physical, psychological, cultural, social, and cognitive aspects of a patient (a holistic approach). The professional nurse who critically thinks and processes all elements of information provided and uses the information gathered in a proficient manner will be able to develop and coordinate care that is safe and effective (Lilley et al. 2017).

Nurses are required to listen to people and respond to their preferences and concerns and to also work in partnership with people to make sure that care is delivered effectively (NMC 2018). There is a requirement for nurses to consider how an analysis of a patient's experience of healthcare can and should inform service improvement and development (Buckley et al. 2016). What the nurse and the patient say during the interaction affects them both, it is a reciprocal relationship.

For Orlando (1961), if the problem has not been discovered it cannot be solved and this is why the therapeutic nurse/patient relationship is so important when implementing the nursing process. Within each phase of the nursing process, the patient's (and if appropriate the family's) story is key and is used as the basis for knowledge, judgement, and actions that will influence the patient care experience. The 'patient's story' is a term used to describe objective and subjective information about the patient that describes who the patient is as a person in addition to their usual medically focused history. Hamilton and Price (2013) suggest that historically, the medical model was where a diagnosis was made by a doctor, with care prescribed based only on the medical symptoms. Focusing on medical needs has the potential to ignore the person's holistic needs (Stonehouse 2017). Aspects of the patient's story will include physiological, psychological, and family characteristics; available resources (and these include human and material resources); any environmental issues; and the person's social context, knowledge and understanding, and motivation. Care is influenced, and is often driven, by what it is the patient states (verbally and non-verbally), and this will also incorporate their physiological state. The patient's story should be seen as something that is dynamic (fluid) and is to be shared appropriately and understood throughout all interactions.

Ida Orlando's theory is clearly concerned with the patient and how the patient affects the nurse's decision making. When there are good assessments and astute observations are performed then good outcomes result, and in so doing care becomes more individualised (Black 2016). However, the theory has some potential limitations; there is much focus on the theory of problems (problematic), with too much focus on the here and now, and there seems to be little on prevention, on taking action prior to the problems appearing.

So far

Understanding and having an awareness of the nursing process is essential if the nurse is to adhere to the tenets of the Code (NMC 2018). This also allows the nurse to recognise and respect the role the nurse has to play in the provision of patient-centred care. Throughout the process the patient's needs are assessed, a nursing diagnosis is made, care is planned and goals are set, care is implemented, and evaluation of interventions is ongoing. The evaluation stage ensures that quality has been delivered.

The stages of the nursing process

The five stages of the nursing process will be discussed in this section. Chapter 7 will specifically address the principles of assessment and the planning stage.

Assessment

Assessment is considered to be the first stage in the planning of nursing care, as it starts the process of gathering information in order to make decisions about appropriate interventions (Ballantyne

2016). It is at this stage when we hear the patient's story. Two types of data are collected during the assessment phase:

1. Objective data
2. Subjective data

These types of data are very different but equally important.

Objective data

This type of data is the type of data that is collected when using one or more of the senses (for example what is seen, smelt, heard, and felt) it is a measurement or it is an observation. A good example of objective data collection is blood pressure. The nurse uses a sphygmomanometer (or an electronic blood pressure measuring device), the device tells us objectively what the measurement of the person's blood pressure is.

Review

Think of some other types/examples of objective data that you collect (but remember, for it to objective it needs to be measurable or an observation).

Oxygen saturation is another example of objective data (Did you include this in your list in the review box?), the pulse oximeter measures the amount of oxygen in the blood and this is then displayed on a screen for the nurse to see. Of course, the pulse oximeter can only be relied upon if it has been deemed to be working correctly and if it has been calibrated. Another important factor to determine is if the objective data is reliable if the nurse using the equipment knows how to use it, interpret the findings, and act on them safely and effectively (user reliability). Objective data is part of the patient's story.

The best way to document objective data is to be precise and factual and whenever possible use measurable data, for example, 'capillary nail bed return is less than two minutes'.

Subjective data

This kind of data is associated with data that is spoken or shared by the patient, it is the type of data that cannot be measured by one of the senses. Subjective data is what the patient says that their symptoms are, these include feelings, perceptions, and their concerns.

This kind of data is crucial as it provides the background as to what the patient's needs are, and why they came into the hospital or the general practice. Listening to them is essential so as to understand the whole picture. Taking notes provides an overall view of the patient and can also help to tell the patient's story. Listening to what it is that troubles the patient will ultimately make their outcome better. Listening also allows the nurse to act as a true patient advocate.

Whenever possible the best way to document subjective data is to put the statement in quotation marks, for example: 'I feel like my heart is racing and missing a beat.' In Box 4.1, the patient scenario considers both objective and subjective data.

Box 4.1 Breaking down objective and subjective data

Sanjay is a 58-year-old male patient who you are looking after with an infected pilonidal sinus. He returned from theatre four hours ago after having had the abscess drained. He says to you, 'I feel like I can't breathe.' His respirations are 28 breaths per minute and his heart rate is 115 beats per minute. Sanjay then grabs his chest and says, 'My chest hurts so bad, please help!' You ask the patient to rate the pain on a scale from 0 to 10, 10 being the worst pain ever. He replies, '10, it hurts so bad!' You then ask him to describe what the pain feels like, the patient reports that his pain feels like pressure. Sanjay then starts to become diaphoretic and pale. You take an electrocardiogram (ECG) that shows sinus tachycardia. The pulse oximeter (oxygen saturation) shows 100% on room air and the patient's blood pressure is 120/80 mmHg.

Breaking this down into objective and subjective data:

Objective data:
- 58-year-old male
- Respirations 28
- Heart rate 115
- Patient is diaphoretic and pale
- ECG showing sinus tachycardia
- Oxygen saturation 100% on room air
- Blood pressure 120/80 mmHg.

Subjective data:
- Sanjay experiencing shortness of breath
- Chest pain that is a pressure feeling and is 10/10

Shortness of breath is classified as subjective as it is Sanjay who is telling you that he feels this way. If the nurse had observed accessory muscle use then use of accessory muscles would be objective, but the feeling of shortness of breath would still be subjective. The diaphoresis and pale skin condition is objective as this is a visible observation.

So far

Subjective	Objective
• Anything that cannot be verified • Feelings • Pain • Nausea • Sensations	• Measurements (metrics) • Observed data using the senses • Vital signs
• Patient feels 'low' • Patient say she has fallen from her bed • Patient reports that their heart is 'galloping' • Patient says 'feel like I cannot breathe'	• Glasgow Coma Score • Body Mass Index (BMI) • Blood pressure • Epistaxis • Sweating • Smell of 'acetone' on the breath • Accessory muscles of respiration being used • Cyanosis

Signs and symptoms

Sometimes people use the term 'sign' and 'symptom' interchangeably. There are, however, important differences that affect their use in the assessment of patients' needs. Whilst there are technical differences between the two words, the important thing for the nurse to note is the information that surrounds them. The nurse has to take heed of both signs and symptoms.

Symptoms can only be described by the person who is feeling them. If the person is experiencing pain, no one knows unless until the person tells the nurse. This is the same with feeling nauseous, feeling dizzy, experiencing numbness, feeling persecuted, and a number of other feelings. Nobody knows about these experiences until they are described.

This does not mean that other people (i.e. the nurse) do not notice when a person is not feeling well. If the person's face is pale, they appear cyanotic, they seem unstable when they are walking, or the person is sweating, then that person is displaying signs. Signs have to be seen and read by someone (e.g. a nurse, family member) as opposed to being felt. Signs are indicators of a problem, abnormal vital signs are indicators of potential problems. 'Danger, keep out' is a sign to warn you that there are potential problems ahead.

Review

In the patient scenario below, use a red highlighter for what you think is subjective (symptom) and a yellow highlighter for what you think is objective (sign) data.

Georgie is 30-year-old female who came into the emergency department accompanied by two friends, with acute mental status changes that began around 1600h this afternoon. The two friends who brought her to the ED state that she has been under a lot of stress lately. They state that she started acting bizarre and unusual from her normal activity and there is a chance that she could be pregnant, she was 'weird' said one friend. They also say that work has been really challenging for her lately and she has been really 'low in mood'. She is in and out of verbal response and in and out of combative behaviour at this time (now 2010h).

Georgie is a doctor and lives locally with the two friends that brought her in today. She has no other family in town, they all live overseas. The patient denies any alcohol, tobacco, or recreational drug use.

The patient has no medical history. The only medication she is taking is birth control and she has no allergies to medications, just an allergy to eggs. When Georgie presented to the accident and emergency department initially with an altered mental status, she was not willing to follow any commands. It was noted that she had an eye flickering (Alert Voice Pain, Unconscious check (AVPU)) and she was responsive to painful stimuli. She had a normal gag reflex. Her vital signs were as follows: blood pressure 102/56 mm/Hg, pulse rate 108 beats per minute, respiratory rate 20 breaths per minute, SaO_2 was 99% on room air, temperature 37.2 °C, skin warm, diaphoretic, good capillary refill less than two minutes, Glasgow Coma Score 13, electrocardiograph sinus rhythm.

During the initial assessment phase the nurse usually starts by talking to the patient, seeing how they are, how they are getting on, and the reason for their visit (to the hospital, emergency department, general practice). Listening attentively and respecting the person's point of view is essential as this allows them to tell their story and for the nurse to appreciate their understanding of what is going on, receiving the information can help the nurse identify what the problem is. Once the subjective data is collected the nurse goes on to gather objective data (for example, vital signs, requests blood specimens or other diagnostic tests). In reality, however, a skilled nurse may be gathering objective and subjective data simultaneously.

Subjective and objective data are required to make a full assessment of the patient – both types of data are needed as they work together, allowing the nurse to reach a more accurate clinical picture. When the patient is able to provide data this is called primary data. When the patient is unable to do this, for example if the person is unconscious, then the nurse may need to revert to accessing data from other sources, and this is known as secondary data collection.

Review

Can you list potential sources of secondary data if the patient is unable to provide you with primary data?

Which type of data is more reliable: primary data or secondary data? Why?

Take note

In order to undertake an assessment that is effective and meets the holistic needs of the patient, Abdelkader and Othman (2017) make clear that time is required for this stage of the process to be effective. A lack of knowledge, high patient/nurse ratios, and lack of motivational factors and appropriate education and training can put this essential active in jeopardy.

When this stage is completed, although the nurse may be adding aspects of data collection to the data already collected, the next stage – making a nursing diagnosis – can begin. The nurse then undertakes an analysis of the data.

So far

Assessment is the first step of the nursing process. It is during this phase that the nurse gathers information about a patient's psychological, physiological, sociological, and spiritual status. This data can be collected in a number of ways. Usually, the nurse conducts a patient interview. A physical examination is performed, referencing a patient's health history, obtaining a patient's family history and overall observation can also be used to gather assessment data. Patient interaction is usually most predominant during this phase; the nurse seeks subjective and objective data and obtains this through the primary source (the patient) or, if this is not possible, through a secondary source (for example the patient's family).

Nursing diagnosis

A nursing diagnosis according to Herdman and Kamitsuru (2017) is a clinical judgement that is concerned with a human response to health conditions/life processes, or a vulnerability for that response, by an individual, family, group, or community. The nursing diagnosis needs a nursing assessment so the patient is correctly diagnosed. Sometimes there is confusion between a nursing diagnosis and a medical diagnosis – the problems identified when making a nursing diagnosis may be linked to a medical diagnosis. The nursing diagnosis will take into account the consequences of the patient having to live with their condition (their signs and symptoms) and how they interact with others, for example their family, friends, their work environment. A nursing diagnosis is the basis for selection of nursing interventions so as to achieve outcomes for which the nurse is accountable. Nursing diagnoses are used to establish the most appropriate plan of care, promoting positive patient outcomes and safe, effective interventions. Nursing interventions will be more than just treating signs and symptoms of the illness, they will address the physical, psychological, social, and spiritual consequences of the condition; a holistic approach (see Box 4.2).

Take note

A 'one size fits all' approach to care provision is unacceptable in contemporary nursing practice.

Valuing equality and diversity are not to be seen as 'add-ons', they must be seen as essential components of how services are delivered and how we work together with individuals and communities and in their communities. Good equality and diversity practice guarantees that our services are accessible to everyone, ensuring that everybody is treated with dignity and respect, encouraging participation and self-management, and supporting improved outcomes for all.

Box 4.2 Daniel Canilla

Daniel Canilla is a 64-year-old man who recently had a pacemaker fitted as he was experiencing cardiac arrhythmias. He has told the district nurse that he is anxious and scared about his life in the future. Being at home, he has not wanted to go out since he had the pacemaker: 'Will it, can it run out of battery? It is as if my life depends on it, what if it fails and if it fails when I am asleep? I just cannot sleep at all, I will just die in my sleep. What about going through X-ray machines at the airport and those security things in shops?' He is clearly worried and distressed. 'I am taking the medication they have given me for my heart but I am truly petrified, my poor wife is worried sick also.'

In Box 4.2, it is evident that Mr Canilla is concerned about his recent treatment for a cardiac arrhythmia. The pacemaker is a medical device that can help to control the arrhythmias, as is the pharmacological treatment that was prescribed by the cardiologist. The presence of the pacemaker is having a significant impact on other human responses such as disturbed sleep pattern, anxiety, and social isolation. Whilst the issue regarding his pacemaker and his medication should not be overlooked, Daniel's fears and anxieties, the stress he is experiencing, his concern for his wife (as a consequence of having the pacemaker fitted), and his lack of understanding are undoubtedly nursing diagnoses. The district nurse needs now to formulate a plan of action (provide a set of goals), then implement that plan and put in place evaluation strategies so as to determine if the interventions have been effective.

Review

Take some time out and learn a little more about cardiac pacemakers (there are several different types). How do they work and what advice can be given to patients to alleviate any anxieties they and their family may have?

In the UK the term 'nursing diagnosis' is not commonly used. There are no definitive classifications or common language in general use with regard to nursing diagnoses. However, the adaptation and implementation of standard nursing languages within clinical practice in the UK are moving forward, particularly with the increasing use of electronic documentation and electronic care planning. However, Ballantyne (2016) argues that nursing diagnoses are used implicitly throughout the nursing process since the patient's needs have been identified and addressed, suggestive of a 'built-in' approach as opposed to a separate entity. She considers, for example, a patient handover, where nursing diagnoses are frequently made following a formal assessment, and numerous nursing diagnoses, for example anxiety, risk of impaired skin integrity, and disturbed sleep pattern, may be used routinely.

Making a nursing diagnosis begins when the nurse has gathered the subjective and objective data. The data is critically analysed and a nursing diagnosis can be made. The diagnosis may be tentative or definitive. The nursing diagnosis is the nurse's clinical judgement regarding the person's response to an actual or potential health condition or needs. Hogston (2011) considers actual problems as those that emerge during or directly after assessment, for example new wounds (biting, abrading) occurring as a result of self-mutilation. Potential problems are those that may arise as a result of the current problem, such as a potential for a self-mutilated bite to become infected. A nursing diagnosis describes a combination of a clinical judgement made about a person's response to health or illness as well as the process of decision making that leads to that judgement. A thorough assessment is an absolute requisite and cannot be overemphasised. Collecting comprehensive and appropriate data from patients (or others when the patient is unable to give information), including those meanings the person attributes to events, is, according to Alfaro-Lefevre (2014) and Alfaro-LeFevre (2017), associated with more diagnostic accuracy and thus will result in more timely and effective interventions.

When the assessment is made and the nursing diagnosis formulated, it needs to be written in a clear way so that it reflects the patient's needs (not the nurse's needs, not the doctor's needs, but the patient's needs). In a needs statement, the nurse has to remember that nursing diagnoses are individual responses to health difficulties or life courses. Return to Daniel in Box 4.2; he expresses that he is 'just not sleeping'. Taking this need and turning it into a needs statement, it would read: 'Mr Canilla is finding it difficult to sleep, 2–3 hours per night due to anxiety and worry as a result of recent pacemaker insertion.' This is different to what a medical diagnosis might read: 'Patient suffering from insomnia due to insertion of ICD 2/7.'

The needs statement is patient-centred (specifically for Mr Canilla), it does not use any technical terms or jargon and could easily be understood by the patient. The nursing diagnosis focuses on how the insertion of the pacemaker is causing Mr Canilla anxiety and thus lack of sleep. The nursing diagnosis also provides a baseline. The baseline offers information about where the patient is now and helps the nurse plot the direction of travel, i.e. after the nursing intervention is Mr Canilla sleeping more than two to three hours a night or less, it provides a parameter that can be measured. The data collected during the assessment provides baseline information. Mr Canilla's needs statement contains objective and subjective data as well as a baseline.

It could be suggested that the focus is on the medical problem, the insomnia, it is generic and not specific (patient), it is technical it uses abbreviations: ICD (implantable cardioverter defibrillator), 2/7 (two days) and may not be so easily understood by the patient (or some other health and social providers for that matter).

Patients may have more than one needs statement and the nurse needs to decide (preferably with the patient) what the priority of needs is. Priority of needs may be clearly obvious, for example a patient with a haemorrhage as the result of a knife attack or person in a state of unconsciousness, and prioritising needs in these situations is associated with safety and maintaining a safe environment.

So far

Having amassed the data, the diagnosing phase requires the nurse to make an educated judgement concerning a potential or actual health problem with a patient. A theory or hypothesis regarding the patient's situation is based on the information that has been collected during the performing of a holistic assessment.

Multiple diagnoses are sometimes made for a single patient. These assessments not only include an actual description of the problem (e.g. sleep deprivation) but also whether or not a patient is at risk of developing further problems (actual and potential). These diagnoses are also used to decide a patient's willingness for health improvement, the diagnosis phase is an important step as it is then used to help the nurse and the patient to determine the course of treatment.

Planning

Many job descriptions require nurses to be able to plan care. This is usually listed an essential skill, regardless of the care setting. The NMC Pre-registration proficiencies (NMC 2018) state that the student nurse must demonstrate proficiency in the planning of care.

In this stage, the nurse intervenes on behalf of and with the patient to address specific problems and needs. This can be done in a number of ways, through independent nursing actions, collaborative activities (with, for example, occupational therapy, physiotherapy) and the administration of prescribed medications

Writing the patient's care plan commences when the nurse and the patient plan achievable goals (these can be long- or short-term). Working with the patient, the nurse and the patient discuss ways in which goals can be achieved. When the nurse gathers data (assessment) and compiles a needs statement (a nursing diagnosis), this begins the care planning process.

During the planning stage interventions are identified in order to diminish, alleviate, or prevent problems identified and at the same time offer the patient support in achieving the goals that have been set (Kozier et al. 2012). There are two components associated with this stage:

1. Setting goals
2. Identifying actions

It is essential during this stage that the goals set are realistic and achievable. The care that is going be implemented (the identification of actions to be taken) must be clearly communicated, whether in a handwritten care plan or an electronic care plan. Whatever the format, the actions need to be clearly stated. Chapter 7 of this text will address the principles that are associated with the planning stage in more detail.

Box 4.3 The five rights of delegation

- The right person must be assigned the right task.
- The right task should be assigned to the right person that is relevant to their scope of practice.
- The right circumstances for delegation to be activated.
- The right directions and communication. The registered nurse has to communicate with and direct the person undertaking the task.
- The right supervision and evaluation with ongoing supervision and evaluation are essential, determining whether or not the task was carried out in the correct, appropriate, safe, and competent manner.

So far

When the patient and the nurse have agreed on the diagnosis, it is at this stage that a plan of action can be developed. If multiple diagnoses need to be addressed, then these needs need to be prioritised, focusing attention on severe symptoms as well as high risk factors. Each problem receives a clear, measurable goal/aim for the expected beneficial outcome. Goals can be long-term or short-term and reflect the individual needs of the patient.

Implementation

This stage of the process could also be considered as the 'doing' stage, the action part. The nursing diagnoses have been made and a plan of action decided on (with the patient if possible), the goals set and the strategies that are intended to be used are now put into place, and the care plan is actioned. Ballantyne (2016) notes that different groups of patients are likely to require different interventions and different care goals.

This hands-on stage requires more involvement with the patient. Here the nurse (and there may be a need for other members of the multidisciplinary team to become involved) uses planned interventions and critical thinking skills as they solve problems and set proprieties. The delegation of care to others has been discussed in Chapter 1 of this text and should always be undertaken with the best interests of the patient in mind (the five rights of delegation are highlighted in Box 4.3).

When there is improper and inappropriate delegation this can lead to poor quality of care, unsatisfactory outcomes of care, and a risk to patient safety.

Take note

When a registered nurse delegates aspects of patient care, for example, that are outside the scope of practice of that healthcare worker, this puts the patient at potential physical and/or psychological risk because this delegated task, which is outside the scope of practice for healthcare workers, is something that this member of staff was not prepared and educated or trained to perform. When the health care worker accepts this delegated activity, it is considered practising outside their scope of practice. All staff should refuse to accept any assignment that is outside their scope of practice.

Delegation on the face of it is the transfer of the registered nurse's responsibility for the performance of a task to another staff member, but the registered nurse always retains accountability for the outcome. Responsibility can be delegated whereas accountability can never be delegated.

There must also be an important element of ensuring that the patient's responses to the intervention are continually reassessed; the goals that have been set may need to be adapted after the nursing intervention has been implemented, and for this reason it is key to continually reassess. When staff come on duty they should be consulting the care plan to determine if there are any changes in the patient's condition or changes to the implementation strategy. It is absolutely essential that all care interventions are evidence-based and documented according to local policy and procedure. Documentation aids effective communication.

Implementing care requires the care plan to provide specific instruction, frequency of care interventions, and other relevant information. Lilley et al. (2017) refer to the nine rights of drug administration (see Table 4.1) as a clear example of the provision of specific instruction when administering prescribed medication.

As with other stages of the nursing process, there are some key skills the nurse needs to possess in order to carry out this stage safely and effectively. The nurse has to be able to demonstrate expertise with regard to psychomotor skills as this is a necessary prerequisite to safely and effectively undertake nursing activities. The nurse has to be proficient in handling technical/medical equipment as well as being able to perform skills, for example administration of medications and assisting the patient with maintaining a safe environment. Therapeutic communication skills have to honed and applied in accordance with the care plan.

So far

The implementation stage requires the nurse to reassess (throughout the whole stage) the implementation of the predefined (after the assessment and diagnosis) nursing intervention, in order to determine the need for nursing assistance. If care is to be delegated to another health care worker this must adhere to the five rights of delegation. It is essential that care is documented according to local policy and procedure so as to enhance communication and record the patient's response to care delivered.

Certain skills influence the implementation of the nursing care plan, including your ability to perform intellectual, interpersonal and technical skills. Intellectual skills involve knowing and understanding essential information prior to caring for patients. Critical thinking is one intellectual skill vital for making quick decisions and taking immediate action. Interpersonal skills involve believing, behaving, and relating to others. Effective communication techniques promote the development of trusting relationships. Acting in a professional manner also involves interpersonal skills. Technical skills, such as changing a sterile dressing or administering an injection, demand safe and competent performance.

All nursing activities performed have to be fully explained to the patient and undertaken with competence and confidence. Explanation has to include what procedures are to be carried out, what sensations may be expected, recommendations as to how to deal with expected sensations, and what the expected result is.

Evaluation

Evaluation is the final stage of the nursing process. However, in reality this stage could begin the cyclical process all over again (it is systematic and dynamic), as many of the skills required to evaluate care interventions can also be found in the assessment stage, and care interventions may need to revised, to continue with the same plan of action or, if the goal/aim has been achieved, to discontinue it. It is important at this stage to use words such as 'monitor', as monitoring requires the nurse to observe for the therapeutic effects of the care that has been delivered as well as for any side effects or untoward events. There are a number of indicators that can be used to monitor impact of care. Subjective and objective data should be collated in a systematic manner in order to evaluate the patient's health status, ask the patient to say how they feel (subjective data), observe the patient, and take note of vital signs, blood values, and other observable data.

55

Table 4.1 The nine rights of drug administration.

Right	Description
1. Right drug	Administration of the prescribed correct drug, requires careful review of the medication as a number of medications have similar names.
2. Right dose	The nurse needs to ensure that the prescribed dose is correctly transcribed and administered. Nurses also have a responsibility to ensure that the dose prescribed is within the appropriate dose range.
3. Right time	Administration of prescribed medication at the correct time can ensure that therapeutic serum levels, local policy and procedure must be followed.
4. Right route and form	Administration of the medication using the prescribed route and form, for example oral, liquid suspension.
5. Right patient	The proposed medication must be administered to the patient for whom it is prescribed. Patient identity has to be confirmed using local policy and procedure.
6. Right documentation	Adherence to local policy and procedure and the timely and accurate documentation of medicines administered.
7. Right reason	The right reason or right action. It is important that the nurse understands the rationale for the medications being prescribed (the nurse will need an understanding of the patient's history). If the medication that has been prescribed is at odds with the patient's condition and the reason for its use are not clear, then it is appropriate for the nurse to gather more information before administering it. There must always be a rationale for long-term use of medication.
8. Right response	This refers to the prescribed medication's desired response (the nurse may be required to evaluate the impact of the drug, for example by measuring a peak flow after the administration of a bronchodilator) and any untoward or undesired responses. These responses should be documented and appropriate actions taken.
9. Right of the patient to refuse	It is the right of the patient to refuse medication and there may be many reasons for this, the nurse should respect the patient's right to refuse. The nurse should attempt to determine the reason for refusal, document this and inform the prescriber, administration involves an evaluation of the effectiveness of the medication's intended purpose through patient assessment and monitoring.

Source: Adapted Lilley et al. (2017) and Elliot and Liu (2010).

Review

Make notes about the subjective and objective data that you should collect to ascertain if the nursing interventions that have been implemented have made a difference to the person's health status:

Subjective	Objective

The nurse working with the patient is a mutual process, evaluating whether care interventions have been successful in reaching the goals/aims set in the planning stage. However, to reiterate, evaluation should take part throughout the implementation stage (constant reassessment) (Yildirim and Ozkahraman 2011). This determines whether the individual is making progress towards the goals set and is achieving the desired outcomes. The NMC (2018) requires nurses to work with their colleagues and to evaluate the quality of their own work and also that of the team. See Box 4.4 for an outline of the purposes of evaluation.

Box 4.4 Some of the purposes of evaluation

- To ascertain the patient's progress or lack of progress as they are working towards the achievement of expected outcomes
- To establish the effectiveness of nursing care as the nurse assists the patient to achieve the expected outcomes
- To consider the overall quality of care provided and to make a judgement on whether change has occurred
- To promote nursing accountability and to share any reasons behind the success or failure of the plan of care.

This stage can also be seen as a component of the quality assurance process. See Moule et al. (2017), who point out that evaluation of service delivery is an important aspect of nursing practice. Service evaluation is being used and led more and more by nurses, who are ideally placed to undertake this important activity. Nursing audit is the process of collecting and analysing data so as to evaluate the effectiveness of nursing interventions. This has the potential to focus on the implementation phase of the nursing process, patient outcomes, or both, with the aim of evaluating the quality of care provided. Nursing audits usually consider data that is related to:

- Safety measures
- Treatment interventions and the responses that patients make to the interventions
- Pre-established outcomes that are used as a basis for interventions
- Discharge planning
- Patient teaching
- Patient staff ratios

When an audit has been undertaken, this can assist in identifying strengths and weaknesses which have the potential to offer direction for areas that may require revision and remediation. Action plans can then be developed as a result of the audit.

The nurse concludes, in a systematic way, if the resources, be these human and or material, have been used effectively in care delivery. Documentation of findings are related to goals and outcome criteria that have been set previously (they must be clear and concise), any revisions made, and any new interventions required. If the evaluation data has indicated that there has been a lack of progress towards achieving the goal/aim, then the plan of care must be modified. Modification occurs through:

- Patient reassessment
- The formulation of nursing diagnoses that are more appropriate to the needs of the patient
- Improvement or development of new or revised goals/aims
- Undertaking different nursing actions or a repetition of particular actions to enhance their effectiveness

Evaluation of care can only occur in an effective and worthwhile manner if during the nursing diagnosis stage a baseline has been set or agreed upon. This then allows the nurse and the patient to compare and contrast. There are other standards that can be used to assist in the evaluation of care, from a personal and institutional perspective, for example Codes of Conduct, patient constitution statements, patient surveys, local policy and procedures, professional body standards frameworks, statutory commission standards.

Consider the patient scenario of Maria Gonzales. The nursing diagnosis of risk of falling due to unsteady shuffling gait and legs and arms asymmetry has been chosen to demonstrate how all phases of the nursing process have come together, culminating in the evaluation stage.

Scenario

Maria Gonzales is a 72-year-old woman who lives alone in sheltered accommodation on the outskirts of the city. Mrs Gonzales' husband died four years ago. Her daughter, Donna, lives locally. She was admitted to the stroke unit with a left-sided weakness as a result of a right-sided ischaemic stroke. She is doing well but, being left-handed, she has reported that she can only use the fork in her left hand with difficulty and this is frustrating her.

Nursing assessment

- 'I am unable to lift a beaker with only the one hand.'
- 'I am struggling to use the walker the OT gave me, it just seems to be getting in my way.'
- She has unsteady gait and in order to get around the bed space is shuffling
- There is asymmetrical strength in her arms and her legs
- Unable to lift the beaker with just her one hand

Nursing diagnosis

At risk of injury due to falls that are related to unsteady shuffling gait and legs and arms asymmetry.

Goals/aims

Maria will:

1. Take part in physiotherapy and occupational therapy evaluation with regard to mobility and weakness on 11/2 at 1530 h
2. Attend subsequent rehabilitation sessions to strengthen muscles 12/2 at 1600 h
3. Carry out all strengthening exercises as prescribed twice daily at 1000 h and 1600 h commencing 13/2

Interventions with rationale

1. Refer to physio and OT for assistive devices to strengthen and enhance gait 11/2. This will engage the assistance of other health care experts, offering Maria the most appropriate care.
2. Provide an escort for Maria to attend classes 12/2 at 1600 h. This offers safety and support.
3. Healthcare assistant to record each exercise/activity twice daily, number of repetitions and the response Maria makes to carrying out these exercises. Documenting the progress Maria is making as she works towards the achieving the goals/aims will help in outcome achievement and evaluation of care.

Evaluation

1. Goal has not been achieved. Appointment 11/2 Maria needed to have a hearing aid assessment at audiology clinic. Continue and re-evaluate 15/2.
2. Goal not met. Unable to evaluate 12/2. Continue and re-evaluate 15/2.
3. 15/2 goal met. Maria attended classes for muscle strengthening and is performing the exercises twice daily as prescribed.

Conclusion

The nursing process has the potential to actively encourage the nurse–patient relationship, ensuring that the patient is at the heart of all that is done and can be applied to all fields of nursing. The nursing processes is a systematic, evolving, dynamic approach to nursing care and comprises five stages. This chapter has addressed each stage under each of the five headings, adopting a linear approach. However, in reality, the nurse oscillates between all stages, often returning to one stage and then moving on again.

The nurse gathers, analyses, organises, provides data and acts upon the information gained, using critical thinking skills and mobilising resources to achieve goals and outcomes that have been set. Nursing diagnoses are formulated based upon the retrieval of objective and subjective data collected from primary and, if appropriate, secondary sources. Whenever possible this is always done in partnership with the patient. The novice nurse is continually developing skills that will enable them to become more astute in assessment, formulating a safe nursing diagnosis, planning care that is related to the needs that have arisen from assessment, delivering that holistic care using critical thinking skills as well as acting in a competent and confident manner, and finally evaluating all that has been done in the best interest of the patient to determine efficacy.

All nurses have a professional obligation to ensure that they provide safe and effective care to those they offer care to (NMC 2018). As well as professional obligations, there are also requirements that must be given due diligence in order to ensure that patient safety is paramount.

References

Abdelkader, F.A. and Othman, W.N. (2017). Factor affecting implementation of nursing process: nurses perspective. *Journal of Nursing and Health Science* 6 (3): 76–82.

Alfaro-LeFevre, R. (2014). *Applying Nursing Process: The Foundation for Clinical Reasoning*. Philadelphia: Lippincott.

Alfaro-LeFevre, R. (2017). *Critical Thinking, Clinical Reasoning, and Clinical Judgment: A Practical Approach*, 6e. Philadelphia: Elsevier.

Ballantyne, H. (2016). Developing nursing care plans. *Nursing Standard* 30 (26): 51–57.

Black, B.P. (2016). *Professional Nursing: Concepts and Challenges*, 8e. Maryland Heights: Elsevier/Saunders.

Buckley, A., Corless, L., and Mee, S. (2016). Patient narratives 1: Using patient stories to reflect on care. *Nursing Times*. 112 (10): 22–25.

Elliot, M. and Liu, Y. (2010). The nine rights of medication administration: An overview. *British Journal of Nursing* 19 (5): 300–305.

Hamilton, P. and Price, T. (2013). The nursing process, holistic assessment and base line observations. In: *Foundations of Nursing Practice: Fundamentals of Holistic Care*, 2e (ed. C. Brooker and A. Waugh), 303–336. Edinburgh: Elsevier.

Herdman, T.H. and Kamitsuru, S. (2017). *NANDA International Nursing Diagnoses, Definitions and Classification, 2018–2020*, 11e. New York: Thieme.

Hogston, R. (2011). Managing nursing care. In: *Foundations of Nursing Practice: Themes, Concepts and Frameworks*, 4e (ed. R. Hogston and B. Marjoram), 2–21. London: Palgrave.

Kozier, B., Harvey, S., and Morgan-Samuel, H. (2012). *Fundamentals of Nursing: Concepts, Process and Practice*, 2e. Harlow: Pearson.

Lappin, M. (2018). The nursing process. In: *Nursing Practice: Knowledge and Care*, 2e (ed. I. Peate, K. Wild and M. Nair), 111–128. Oxford: Wiley.

Lilley, L., Rainforth-Collins, S., and Snyder, J.S. (2017). *Pharmacology and the Nursing Process*, 8e. St Louis: Elsevier.

Moule, P., Armoogum, J., Douglas, E. et al. (2017). Evaluation and its importance for nursing practice. *Nursing Standard* 31 (35): 55–63.

Nursing and Midwifery Council (2018). The Code. Professional Standards of Practice and Behaviour for Nurses, Midwives and Nursing Associates. https://www.nmc.org.uk/globalassets/sitedocuments/nmc-publications/nmc-code.pdf last accessed 8 May 2019.

Orlando, I.J. (1961). *The Dynamic Nurse-Patient Relationship Function, Process and Principles*. New York: Putnam.

Stonehouse, D. (2017). Understanding the nursing process. *British Journal of Healthcare Assistants* 11 (8): 388–391.

Yildirim, B. and Ozkahraman, S. (2011). Critical thinking in nursing process and education. *International Journal of Humanities and Social Sciences* 1 (13): 257–262.

Yura, H. and Walsh, M.B. (1967). *The Nursing Process: Assessing, Planning, Implementing and Evaluating*. Washington: Catholic University of America School of Nursing.

Chapter 5

Care plans

Aim

This chapter aims to introduce the reader to different types of care plans that are in use in healthcare settings.

Learning outcomes

By the end of the chapter the reader will be able to:

1. Discuss care plans that are used in healthcare settings
2. Describe the key purposes of care plans
3. Discuss the content of the care plan and the importance of choosing the correct care plan
4. Highlight the advantages and disadvantages of each

Introduction

Most care areas or organisations will provide local protocols for a care planning activity. A protocol is a document that has been developed to help the nurse with regard to decision-making related to specific issues. A protocol should set out in a step-by-step manner detailing what actions should be taken, providing an explanation for the reason and also justification for each action contained within it. You should make yourself familiar with any protocols, local policies, and procedures that are available in your care area or the organisation where you are working.

Care plans

Being involved in the various aspects of the care planning process will enable you to gain confidence and competence towards becoming a registered nurse. As a student under supervision, you will be required to make entries to the care plan. You will also be required to provide registered nurses with verbal reports about those people you have provided care and support to. The verbal contribution you make will also influence how the care plan develops. Your contribution is important and as such it is key that you know something about how care plans are developed as well as how to use them. The usual way of writing goals with the patient for them to achieve and to itemise the ways in which the patient can be helped is through the use of the individualised care plan (entirely aimed at seeing the patient as an individual). This enables the nurse to document problems. The individualised care plan means that the nurse, working very closely with the patient, must be able to tailor care provision.

Fundamentals of Assessment and Care Planning for Nurses, First Edition. Ian Peate.
© 2020 John Wiley & Sons Ltd. Published 2020 by John Wiley & Sons Ltd.

Over the years, the care plan has evolved (and will continue to change), from blank paper-based care plans (manual) to a pre-printed word-processed care plan to an electronic care plan that is located on a computer or on a hand-held mobile data collecting system.

Review

Can you think of some of the advantages and disadvantages of using paper-based/manual care plans?

Individualised care plans are grounded on a complete holistic assessment as well as reflecting all the stages of the nursing process (ADPIE). The compilation of a handwritten care plan does take time, as well as the time needed to compose the care plan, and this needs to be acknowledged. Time needs to be set aside for this important activity as a rushed or poorly constructed care plan (which in effect is a prescription for care) may result in substandard care delivery and this will result in a negative impact on patient outcomes. Time is also needed to write and maintain the content within the care plan as the patient's condition changes (to update them), as they meet (or do not meet) the goals set. Do not cut corners with this essential nursing activity in order to save time; it could be tentatively suggested as being tantamount to professional misconduct.

The electronic care plan may save the nurse some time but – and this is important – the skills required for the production of a holistic, bespoke written or electronic care plan are exactly the same. The electronic care plan should not be seen as a panacea for all issues associated with care planning.

Barrett et al. (2012) report that there is limited evidence to suggest producing an individual care

Review

In the area where you are working, find out about:

- Electronic care plans
- The Electronic Patient Record

What are they and how do they complement each other?
Now make a list of the advantages and disadvantages of using:

- Handwritten care plans
- Electronic care plans

plan improves health outcomes or that it helps the patients make a quicker recovery. It should also be noted that it is also the case that there is a dearth of evidence that nursing care plans have any detrimental effect on the patient experience. It may be this that promotes the negative attitude that care plans are a bureaucratic and/or meaningless paper exercise that takes the nurse away from providing hands-on nursing care.

Chapter 4 of this text emphasises that care plans can also be used to provide quality indicators with regard to the standards of care offered, helping to determine whether the interventions and resources used have had the desired effect or produced the desired outcomes. Without the use of care planning this process of ongoing quality assurance may be more difficult to establish. Analysis of care plans can reveal patient outcomes in terms of their achievements related to the goals they have set with the nurse about their health. They can also be used to assess patient satisfaction and the impact of the nurse–patient relationship. Without individual care plans, other methods of analysis would be required.

In an attempt to combat the time taken up by writing care plans with nothing pre-written (non-populated), there are alternatives available. The standardised, pre-written care plan is one example, it is a kind of template. Standardised, pre-written care plans can help to provide consistency of care, helping to ensure that important interventions have not been omitted or forgotten. Such care plans are based on the assumption that different patients will often have similar problems (Ballantyne 2016). See Table 5.1, which provides an example (and there are many) of the use of a standardised, pre-written care plan for a patient with an indwelling urinary catheter.

Indwelling urethral catheter

This type of care plan may not be appropriate for every patient, as they are often single-problem plans or they are used in conjunction with a specific medical diagnosis, and, indeed, it could be suggested that it contradicts the notion of holistic, tailored, individual care. The nurse needs to be judicious and remember that there is no 'one size fits all' solution when providing individualised care; the use of the core care plan as a means of saving time should be given serious thought.

The pre-populated care plan (standardised, pre-written care plan) can also be called a 'core' care plan. Core care plans will include a number of pre-written problems, goals and nursing interventions that are associated with a specific issue(s).

According to Barrett et al. (2012), care plans can be described as the written records of the care planning process, as written reflections of the nursing process. Care planning is the action and a care plan is a record of that action (Ballantyne 2016). Care plans provide a means of communication amongst nurses, patients, and other healthcare providers, as we all work together to achieve positive health care outcomes for the people we offer care to. The contents of care plans (and there are several types) include a number of components as well as the interventions required by the nurse to consider the patient's nursing diagnoses and to produce the desired outcomes.

Padmore and Roberts (2013) suggest that working with the patient, gathering data, and formulating care plans can assist in establishing a trusting partnership between the nurse and the patient that may afterwards permit a shared understanding and respect for the individuality of the person and their needs. Bloomfield and Pegram (2015) provide an example of the systematic, holistic assessment of a patient with a mental health condition, which would involve the collection of subjective and objective data.

Review

Where you work, are patients involved in care planning activities, are they involved fully, partially, or maybe not at all? What strategies might be used to engage the patient more in care planning?

In the UK there are many types of care plans that are in use across various health care settings. Regardless of the variety, each of them, according to the Royal College of Nursing (RCN) (2016), will strive to meet the same three purposes:

1. To ensure that the patient receives the same care irrespective of which members of the care team are on duty
2. To ensure that the care that has been delivered has been recorded
3. To offer support to the patient, to identify, manage, and aim to solve or alleviate problems.

A care plan is a written document that can be either electronically produced or handwritten (paper-based) throughout the day as it is continually used and altered. Templates are used to provide a basis for the nurse to write the care plan, the starting point, it provides areas the care plan will cover. There are some templates that are very rudimentary, and these often tend to emphasise the essentials of care, for example the essential skills clusters:

- Nutrition and fluid management
- Elimination
- Mobility
- Sleeping
- Patient positioning
- Skin care
- Oral care

Table 5.1 An example of a standardised, pre-written care plan for a patient with an indwelling urinary catheter.

	Patient's name:	Date of Birth:	ID/Hosp Number:	
Date	**Assessed Need**	**Goal**	**Intervention**	**Evaluation of intervention/ Goals and review date**	**Signature**
	_____ has an indwelling urethral catheter in place due to • Acute retention of urine • Chronic retention of urine • For comfort/palliative care • Healing of sacral/perineal wounds Therefore, _____ is at increased risk of acquiring a catheter-associated Urinary Tract Infection (CAUTI).	To minimise the risk to _____ of acquiring a CAUTI Early recognition of the signs and symptoms of UTI enabling prompt treatment	• Review the ongoing clinical indication for use. • Ensure _____ is provided with information regarding the rationale for insertion of the catheter, plan for review and replacement. • Before insertion of the urinary catheter explain and discuss the procedure with _____. Obtain consent and always check for any known allergies (latex/ anaesthetic gel). • Ensure that evidence-based principles of hand hygiene are adhered to prior to and after direct care • At all times maintain _____ dignity and respect by ensuring a comfortable position and _____ is not exposed before the insertion procedure commences. • Maintain a sterile closed drainage system with the choice of urine bags based on individual assessment and in line with local protocol.	Urinary catheterisation should be a last resort after all other options have been considered and continued clinical need reviewed. Offering information reduces anxiety. Effective hand hygiene reduces risk of cross-infection.	

Other kinds of care plans can be more complex and could include aspects related to the following issues, such as:

- Falls prevention
- Infection prevention and control
- Wound care
- Psychological, emotional, and spiritual needs
- Recording of clinical signs
- Communication and provision of information
- Sex and sexuality

Each patient should have an individual care plan specifically prepared for that person. When possible, the care plan is developed along 'with' the patient, as opposed to 'for' the patient. The nurse must accept that patients and their families can become expert in their own care and they need to have the resources available to assist them to make informed decisions and that plans for intervention, care, and support are tailored to individual needs and preferences.

Review

Can you think of any instances where the patient would not be able to contribute to the development of their care plan?

The care plan must be read and then used to guide practice. It is updated and amended as care needs change, ensuring the ongoing applicability of the nursing care plan to identify whether a further assessment of the patient and a care plan review is required. Updating of the care plan may be the responsibility of one individual in the team, or this might be the responsibility of all team members.

As with any other written record that concerns a patient's health and wellbeing, care plans are subjected to standards and local policy requirements regarding regulation and legislation around record keeping, confidentiality, and consent. The nurse must adhere to those rules that govern documentation including those within the Code (NMC 2018). Care plans have to be written clearly and this means that any abbreviations used, for example, have been agreed so that everyone (including the patient) understands them and there is less risk of confusion arising. There is no definitive definition of what a care plan is. Box 5.1 makes some suggestions as to what a care plan is and what it is not.

Box 5.1 What a care plan is and is not

A care plan is:

- Based on a thorough assessment of need
- The written record of a plan of action (or elements of care) that has been negotiated with the patient to meet their needs
- Something which people feel they own
- A clear record of needs, actions and responsibilities
- A tool that can be used for managing risk
- A plan which can be used and understood by patients, families and carers and other agencies
- Something that can be a multi-professional, multi-agency activity
- Produced in the most appropriate form
- Shared effectively with those who are a part of it

- An essential element in engaging patients and communicating with them what the service can and will do as well as what responsibilities they, their family and carers, and the patient will have

A care plan is not:

- A paper exercise
- A wish list
- Written once and never revisited

Review

Go to the NMC website (www.nmc.org.uk) and find the menu option 'Hearings'. Here you can read how registrants are called to account for their actions or omissions. In one case the registrant was alleged to have '…failed to ensure that Patient A and/or B's care plan(s) around blood sugar monitoring were clear'.

Review

Choose a nursing care plan that has been used in practice and make a critique of the care plan:

- What do you think are its strengths and limitations?
- Do you think the care plan provides evidence that it is patient-centred?
- Is there anything that might be missing?
- Is the way it was laid out (its format) easy to use?
- If you had to, how might you change it?
- Share your discussions with another nurse.

So far

The care plan (and there are various types, for example the manual handwritten care plan and the electronic care plan) is the document that details the prescription of care and has to encompass all aspects of the nursing process. The care that has been agreed must always be echoed in the care plan, this demonstrates how care was approached and how it is being provided in a holistic manner. It is written whenever possible with the patient and, if appropriate, the family. The care plan has to be written in such a way that all of those who use it to deliver the care prescribed can understand it.

Care pathways

Care pathways, first established in the United States of America are also known as integrated care pathways, anticipated recovery paths, and care maps. Watts (2012) suggest that the origins of integrated care pathway models were within the engineering and manufacturing industries. The aim was to ensure consistency as well as decreasing costs whilst also maintaining quality. In the early 1980s the approach transferred into health care, where they were used primarily in secondary care in planned surgery. They celebrated collaboration and a multidisciplinary approach to care (Hayes et al. 2014), and this is why they are sometimes called integrated care pathways.

Their use has now spread throughout almost every aspect of healthcare. The European Pathway Association (n.d.) defines a care pathway as a complex intervention for joint decision making and organisation of care processes for a well-defined group of patients during a well-defined period. These care plans also embed the patient story. Care pathways have defining characteristics, which include:

1. A clear statement of the goals and main elements of care based on evidence, best practice and patients' expectations and their characteristics
2. Enabling communication amongst team members and with patients and their families
3. The coordination of the care process by organising the roles and sequencing the activities of the various members of the multidisciplinary care team, patients, and relatives
4. The documentation, monitoring, and evaluation of any variances in care and outcomes
5. The identification of the most appropriate resources

Similarly, Zerwekh and Zerwekh-Garneau (2018) note that there are four essential elements:

1. A timeline that outlines when care is to be delivered
2. The categories of care or activities and their interventions
3. Immediate and long-term outcomes that are to be achieved
4. A variance record that permits those who are delivering the care with the opportunity to document when and why the patient's progress varies from that outlined in the care pathway

The aim of an integrated care plan in order to meet the needs of patients requires:

- The right people
- In the right order
- In the right place
- Doing the right thing
- In the right time
- With the right outcomes
- With all of the attention focused on the patient experience

These multidisciplinary care pathways are written, used, and revised by all members of the healthcare team (it must also be remembered that patient input is key). A care pathway is usually created for a particular group of patients and multidisciplinary collaboration is a hallmark of high-quality safe and effective care (Stannard 2014). The Liverpool Care Pathway for the dying patient was developed in 2008 by the Marie Curie Institute Liverpool for use by the multidisciplinary team (DH 2008). This tool fell from grace in 2013 and was replaced by a dying care pathway for individuals in England (Hayes et al. 2014). The Royal College of Anaesthetists (2015) provide cardiac surgery as an excellent example of an efficient patient-centred care pathway that is led by a multidisciplinary team and is achieving better outcomes than a number of other types of major surgery. There is a need, they suggest, to adopt a similar approach for patients who are undergoing all other forms of surgery.

Review

Are there any care pathways, integrated care pathways, anticipated recovery paths, and care maps used where you are working? What aspects of care provision are they mainly related to?

Clear communication of the patient's story (their journey) along with evidence-based clinical practice guidelines, standardised assessments, and processes across care environments results in one patient-centred plan to which the whole interprofessional team is aligned. The patient's well-documented history becomes their story, significantly improving communication through the various stages of care transition. If complications or unexpected events occur during the patient journey (the provision of health care and how a patient responds can be unpredictable), for example the patient is not recovering as outlined in the care pathway or there is a setback in their condition

Box 5.2 The purpose of good nursing documentation

- Provides continuity and quality of care
- Provides legal evidence of the process and the outcomes of care
- Supports the assessment of the quality, efficacy, and effectiveness of patient care
- Provides evidence for research, financial, and ethical quality assurance purposes
- Provides the database infrastructure to support the development of nursing knowledge
- Helps to formulate standards for the development of nursing education and standards of clinical practice
- Provides the database for other purposes, for example risk management and the upholding of patient's rights

Source: Adapted Welford and Shortt (2014).

(for instance, they develop a thromboembolic event), then there has to be scope and flexibility in the integrated care plan to address these additional needs.

The integrated care plan document becomes all or part of the contemporaneous patient record, and completed activities, outcomes, and any variations between the care that was planned and actual care delivered are recorded at the point of delivery. Box 5.2 provides an overview of the purpose of effective nursing documentation. An integrated care plan provides evidence that up-to-date guidance is being used in care delivery (care based on an evidence base), such as guidance issued by the National Institute for Health and Care Excellence (NICE), Scottish Intercollegiate Guidelines Network (SIGN), and other clinical governance guidelines (for example, the Department of Health and Social Care, the Royal Colleges). Using these benchmarks can aid audit, identify variance, and can contribute to quality and effectiveness agendas.

So far

Integrated care pathways can be used across a range of health care settings, they:

- Put the focus on the patient's overall journey
- Get patients the right care and treatment at the right time
- Ensure that care decisions are evidence-based
- Make sure that different members of a care team (for example a physiotherapist, doctor, nurse, pharmacist, social worker) work together in an effective way
- Empower and inform patients and their carers.

Care bundles

A care bundle is a group of evidence-based best practices related to a disease or set of symptoms that result in improved outcomes when they are implemented together as opposed to being implemented individually. It is the 'togetherness of practice' that lends its name to the care bundle. When these interventions (practices) are performed collectively and consistently Resar et al. (2005) assert that they have been proven to improve patient outcomes. The care bundle binds the changes that are to take place in care provision together into a package of interventions that nursing staff and others know have to be followed every single time for every single patient.

Care bundles were first developed over 20 years ago and have been used in different medical and surgical specialties. The Institute for Healthcare Improvement (2016) were responsible for their creation. Care bundles produced by the Institute for Healthcare Improvement have been created to address a

Box 5.3 Components of a care bundle used to prevent catheter-associated urinary tract infection

1. Is the urinary catheter required?
2. Has the urinary catheter been continually connected?
3. Has a clean container been used to empty the catheter bag?
4. Has daily meatal hygiene been performed by the patient or health care provider?
5. Has the healthcare provider performed hand hygiene and worn an apron and gloves prior to emptying the urinary catheter bag, and on completion has personal protective equipment been removed?

number of issues, for example to reduce ventilator-associated pneumonia in patients being cared for in intensive care units and to prevent the incidence of catheter-associated urinary tract infection. Venkatram et al. (2010) have demonstrated that urinary catheter care bundles have been shown to be effective in reducing the rate of catheter-associated urinary tract infection. A urinary catheter care bundle may include the components identified in Box 5.3.

Review

In the care area where you are working are there any care bundles in use? If there are, what are they and what was the reason for their introduction? Who has responsibility for the care bundles?

Care bundles are used in association with the nursing process as the nurse, with the patient, assesses needs, plans interventions, gathers the equipment required to implement the bundle, and performs the care required with ongoing evaluation. The care bundle is specifically applied to the intervention stage of the nursing process, as the nurse engages in critical thinking and the application of specialist clinical knowledge.

So far

A care bundle is a set of interventions that, when used together, have the potential to significantly improve patient outcomes. When a care bundle is implemented the multidisciplinary team work together to deliver the best possible care that is supported by evidence-based research and practices. The critical aim is to improve patient care.

The are many types of care bundles, a number of them are associated with the insertion of invasive devices, such as a urethral catheter. Many care bundles (but not all) have been formulated for use in the intensive care unit. The essence of a care bundle is that its whole is more important than the sum of its parts.

Discharge planning

The problem-solving process drives the discharge process and is used to develop the plan, the discharge may occur for a number of reasons, for example:

- The patient may have met their goals/aims/objectives
- The patient requires a different level of care
- The patient requires alternative care
- The patient decides they do not wish to continue to receive care (self-discharge)

Zerwekh and Zerwekh-Garneau (2018) encourage nurses to engage in the discharge planning process early. Discharge planning begins early after admission or even before admission, and must always include the patient and where appropriate their family. If a patient is scheduled to have elective knee replacement or any pre-planned procedure, for example, the nurse working in the pre-assessment clinic or the orthopaedic clinic can begin the discharge process prior to the patient being admitted for surgery regarding rehabilitation. The nurse can begin this important process by discussing and explaining (using a number of resources) the care and support that may be required at home after discharge and the need to attend for post-operative physiotherapy.

Review

Is there a pre-assessment clinic running in the place where you work? Who manages the clinic? Is this uni-professional (nurses only) or multi-professional (nurses, physiotherapists, anaesthetists)?

What is the purpose of the pre-assessment clinic, how can this benefit patients in anticipation of their discharge?

If it is possible to plan discharge early, then the patient will have an understanding of how their care is likely to progress, what they are likely to expect and even when they are likely to be discharged. An integrated care plan will have an expected date of discharge included in it. This will facilitate a smoother discharge and potentially reduce the length of stay, the risk of complications, and unnecessary re-admission. Discharge from care has to be safe and coordinated with the patient at the centre of any plans being made. It also has to be remembered that discharge from care may not always be to the person's home, residential care home, or nursing home; in some instances it may be to another place, for example a rehabilitation unit, another hospital, another care provider (a hospice), or a place of detention. Planning for discharge early can help some patients who may need to arrange child care, organise alternative arrangements for the care of a dependent relative, discuss how they are to cope with any economic issues that may ensue as a result of admission, as well as helping them with their employer to prepare for them to return to work. See Box 5.4 for what issues Le May (2017) considers can make discharge effective.

Box 5.4 Components of a successful discharge plan

- The discharge plan has to be formulated in partnership with the patient and if appropriate the family.
- The patient must be fully updated and informed of the plan and any changes, the patient is key to shaping it.
- A key worker should be appointed to coordinated discharge for the service and liaise with another service if required.
- All relevant documents must be updated and information transferred to all appropriate services in a timely manner to ensure that continuity of care is maintained.
- Appropriate services must be introduced into the care package early on so that continuity of care is maintained.
- The plan must be monitored and evaluated.
- Any variation in the plan should be identified, explained and if possible corrected.

Source: Adapted Le May (2017).

Take note

Discharging a homeless patient

Any discharge process for homeless people, as with anyone else, must start on admission to hospital and if possible before admission. Early identification of a housing need is essential to trigger the appropriate responses, within the hospital and with external agencies who are likely to play a key role in ensuring that the housing and health needs of the patient can be properly met during and after their stay in hospital.

Many homeless patients are still being discharged before their wider health needs have been met and without consideration of the likely conditions people are returning to. It is unacceptable that people are discharged without being fit for discharge, with unmet health problems which will often require them to return to acute services once these have met crisis point.

Some homeless people are unable to attend follow-up care due to their homelessness or severity of health problems, for example attending appointments, storing medication, or dressing wounds can be difficult if living on the streets or in a chaotic environment. Discharge of a homeless person late in the afternoon or at night might mean they have no option but to sleep on the streets as they may have missed an opportunity to find secure night accommodation in a hostel or shelter.

Working with multiagency partnerships (and coordinating of services) and with other agencies, local authorities, voluntary sector agencies, housing teams, and night shelters enable care providers to have policies in place to ensure that the homeless are discharged safely and with appropriate support, just as they would do with a person who has a place to be discharged to. There should be a clear process in place for admission through to safe discharge so the person has somewhere to go and with the support they require for their ongoing care.

Engagement working is prequisite to ensuring that the needs of this community are being met safely. Staff may need to be reminded of their duty of care to all people they have the privilege to offer care to, and this also includes the homeless.

Source: Homeless Link and St Mungos (2012) and Cornes et al. (2017).

Review

Put together a file that includes information on local charities and voluntary organisations that offer support to the homeless community in the area where you are working/living.

Self-discharge

Self-discharge occurs when an adult wishes to discharge against medical advice. Most organisations will have policies and protocols that have to be followed if a patient wishes to self-discharge, and this must be adhered to. In this event those staff involved will try to seek the reasons why from the patient and try to provide support for them to remain in hospital. Ensure that all relevant information is made available to assist the patient in this decision-making process.

Review

What policy is in place in the area where you work when a patient informs you that they wish to self-discharge. What does your local policy and procedure require you to do? How and where would you document this request made by the patient?

Those adult patients who may wish to self-discharge can fall into the following groups:

- The adult patient who has the capacity to make the decision to self-discharge against medical advice. These patients are free to leave.
- The adult patient who lacks capacity to make the decision to self-discharge against medical advice. Further consideration must be given as to whether discharge is in the patient's best interests.
- The adult patient with evidence of an acute mental health disorder where there is the potential for the risk of further deterioration or harm to the patient or to others. Discussion has to take place with the mental health team and possible Mental Health Act assessment will be required.

Where a patient expresses a wish to leave hospital, staff should respond appropriately and lawfully. Patients must be treated in a dignified and respectful manner and are offered appropriate support to help them discharge themselves safely. It is paramount (as is the case with all aspects of care planning) that documentation relating to this stage of the process is undertaken in accordance with local policy and in alignment with professional expectations.

So far

Care plans should include the important issue of discharge. The discharge process should begin as soon as the patient has been admitted for an episode of care, and where possible this should occur prior to admission. Effective discharge planning can reduce unnecessary stay and inappropriate re-admission.

Conclusion

This chapter has provided an overview of care plans. Care plans are the vehicles that are used to document and guide the provision of care. All stages of the nursing process are present in a competently constructed care plan. The care plan, the prescription of care, needs to be written in a competent and clear manner, with the recipient of care and those who are implementing care working towards achieving the aims and goals agreed upon.

Time must be set aside for the nurse, working with the patient, and if appropriate the family to construct the care plan. There are several types of care plans which can be used, and each type has advantages and disadvantages.

References

Ballantyne, H. (2016). Developing nursing care plans. *Nursing Standard* 30 (26): 51–60.

Barrett, D., Wilson, B., and Woollands, A. (2012). *Care Planning: A Guide for Nurses*, 2e. Harlow: Pearson.

Bloomfield, J. and Pegram, A. (2015). Organisational aspects of care. *Nursing Standards* 29 (27): 35–40.

Cornes, M., Whiteford, M., Mathorpe, J. et al. (2017). Improving hospital discharge arrangements for people who are homeless: a realist synthesis of the intermediate care literature. *Health and Social Care in the Community* 26: e345–e359.

Department of Health (DH) (2008). End of life care strategy: Promoting high quality for all adults at the end of life. https://assets.publishing.service.gov.uk/government/uploads/system/uploads/attachment_data/file/136431/End_of_life_strategy.pdf (accessed April 2018).

European Pathway Association (n.d.) Definition of care pathway. http://e-p-a.org/care-pathways (accessed April 2018).

Hayes, A., Henry, C., Holloway, M. et al. (2014). *Pathways through Care at the End of Life: A Guide to Person-centered Care*. London: Jessica Kingsley Publishers.

Institute for Healthcare Improvement (2016). What is a bundle? www.ihi.org/resources/Pages/ImprovementStories/WhatIsaBundle.aspx (accessed April 2018).

Le May, A. (2017). *Rapid Adult Nursing*. Oxford: Wiley.

Homeless Link and St Mungos (2012). Improving hospital admission and discharge for people who are homeless. www.homeless.org.uk/sites/default/files/site-attachments/HOSPITAL_ADMISSION_AND_DISCHARGE._REPORTdoc.pdf (accessed April 2018).

Nursing and Midwifery Council (2018). The Code. Professional Standards of Practice and Behaviour for Nurses, Midwives and Nursing Associates. https://www.nmc.org.uk/globalassets/sitedocuments/nmc-publications/nmc-code.pdf last accessed 8 May 2019.

Padmore, J. and Roberts, C. (2013). Care planning. In: *The Art and Science of Mental Health Nursing: A Textbook of Principles and Practice*, 3e (ed. I. Norman and I. Ryrie), 220–232. Maidenhead: McGraw-Hill Education.

Resar, R., Pronovost, P., Haraden, C. et al. (2005). Using a bundle approach to improve ventilator care processes and reduce ventilator-associated pneumonia. *Joint Commission Journal on Quality and Patient Safety* 31 (5): 243–248.

Royal College of Anaesthetists (2015). Perioperative medicine: The pathway to better surgical care. www.rcoa.ac.uk/sites/default/files/PERIOP-2014.pdf (accessed April 2018).

Royal College of Nursing (RCN) (2016). Nursing care plans. https://rcni.com/hosted-content/rcn/first-steps/care-plans (accessed April 2018).

Stannard, S. (2014). Evidence in perioperative care. *Nursing Clinics of North America* 49: 485–492.

Venkatram, S., Rachmale, S., and Kanna, B. (2010). Study of device use adjusted rates in health care-associated infections after implementation of 'bundles' in a closed-model medical intensive care unit. *Journal of Critical Care* 25 (1): 174–178.

Watts, T. (2012). End of life care pathway tools to promote a good death: a critical commentary. *European Journal of Cancer Care* 21 (1): 20–30.

Welford, C. and Shortt, S. (2014). Innovations in care planning documentation. *Nursing and Residential Care* 16 (4): 451–453.

Zerwekh, J. and Zerwekh-Garneau, A. (2018). *Nursing Today: Transition and Trends*, 9e. St Louis: Elsevier.

Chapter 6

Models of nursing

Aim

This chapter aims to provide the reader with an overview of various models of nursing, their philosophies and principles.

Learning outcomes

By the end of the chapter the reader will be able to:

1. Describe the principles underpinning nursing models
2. Compare and contrast a nursing model and the medical model
3. Explain what is meant by a model and a theory of nursing
4. Discuss the attributes of the Activities of Living model

Introduction

There is a close relationship between nursing models and the nursing process. Nursing models were developed to offer a definition as to what nursing is and could be. A nursing model (a framework to guide practice and education) describes the beliefs, values, and goals of nursing and the knowledge and skills that are required to practise nursing. Nursing models have received criticism, it has been suggested that they are irrelevant, confusing and their implementation was poorly managed (Murphy et al. 2010).

In the late 1990s Walsh (1998) explained that the nursing process is a tool that is used to provide structure to the delivery of care delivery and models of nursing are used as tools to inform us on how care should be provided. Nursing models very often refer to their use in the nursing process, this demonstrates how they are both very closely if not inextricably linked. Models provide detail, and this detail is to be used alongside the nursing process in order to aid care delivery. Most nursing models fit into one or more of the five stages of the nursing process. This chapter will discuss three nursing models: Orem's Self-care Deficit Theory (Orem 1980, 1990), Roy's Adaptation Model (Roy 1981; Roy and Andrews 2008), and The Roper, Logan, and Tierney Activities of Living model (1983, 1996).

Fundamentals of Assessment and Care Planning for Nurses, First Edition. Ian Peate.
© 2020 John Wiley & Sons Ltd. Published 2020 by John Wiley & Sons Ltd.

Nursing theories

The use of a formalised framework to guide practice (the nursing process) is valuable in providing a systematic prescription for action. This has to encompass a sound theoretical base as well as acting as a learning tool, as is the case when developing problem-solving skills and applying evidence to practice. Nursing theories can be complex.

Nursing theories are seen as well-thought-out and systematic expressions of a set of recommendations that are related to questions on the subject of nursing. There has been much written about nursing theories (Lappin 2018), he cites the early renowned theorists such as Virginia Henderson, Hildegard Peplau, Betty Neuman, Martha Rogers, Sister Callister Roy, and the most famous of all theorists, Florence Nightingale. A nursing theory is a compilation of ideas, definitions, relationships and expectations or suggestions that have been derived from nursing models or from other disciplines, offering a purposive, methodical outlook of phenomena by bringing together certain interrelationships so as to describe, explain, forecast, and/or recommend.

Nursing theory according to Alligood (2017) helps the nurse to provide knowledge in order to advance practice by describing, explaining, predicting, and controlling phenomena. The role and function of the nurse working alongside other health care professionals can advance their contribution to health care even further as a result of theoretical knowledge as systematically developed methods (theory) are more likely to be successful. Nurses will also act and feel more confident and competent in what they are doing and why they are doing it if they are challenged by patients or other health care professionals. Nursing theory, knowledge, and understanding present nurses with a sense of professional autonomy by steering their clinical practice, their learning, and their research function (Lappin 2018).

Review

Reflect on an area of care where you have worked. Did that area of care have an explicit nursing philosophy, and if so, what did it say about nursing?

Torres (1990) considers a theory might identify the two concepts, need and nursing. The concept of need could be described in relationship of genuine experiences that a person might come across that could interfere with an ideal health state. The second concept, the concept of nursing might be defined in terms of actions that may be needed to achieve an optimal health state, for example touch, listening, or teaching. The theory could connect the two concepts of need and nursing so that nursing actions can be consciously viewed as addressing needs and as such reach a goal of optimal health.

Lappin (2018) notes that without the theory, we may not be able to perceive the relationship that exists between a need and a nursing action: the theory, according to Torres (1990) should provide a unique way of viewing nursing actions as responding to and meeting a particular goal, a specific relationship. Generally, nursing theories can be divided into different categories related to their function. It is also possible to classify theories according to the extent their principles can be generalised. Categories may include:

- Needs theories
- Interaction theories
- Outcome theories

These categories denote the essential philosophical underpinnings of the theories.

Theories should be relatively simple but generalisable, consider the theories in Table 6.1.

Nursing theory according to Walker and Avant (2011) enables the development of nursing knowledge and this provides the principles to support nursing practice. Theory shapes practice and provides a method for articulating key ideas that are associated with the essence of nursing practice.

Table 6.1 Theories.

Theory	Description
Nightingale's Environmental Theory	The focus is predominantly on the patient and the environment. Nursing according to Nightingale is an act of utilising the environment of the patient to assist in recovery that requires the nurse's initiative to arrange environmental settings appropriate for the gradual restoration of the patient's health. External factors associated with the patient's surroundings can impact (positively and negatively) on life or biological and physiological processes and development. The nurse manipulates the environment to manipulate recovery.
Needs Theory	The theory emphasises the importance of increasing the patient's independence so that progress after hospitalisation will not be delayed. Virginia Henderson's (1966) theory sees individuals as having basic needs (she identifies 14 of them) that are components of health. Her emphasis on basic human needs as the central focus of nursing practice has led to further theory development regarding the needs of the patient, and how nursing can assist in meeting those needs. The Roper et al. (1996) model considers 12 activities of living.
Body Image Theory	Body image is a multifaceted psychological experience of personification that greatly impacts on the quality of human life (Cash and Pruzinsky 2002). When there is an alteration in body image the nurse working with the patient needs to determine how the patient is going to manage this new set of circumstances; a robust individual and holistic assessment will help with this. The theory can make the nurse (and the patient) think about and put into action how it is they may deal with the physiological and psychological aspects of their situation.
Interaction Theories	Interaction theory is about the relationships that nurses form with patients and how people relate to each other. Part of the nurse's role involves an attempt to enter into the subjective world of patients in order to see things as they do. Only by doing this can a nurse make an accurate assessment of an individual's needs and plan an appropriate series of nursing interventions (Peplau 1988). The therapeutic, interpersonal process; the nurse–patient relationship is the centre of nursing.
Outcomes Theories	The nurse as the changing force, enables individuals to adapt to or cope with ill health, people are seen as adaptive systems that are continually interacting with internal and external environments. Whilst doctors focus on biological systems and disease processes, the specific role of the nurse is to promote adaptation in health and illness (Roy 1981). The goal of nursing is to foster successful adaptation.

Source: Adapted Lappin (2018).

75

Theory describes, explains, predicts, and prescribes and is used in all facets of nursing care helping the nurse in organising, understanding and analysing patient data. Theory provides a systematic, reliable way of thinking about nursing care to help direct the decision-making process. Theory-based nursing is evidenced when nurses deliberately structure their practice around a specific theory to guide them as they offer care to the patient.

Take note

Evidence-based nursing

The Royal College of Nursing has provided a resource to help nurses understand what it means to practise in line with best available evidence. The resource highlights evidence-based practice guidelines, research and other tools, as well as updates on evidence-based techniques and processes from across the UK. Included in the resource is international content collected from credible resources.

www.rcn.org.uk/professional-development/quality-and-safety/evidence-based-practice.

So far

Nursing theory is developed from groups of concepts and describes their interrelationships and as such presents a systematic view of nursing related events. The purpose of theory is to:

- Describe
- Explain
- Predict
- Prescribe

Nursing theory assists with the development of nursing knowledge, providing the principles to support nursing practice, shaping practice, and providing a method for communicating ideas that are related to the essence of nursing practice.

Nursing models

There are various conceptual models that have been devised to articulate beliefs about nursing's essential components and the underpinning theory. In representing the reality of practice there are four central concepts:

1. The person who is the recipient of care
2. The environment within which the person exists (this can be internal and external)
3. The health illness continuum within which the person finds themselves in at the time of contact with the nurse
4. The nursing interactions, used to alter or manage the environment

See Figure 6.1.

Nursing models are a set of theoretical and wide-ranging statements about the concepts that serve to provide a framework for organising ideas about patients, their environment, health and nursing (Lappin 2018). Nursing models offer a foundation for the development of nursing as a discipline (Fawcett and Desanto-Madeya 2013) and, if adopted by a nursing team, promote consistency

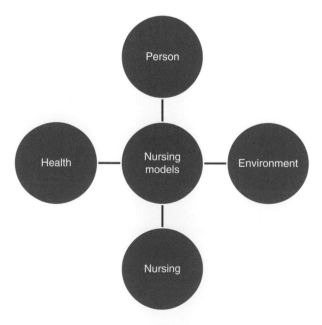

Figure 6.1   Four central concepts representing the reality of practice.

Box 6.1 One-, two-, and three-dimensional models of the kidney

- A one-dimensional model of the kidney would be a verbal description of the organ, its structure and function
- A two-dimensional model would be a drawing of the kidney and its various components and how they relate to each other. You would glean more information from the two-dimensional model than you would from the one-dimensional model
- The three-dimensional model of the kidney will provide you with most information about the organ. This model would be a replica of the kidney, it would mimic its size, its colour, its position in the body, its close relationship with other structures. You can touch the three-dimensional model.

and continuity of nursing action. The selection of a particular model for practice depends largely on the extent to which it reflects the nursing team's own values and perceived goals.

Murphy et al. (2010) explain that in very simple terms, a model can be said to be one way of representing reality. For example, model cars or airplanes are representations that help people to familiarise themselves with an object, they help people understand it and deconstruct it to see how it works and to see how it might be applied. Models are also capable of representing abstract and complex situations, for example economic models, health beliefs, or grief and bereavement.

A one-dimensional model is usually abstract in nature. These types of models cannot be taken apart or explicitly observed, they can be thought about, mulled over, and manipulated mentally (this is why they are classified as abstract). A two-dimensional model includes diagrams, graphs, and drawings. An example of a two-dimensional model would be the map of the London underground system or a map of a bus route, the number 36 bus route. Generally, most nursing models began as one-dimensional and abstract and then developed into a two-dimensional model. Three-dimensional models are physical models, for example scale models (see Box 6.1).

Review

Think about some examples of:

- One-dimensional models
- Two-dimensional models
- Three-dimensional models

All three-dimensional models will provide much information about the phenomenon being studied. They help in understanding by providing a simple but structured view allowing you to appreciate the relationships between various concepts they seek to illuminate and explain.

So far

Most models consider the following key issues:

1. The person who is the recipient of care
2. The environment within which the person exists (this can be internal and external)
3. The health illness continuum within which the person finds themselves in at the time of contact with the nurse
4. The nursing interactions, used to alter or manage the environment

Models of care can only help nurses direct practice. They work hand in hand with the nursing process and if used appropriately will enable the nurse to provide care that is individual and takes into account holistic needs.

Orem's self-care deficit theory

The key feature of Orem's model (Orem 1980) is to help people and communities who have or may have a health-related self-care deficit (see Table 6.2 for Orem's key concepts). Orem's model can be used in a variety of settings. The importance of partnership with patient and carers is acknowledged and respected and their involvement in planning nursing interventions is seen as essential. The notion that people are active in learning to live with the effects of their condition temporarily or long-term is key, and the nurse working with the patient though all stages of the nursing process encourages this.

The model emphasises patient autonomy. This emphasis will resonate with nurses whose aim is to help individuals and communities to accept responsibility for themselves. Given the role people with long-term conditions play in managing their condition, who are seen as experts in their own care, further stresses the alignment with this model and the various long-term conditions.

Self-care is the contribution that people make to their own lived experience of their condition and involves undertaking activities to maintain health and wellbeing. Nurses assist patients to achieve self-care recognising the person's individual ability. The model requires the nurse and the patient to work together and entering into negotiation (this will also include other members of the multidisciplinary team and if appropriate family), care is organised in terms of one of three nursing systems (see Figure 6.2). The nurse, for example, may perform activities for the patient, assist the patient in

Table 6.2　Key concepts of Orem's Self-Care Deficit model (Orem 1980).

Self-care requisites	Self-care	Nursing system
• Universal self-care • Developmental self-care • Health deviation self-care	• Demands • Capabilities • Deficits	• Wholly compensatory • Partiality compensatory • Supportive-educative

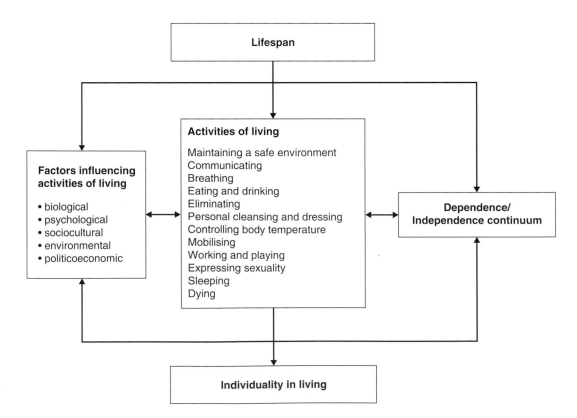

Figure 6.2　Roper et al.'s Activities of Living model (Source: Holland et al. 2008).

carrying out shared activities, or help them in developing the ability to act on their own behalf, through support and education. The decision to use a nursing system or a combination of systems changes in response to patient need over a period of time.

Roy's adaptation model

Roy's adaptation model (Roy and Andrews 2008) considers human behaviour as being influenced by a set of interrelated biological, psychological and social systems, each of which is directed towards achieving a state of relative balance. This (as far as possible) promotes regularity of function, assisting the individual to adapt positively to environmental stimuli or stressors (this can be internal and external). There are three types of stimuli identified by Roy to which people are exposed:

- Focal
- Contextual
- Residual

A focal stimulus is seen as something that has an immediate effect on the person, a contextual stimulus is a contributory circumstance and a residual stimulus comes about from beliefs or attitudes that are associated with past experiences. Maladaptation happens when the effect of any stimulus exceeds a person's capacity to provide a positive response. When this occurs, there will be a threat to continued health and wellbeing. This model appreciates that people possess a unique capacity to manage stimuli, in so far as people respond differently when faced with the same events, the ability to adapt will vary from person to person.

The nurse intervenes when required, when a person's normal methods of coping with stressors have proven ineffective. The role of the nurse and the nursing interventions prescribed focus on promoting adaptation in maintaining health, and throughout periods of illness the aim is to manipulate stimuli, supporting people to respond positively.

There are several areas of practice where this model is and can be used. As the focus of Roy's model is on the belief that individuals manage and adapt to the same events differently, this requires the person to develop the ability to live with the consequence of their condition, engaging them to work in partnership in their care. The model assists nurses working with the patient to identify successful past coping mechanisms and elements that are likely to hinder future adaptation, intervention can then be planned with goals that can be achieved and tailored in relation to individual resources.

Roper, Logan, and Tierney activities of living model

This model, the Activities of Living model (Roper et al. 1996) (ALs) has been widely adopted and adapted in the UK. The Roper, Logan, and Tierney model is a theory of nursing care that is based on ALs, it provides the portrayal of an uncomplicated view of nursing that can be applied across settings. The model is based on the work of Henderson (1966) (see Chapter 1). The model provides the nurse with a clear framework that can guide the nurse when assessing the patient and can be used throughout the patient's care. The model assesses how the patient's life has changed as a result of illness, injury, or admission to a care facility. There are a number of components associated with the model (see Figure 6.2).

The model should not be used as a checklist, with boxes to be filled in and ticked off, it assists the nurse with their approach to the organisation of care. When the patient is admitted, assessment should take place using the various components of the model and the care plan formulated on the findings of assessment. The model provides for the patient's dependence and independence to be reviewed throughout their stay. Considering changes in the dependence–independence continuum, permits the nurse working with the patient to determine if the patient is improving or not and to make changes to the care provided.

In this model, the focus of nursing intervention is on assisting individuals in the prevention, resolution, and management of problems. The model defines problems as actual or potential focusing on nursing interventions to assist the individual in prevention, resolution, and the management of the problems. Nurses are aware not only with those problems that actually exist but, also, with preventing others from developing. The model can be applied to an acute care episode or to long-term conditions, health status, and lifestyle feature in the model, this can help the nurse to perceive their role in terms of addressing immediate needs but also focusing on health promotion.

Holland et al. (2008) provide an introduction to the model, describing how to apply it in practice, addressing the underlying beliefs of model. The nature of the individual receiving care, the environment, health and illness, and nursing have been articulated by Roper et al. (1996).

The person

The person is seen as an individual who engages with the complex process of living in a unique way doing this through a number of activities. These activities are influenced by where it is the person is on the lifespan continuum, physical, psychological, sociocultural, environmental, and politico-economic factors, and the degree of independence/dependence the individual enjoys (Roper et al. 1996).

The environment

Essentially the environment is seen principally in terms of its influence on the person's ability to carry out the ALs. How the environment influences the person is wide and varied and can include where a person lives, the condition of their housing, and their place of employment. Global issues, for example the availability of food supplies, having to go into hospital, and the effects that illness can have on an individual's routine, can be seen as influencing factors.

Health

This is a dynamic, fluid process with various components. There is no clear distinction between health and ill health. The health status of a person is related to the person's capacity to adapt to and cope with challenges they face throughout their life. Health or what health means has to be considered in a holistic way, for example a person who feels well and lives in a way which they find satisfactory may be considered by that person to be 'healthy' despite the fact they have a significant disability. A person with no signs or symptoms of physical illness may be said to be 'unhealthy' because they feel 'unwell'.

The five key components

There are five key components associated with this model:

1. The 12 activities of living
2. The five influencing factors
3. The lifespan continuum
4. The independence-dependence continuum
5. Individuality in living

The activities of living

Living is a complex process. Living can be described as a combination of the 12 ALs (see Figure 6.3) which are undertaken using a number of actions to ensure survival. Each person will experience the activities differently and will carry out these activities in a unique way. In particular circumstances, people are able to perform the activities of living independently. However, when disease or difficulties occur, the nurse can use these ALs to assess the patient and identify interventions that may promote independence in areas that may be difficult or impossible for the individual on their own. The model helps to assess the individual's relative independence (on a continuum ranging from complete dependence to complete independence) and potential for independence with regard to the ALs. This takes into account their lifespan, age (development), and five key influencing factors in order to determine the interventions that will lead to increased independence, as well as ongoing support that will be needed to compensate for dependency.

The ALs are assessed on admission, assessing each person, using the ALs as a framework, to determine if there are changes that have occurred as a result of any health condition, and a review is undertaken as the patient progresses and as the care plan changes. It is erroneous to use the ALs as a checklist and to neglect the other four key components of the model.

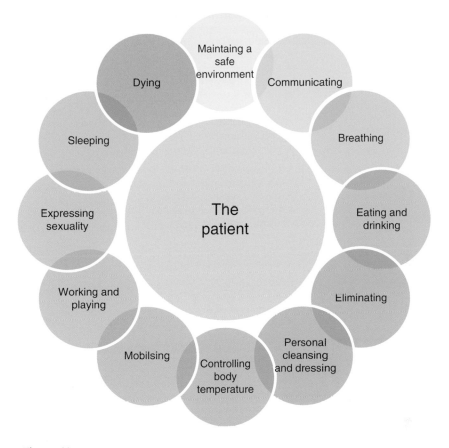

Figure 6.3 The 12 ALs.

Whilst the ALs are identified individually, in reality when using the model to undertake patient assessment, often more than one AL can be assessed, for example mobility (or the inability to mobilise) is linked to other activities such as maintaining a safe environment, the ability to eliminate, eating and drinking, and so on. Table 6.3 provides a start with relation to some of the prompts that may assist with the assessment of each activity (to reiterate, one AL cannot be seen in isolation).

In Table 6.3, it can be noted that some of the prompts appear for more than one of the ALs. The key issue is to ensure that a detailed assessment is undertaken using the ALs as a framework. When assessing pain, if a person has pain (bone pain, for example), this can impact on nearly all of the ALs. On the other hand, if a person is being admitted for the removal of a sebaceous cyst under local anaesthetic, then not all of the ALs will be relevant. The nurse needs to be judicious.

Take note

An older man who has prostate cancer with bony metastases is admitted to hospital after falling and it may be seen as simply 'having problems with mobilising'. This may not take into account the systemic influences of his condition, the effectiveness of his current long-term pain management strategies, the psychological impact of him not being able to go out and work as previously, having to come to terms with the idea of taking medical retirement and potentially having to accept help despite being fiercely independent and a caregiver to his partner, and difficulty paying bills and having to consider claiming benefits, something he has always thought of as 'handouts'.

The ALs works with other components of the model; the model should not be seen as a mere checklist.

Table 6.3 Some prompts that may assist with the assessment of each Activity of Living (AL).

Activity of living	Possible prompts
Maintaining a safe environment	• Ability to maintain patent airway • Physiological measurements, such as blood pressure, temperature, pulse, respiratory rate, oxygen saturations • Ability to see and hear • Cognitive status • Sensory deficits • Pain assessment • Falls assessment (balance)
Communication	• Language spoken, is an interpreter needed • Ability to see and hear • Need for hearing aid (sound amplification device) • Need for visual aids (reading and writing systems without the use of sight) • Ability to speak • Aphasia, dysphasia • Communications aids
Breathing	• Patent airway • Respiratory rate, depth, rhythm • Oxygen saturations • Dyspnoea • Smoking history • Environment (polluted atmosphere)
Eating and drinking	• Hydration status • Nutrition status (malnutrition universal score tool score) • Ability to chew and swallow • Food and drink preferences • Specific dietary requirements (therapeutic and cultural) • Aids used to assist with eating and drinking • Alcohol consumption • Weight and Body Mass Index • Waist:Hip ratio • Known allergies
Eliminating	• Elimination routines/habits • Continence • Frequency of micturition (day/night) • Constipation • Diarrhoea • Presence of urinary faecal diversions (colostomy/ileostomy) • Elimination aids (indwelling and external catheter, use of commode, urine bottle)
Personal cleansing and dressing	• Hygiene routines/habits • Ability to dress/undress • Personal preferences
Controlling body temperature	• Body temperature • Ability to maintaining own temperature • Methods usually used to maintain own body temperature
Mobility	• Usual gait/posture • Cognitive status • Falls assessment • Aids used to assist with mobility • Moving and handling assessment • Pressure risk assessment score
Working and playing	• Current employment • Previous employment • Hobbies/leisure activities • Sporting activity

Table 6.3 (Continued)

Activity of living	Possible prompts
Expressing sexuality	• Personal choice • Self-image • Menses • Sexual function • Libido • Use of sex aids
Sleeping	• Usual sleep pattern • Number of pillows used and type • Use of sleeping aids (medication and activities) • Work pattern (night duty)
Dying	• Fears and anxieties • Cultural/religious beliefs • Preferences

Performing any one of the ALs demands the organisation of a complex pattern of behaviours. To be able to carry out the ALs, the person relies on skills including the receiving and clarification of information and when responding to this there is a need to articulate appropriate responses. There are a number of variables that influence a person's ability to carry out the ALs effectively, for example the ability to physiologically and psychologically function in an effective manner. As a result of this there is much potential for fault (error) to occur, resulting in actual and potential problems.

Take note

For many people (particularly those with long-term conditions) disruption in their ability to carry out one AL can lead to difficulty in the ability to carry out others. For example, a person who has had a stroke might also find that their ability to maintain a safe environment, communicate, eat and drink, use the toilet, carry out personal hygiene, to mobilise, work, socialise, and sleep may be negatively impacted.

Lifespan continuum

The lifespan continuum is indicated by a line. The lifespan continuum is a representation of the passage of life from conception to death (note this is not from birth to death, this is from conception to death); see Figure 6.4.

When an individual traverses the lifespan this is punctuated by recurrent change, as the person progresses through a number of developmental stages, each stage is accompanied by various levels of physical, intellectual, and social functioning. Adulthood is usually described as self-reliance, and tends to focus on work and family. However, this is not true for everyone, and there are many permutations and much diversity in personal lifestyle and behaviour during adulthood. Using age only will not offer the nurse enough information to understand the potential impact that acute illness, disease, and long-term conditions will have on the person (what they are facing or may face). The nurse is required to understand which developmental tasks a person is already achieving, those that they have a desire to achieve and how much they and their family value these aspirations. When the nurse determines where the patient is on the lifespan and is able to establish the ALs that the person is able to do for themselves independently and those they cannot do, this then demonstrates actual or potential problems that require nursing interventions.

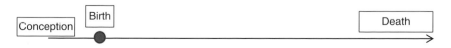

Figure 6.4 The lifespan continuum.

Dependence/independence continuum

The second continuum is the dependence/independence continuum (see Figure 6.5). Holland et al. (2008) remind us that this component of the model highlights the fact that not all people are able to carry out each AL unassisted. The person may not have the physical or cognitive means to carry out the ALs, there may be an inability to perform them which can be temporary or long-term (acute or chronic), or the person may no longer have the abilities that they once had. There are some people who have not acquired the necessary skills or do not have the skills to perform the ALs independently.

The notion of a dependence/independence continuum will only be of significance when they are considered in relation to each other. As a result of this, any form of assessment in relation to this continuum will be subjective as this will be determined by the nurse's and patient's interpretation of abilities when compared with clinical, developmental and social benchmarks. There is no valid and reliable single measure that reflects the capacity for independent function in all of the ALs. It can be suggested that there are few people, if any, who are fully independent.

The ALs are interactive and the inability to perform one of them independently will impact negatively on the person's ability to perform others. This can occur if the person is experiencing an acute illness or has a long-term condition. Because of this, it is important that the nurse pays attention to each activity when undertaking an assessment of a patient's dependence/independence status. A patient who has reduced mobility due to a fractured femur, for example, may also be dependent on others with regard to other ALs such as maintaining a safe environment, eating and drinking, and personal cleansing and dressing. The fractured femur can also interfere with the person's elimination needs, their sleep, being able to go to work and to maintain their own body temperature (they may be unable to independently cover themselves with bedding if they are cold or conversely remove bedding if they are too warm).

The five influencing factors

Sometimes the five influencing factors (the influencing factors) are also referred to as the Key Concepts. The influencing factors, the two continua, and the 12 ALs permit the nurse to undertake a holistic assessment. It is essential that the nurse has an understanding of these influencing factors (see Table 6.4 and Figure 6.6).

The influencing factors can have bearing alone (individually) or in a combination and can influence each of the ALs. The influence of each can be interrelated and during the assessment phase of the nursing process the nurse needs to take these factors into account. This has the potential to provide the nurse with a deeper understanding of the cause of a person's needs and also to assist in devising methods and interventions to assist the person.

So far

The five influencing factors are important determinants the nurse must consider when undertaking a holistic assessment. The factors (individually or together) will impact on the person as well as on the person's relationships with others. The person's illness (acute or chronic) determines the degree of independence that person has in performing the ALs. The person's understanding, what they think about their illness, their hopes, feelings, and beliefs are seen as psychological factors influencing a person's ability to perform the ALs. The sociocultural influencing factor concerns expectations and values influenced by societal status, responsibilities, and the person's position in the society. Environmental factors, for example noise, climate, and atmospheric pollution, can modify performance of ALs. The final factor, politico-economic, is associated with how policies are formulated and enacted and how economies around health care can impact on a person's health and wellbeing.

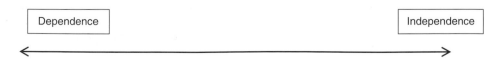

Figure 6.5   The dependence/independence continuum.

Table 6.4   The five influencing factors on the Activities of Living (ALs).

Factor	Description
Biological	Influenced by the person's overall health, current illness or state of injury, anatomy, physiology, and pathophysiology. The patient's illness is considered here and the ways in which the body adapts internally and externally (if it adapts). For example, a patient with chronic obstructive pulmonary disease (COPD) may be easily fatigued, preventing that person from carrying out their ALs in an independent way. However, the person who is living with HIV may still be able carry out the ALs independently, adapting when necessary. Health status has a significant impact on a patient's capacity to act independently. Illness can interfere with a patient's usual functioning, it can suddenly disrupt the patient's competence and confidence to perform the ALs and this can impact on families and communities.
Psychological	This influencing factor incorporates intellectual and emotional factors, cognition and spiritual beliefs as well as the ability to understand and grasp ideas. According to Roper et al. this is described as knowing, thinking, hoping, feeling, and believing.
Sociocultural	The sociocultural influencing factor incorporates spiritual, religious and ethical factors that are influenced by society. It also includes expectations and values that are based on social class or status. It is the effect of the society and culture in the expectations exerted on a person in attaining needs independently. This may be influenced by societal status, responsibilities and the person's position in the society.
Environmental	The ALs are affected by the environment's influence on the patient as well as the patient's influence on the environment.
Politico-economic	Influenced by governments and government policies (local, national, and international) and health and social care programmes, health economics, availability and access to benefits and resources.

85

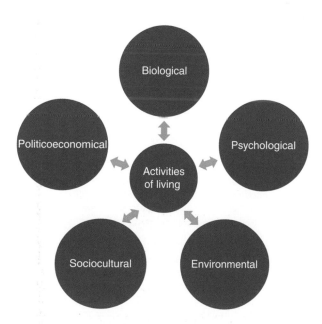

Figure 6.6   The impact of the five influencing factors on the ALs.

Individuality

Each AL that a person performs is unique to that individual. This comes about as a result of the multifaceted interactions that take place between the various components described in the model. When the nurse uses the model as a framework for assessment then person-centred care can emerge through a systematic approach.

So far

Three nursing models have been discussed, with a focus on the ALs model. The models can be used in various care settings. The model of care being used should reflect the philosophy of care in the care environment.

Conclusion

There are various philosophies, conceptual models, and theories that the nurse can and does draw on when formulating a plan of care and providing patient-centred care. These theories relate to practice, they represent different realities and consider different facets of practice. The various theories should not be seen as if in competition with each other. There is no right or wrong one; you can subscribe to one or more than one theory. The theories offer understanding into different ways to explain, describe, predict, and prescribe nursing care. This chapter has offered only a very brief introduction into nursing theories. The reader is encouraged to delve deeper and generate further understanding.

Models of nursing assist the nurse to adopt a systemic approach to care provision. Models of nursing are wide and varied, the most widely used model of nursing used in the UK is the Activities of Living Model (Roper et al. 1996). The ALs model is often misunderstood and is thought to have limited scope. However, the ALs and the various components of the model are complex when used appropriately. The model should not be used as a checklist but as a framework or a theory that can assist the nurse when attempting to offer individualised care that is safe and effective.

References

Alligood, M.R. (ed.) (2017). *Nursing Theorists and their Work*, 9e. St Louis: Elsevier.

Cash, T.F. and Pruzinsky, T. (eds.) (2002). *Body Image: A Handbook of Theory, Research, and Clinical Practice*. New York.: The Guilford Press.

Fawcett, J. and Desanto-Madeya, S. (2013). *Contemporary Nursing Knowledge: Analysis and Evaluation of Nursing Models and Theories*, 3e. Philadelphia: FA Davis.

Henderson, V. (1966). *The Nature of Nursing: A Definition and its Implications, Practice, Research, and Education*. New York: Macmillan Company.

Holland, K., Jenkins, J., Solomon, J., and Whittam, S. (2008). *Applying the Roper–Logan–Tierney Model in Practice*, 2e. Edinburgh: Churchill Livingstone.

Lappin, M. (2018). Models of nursing. In: *Nursing Practice: Knowledge and Care*, 2e (ed. I. Peate and K. Wild), 129–145. Oxford: Wiley.

Murphy, F., Williams, A., and Pridmore, J.A. (eds.) (2010). Nursing models and contemporary nursing 1: their development, uses and limitations. *Nursing Times* 106: 23.

Orem, D.E. (1980). *Nursing: Concepts of Practice*. 3 New York: McGraw-Hill.

Orem, D.E. (1990). A nursing practice theory in three parts, 1956–1989. In: *Nursing Theories in Practice* (ed. M.E. Parker), 47–60. New York: National League for Nursing.

Peplau, H. (1988). *Interpersonal Relations in Nursing a Conceptual Framework of Reference for Psychodynamic Nursing*. Basingstoke: Macmillan.

Roper, N., Logan, W.W., and Tierney, A.J. (1983). *Using a Model for Nursing*. Edinburgh: Churchill Livingstone.

Roper, N., Logan, W.W., and Tierney, A.J. (1996). *The Elements of Nursing*, 4e. Edinburgh: Churchill Livingstone.

Roy, C. (1981). *Theory Construction in Nursing: An Adaptation Model*. Englewood Cliffs: Prentice Hall.

Roy, C. and Andrews, H.A. (2008). *The Roy Adaptation Model*, 3e. Englewood Cliffs: Prentice Hall.

Torres, G. (1990). The place of concepts and theories within nursing. In: *Nursing Theories: The Base for Professional Nursing Practice*, 3e (ed. J.B. George). Upper Saddle River, NJ: Prentice Hall.

Walker, L.O. and Avant, K.C. (2011). *Strategies for Theory Construction in Nursing*, 5e. Norwalk: Appleton Lange.

Walsh, M. (1998). *Models and Critical Pathways in Clinical Nursing: Conceptual Frameworks for Care Planning*, 2e. Edinburgh: Baillière Tindall.

Chapter 7

The skills of assessment and planning care

Aim

The chapter provides an introduction to the skills required to undertake a comprehensive assessment of needs and offers a discussion on how to plan care (including goal setting).

Learning outcomes

By the end of the chapter the reader will be able to:

1. Describe the principles required to conduct an assessment of needs
2. Outline the various components associated with planning care and goal setting
3. Discuss the skills required to assess needs in a competent and holistic manner
4. Explain the importance of assessment and the planning of care when providing high-quality, competent, and confident care.

Introduction

The skills of assessment will require the nurse to include physical and psychological assessment. The nurse has to take a patient history in order to determine needs and make a diagnosis as care is planned, delivered, and evaluated. There are a number of elements associated with assessment and they include:

- Communication
- Measurement
- Observation

All nurses are required to practise in a holistic, non-judgemental, caring, and sensitive manner. Practising in this manner can help avoid making assumptions about people and help recognise and respect individual choice as well as acknowledging diversity (NMC 2018).

Platform three of the NMC (2018) standards for proficiency is specifically related to assessing needs and planning care. At the point of registration, the nurse is required to demonstrate proficiency in prioritising the needs of people they care for when assessing and reviewing mental, physical, cognitive, behavioural, social and spiritual needs. The nurse has to use the information that has been obtained during assessments to identify the priorities and requirements for person-centred and evidence-based nursing interventions and support. Nurses will, according to the NMC (2018), work in partnership with

Fundamentals of Assessment and Care Planning for Nurses, First Edition. Ian Peate.
© 2020 John Wiley & Sons Ltd. Published 2020 by John Wiley & Sons Ltd.

people, developing person-centred care plans that will take into account individual circumstances, characteristics, and preferences.

Assessment and planning care are two stages of a systematic problem-solving approach to care and they are used to help identify, prevent, and treat actual or potential health problems and promote wellness. Assessment has to be used alongside a model of nursing. The model provides a framework for assessment to be undertaken (see Chapter 6).

Assessment

Assessment is described by Le May (2017) as the systematic collection of key information to inform care. Assessment requires the nurse to:

- Observe the patient
- Carry out a clinical examination
- Gather data
- Communicate
- Undertake various measurements

The assessment is, according to Weber and Kelley (2018), the most critical phase of the nursing process. An initial assessment is carried out when the nurse first meets the patient or they are admitted into the care of the nurse. Assessment is ongoing and identifies pre-existing and new problems. An emergency assessment can be either physiological or related to a mental health crisis.

Types of assessment

Nurses and other health care professionals use a variety of types of assessment (see Table 7.1). The nurse chooses the most appropriate type of assessment based on the patient's needs and what part of the patient journey the person is at.

The admission assessment

An admission assessment is undertaken by the nurse with patient (the primary source) or carer (the secondary source), preferably upon arrival to the ward or department. The admission assessment must be completed within 24 hours of admission or as per local policy and procedure. Health care providers have a number of ways of administering the assessment process upon admission, this includes how the assessment is undertaken (electronic or written process) and the format to be used. At all times during the admissions process the nurse must ensure that patient privacy and confidentiality are maintained.

So far

Assessment is the key phase of the nursing process, so much so that it is being revisited in this chapter. There are a number of types of assessment that need to be undertaken. The nurse uses clinical judgement to determine the type of assessment if this is not obvious (for example, an admission assessment is needed when the patient is admitted to the care facility (ward/department)).

Table 7.1 Types of assessment.

Type of assessment	Description
Admission assessment	Comprehensive nursing assessment will include a patient history, an observation of the patient's general appearance, a physical examination and vital signs.
Shift Assessment	Concise nursing assessment that is completed at the commencement of each shift or if the patient's condition changes at any other time during the shift.
Focused assessment	This is a detailed nursing assessment that considers specific body system(s) relating to the presenting problem or current concern(s) of the patient. This can involve one or more body systems.

Patient history

The skills required to undertake a patient history in an effective and competent manner require the nurse to use all of their senses as they listen to the patient. Setting the scene is important, as the patient is giving permission to tell the nurse their story freely; they should not feel as if the nurse is judging them or the lifestyle that they have chosen. When asking questions, these should be as open as possible. Constantly check that what you think is the problem is what the patient thinks is the problem. At all times keep an open mind and always consider: 'Am I making assumptions about this person?' Be aware of this and reconsider your approach.

History taking is but one aspect of the consultation and does not exist in isolation. This key activity demands communication skills that are effective as the nurse gathers information about the patient. This information can often be intimate in nature. History taking is often seen as the most important component of any clinical encounter. Being able to take a clinical history is key to developing, establishing, and sustaining an effective therapeutic relationship with the patient. The process requires collaboration and consultation as well as using a holistic approach. Nurses should discuss the history of current illness/injury, what is the reason for the current admission, any relevant past history, known allergies and reactions to any allergy, the use of medications, the person's immunisation status, family, and social history.

Gaining a patient history is not only about the gathering of information. If undertaken in an effective way, there is much potential to reveal the nature and extent of the problem that the person is experiencing, the antecedent to the problem, and how the problem is impacting on the patient. It can uncover patient concerns, their ideas and their expectations. Therefore, it is important to have structure and order or a framework to guide the process. Most health care organisations provide a pre-determined framework that is to be used when taking a patient history. This can help in consistency when taking a history. It must be noted, however, that this is just a framework, a guide, a focus for discussion, and the nurse may need to add or even delete some elements of that framework in a justified manner.

A systematic approach to history taking has been suggested by Blainey (2014). When used effectively this can offer an ordered approach as opposed to an ad hoc or random approach (see Box 7.1).

A focused approach is required and the specific history-taking framework that is used by the various professional groups may differ. Irrespective of this, the skills that are required for effective history taking are common to all healthcare professions.

Ultimately the ability to undertake a history in an effective way relies on the nurse's communication skills. When these skills are used in the right way, taking into account the context of care, then the outcome can be considered a successful encounter for the patient and nurse. Putting into place effective communication skills has the potential to enable the patient to tell the story of their illness and for them to make known their needs.

It has to be made clear to the patient (and if appropriate family) the reason why there is a need to take a history, for example it may be that the nurse is trying to make a decision on what type of investigations are required or you may be determining a patient's suitability for a specific type of anaesthetic. Other reasons as to why a patient's history may be taken are outlined in Box 7.2.

Box 7.1 A systematic approach to history taking (Blainey 2014)

- Presenting complaint
- History of presenting complaint
- Past medical history
- Drug history
- Family history
- Social history
- Systems enquiry

Box 7.2 Some reasons for undertaking a patient history

- To discover what body the system(s) are responsible for causing the symptom(s) the patient is experiencing
- To help in making a diagnosis
- To determine a differential diagnosis
- Gathering data (subjective and objective) regarding the patient's health
- To provide an explanation for the cause(s) of the disease process
- To consider a patient's fitness to undergo an anaesthetic for surgery
- To begin to understand and appreciate the patient's individual circumstances, their anxieties, hopes, expectations, and beliefs

So far

History taking is just one part of the consultation. Effective communication skills are required as the nurse gathers information about the patient, which can sometimes be of an intimate nature. The history is the most important element of any clinical encounter. Taking a clinical history (and how it is taken) is key to building and maintaining an effective relationship with the patient; the process involves collaboration and consultation.

The skills required to take a patient history require much practice and over time the nurse can perfect this and carry out the activity in a competent and confident manner.

General appearance

Assessment of the patients' overall physical, emotional, and behavioural state begins as soon as the nurse meets the patient (and family). This occurs on admission and continues to be observed throughout the patient's stay in hospital.

Observe the patient when first met and take note of their general appearance, does the person look anorexic, overweight, obese? Does the patient look unwell, anxious distressed, pale or flushed, breathless, cyanotic, lethargic, or active? Is the patient agitated or calm, euphoric, compliant, or combative, what is their mood and effect?

Vital signs

The recoding of baseline observations is undertaken as part of an admission assessment and these are documented on the patient's observation chart or equivalent of this. Ongoing assessment of vital signs are completed as dictated by the patient's condition or according to local policy and procedure observing the trending of vital signs helps to support the clinical decision-making process. More frequent monitoring of some patients will be needed for those with recognised risk factors for deterioration, where there is concern of serious illness/deterioration and those undergoing high-risk treatments such as chemotherapy, blood transfusion, and so on.

Cook and Montgomery (2010) note that the monitoring and measurement of vital signs and clinical assessment are core essential skills for all health care practitioners. The assessment of vital signs is undertaken in a number of care settings:

- acute care
- GP surgeries
- walk-in clinics
- telephone

Box 7.3 Vital signs

- heart rate
- respiratory rate and effort
- blood pressure
- oxygen saturations
- capillary refill time
- level of consciousness and temperature
- weight
- height
- pain

- advice and triage services
- schools
- care homes and other community settings

Vital signs assessment describes the broader process involving visual observation, palpation, listening, and communication to evaluate the patient's condition (NHS 2017). Assessment can include a range of characteristics, interactions, non-verbal communication and the reaction the patient displays to the physical surroundings. Vital signs can include those listed in Box 7.3.

Observing and monitoring the patient accomplishes many functions. It provides a baseline of normal vital signs for those who are attending for a procedure or surgical intervention in order to re-evaluate the patient's health status after completion of the intervention as well as providing a baseline of the ill patient's physiological condition when presentation to hospital or other health care settings. It should be noted that this baseline is not the patient's baseline normal physiological state but, is related to physiological change. The base line trend can assist with an analysis of a person's illness. It provides a rigorous assessment of physiological state on admission to hospital or when there is concern that there is deterioration in a person's condition, to assist in making a diagnosis, to contribute to the consideration of differential diagnoses and to ascertain how unwell a patient is. The baseline assessment of vital signs can help to triage workload and to identify patients who are potentially at risk of deterioration and when risk has been identified planning to manage and mitigate those risks can be put in place.

In some instances, vital signs will be assessed, measured, and monitored by nursing associates, healthcare assistants and nursing students, these members of staff will have received appropriate training to undertake this role. Those undertaking this role will do so under the direction and supervision of a registered nurse and must be aware when it is that they will be required to escalate any concerns.

Family members can also provide a useful context regarding how a patient is in comparison to their normal state. Those undertaking observation and monitoring of patients (regardless of setting) must be aware of this and respond and record any concerns that are raised.

There are a number of validated tools that are available to enable the nurse to track and trigger a patient's condition such as National Early Warning Score 2 (NEWS2) (Royal College of Physicians 2017). These tools are used to assist in the recognition of deterioration in a patient. They highlight the frequency of observations and triggers for escalation. In order to ensure that there is a timely and accurate response to the deterioration in the patient's condition the use of a structured communication tool such as SBAR (NHS Improvement 2018) is used:

S = Situation (a brief statement of the problem)
B = Background (relevant and brief information related to the situation)
A = Assessment (analysis and deliberations of options – what you found/think)
R = Recommendation (action requested/recommended – what you want)

So far

Assessing vital signs means the nurse has to be able to understand what vital signs need to be assessed, interpret the findings and then (if required) act on the data gathered.

What are considered vital signs in one area of care may differ in another area of care. Practising under supervision will enable the nurse to demonstrate proficiency in this key area of care.

Vital signs are only one part of the assessment process, using the skills of observation and physical examination are equally as important.

Physical assessment

The nurse must remember that intimate examinations can be embarrassing or distressing for patients and whenever the nurse examines a patient they must be sensitive to what they may think of as intimate. This is expected to include examinations of breasts, genitalia, and rectum. However, it could also include any examination where it is necessary to touch or even be close to the patient. When undertaking an intimate examination, the nurse must offer the patient the option of having an impartial observer (a chaperone) present wherever this is possible. This will apply whether or not the nurse is the same gender as the patient. A chaperone would normally be a health professional.

A structured and coordinated physical examination permits the nurse to obtain a complete assessment of the patient. Observation/inspection, palpation, percussion, and auscultation are techniques that are used to collect information. Clinical judgement is used to decide on the degree of assessment needed. Assessment information includes, but is not limited to primary assessment (sometimes called primary survey) (airway, breathing, circulation, disability and exposure) and focused systems assessment.

Shift assessment

At the start of each shift an assessment is undertaken on every patient, this information is used to develop the plan of care and make amendments to the existing care plan if needed. Initial shift assessment is documented on the patient care plan and further assessments or changes must also be documented. Clinical judgement is employed by the nurse to decide on the extent of and type of assessment needed.

Assessment information (this reflects the activities of living) includes, but is not limited to:

- Airway: noises, secretions, cough, any artificial airways
- Breathing: bilateral air entry and movement, breath sounds, respiratory rate, rhythm, work of breathing: – spontaneous/laboured/supported/ventilator dependent, oxygen requirement and mode of delivery.
- Circulation: pulses (location, rate, rhythm, and strength); temperature (peripheral and central), skin colour and moisture, skin turgor, capillary refill time; skin, lip, oral mucosa and nail bed colour. If monitored ECG rate and rhythm.
- Disability: use assessment tools such as Alert Voice Pain Unconscious score (AVPU), Glasgow Coma Scale. Identify any abnormal movement or gait and any aids required, for example mobility aids, transfer requirements, glasses, hearing aids, or prosthetics/orthotics.
- Environment: where appropriate, examine the patient properly, full exposure of the body may be needed whilst at the same time respect the patient's dignity and minimise heat loss
- Observation of vital signs
- Skin: colour, turgor, lesions, bruising, wounds, pressure injuries.
- Hydration/Nutrition: assess hydration and nutrition status and check feeding type – oral, nasogastric, gastrostomy, jejunal, fasting, type of diet, intravenous fluids.
- Output: assess bowel and bladder routine(s), incontinence, management urine output, bowels, drains, and total losses. Fluid balance activity must be reviewed.
- Blood sugar levels as clinically indicated.

- Focused Assessment
- Risk Assessment: pressure injury risk assessment (refer to local policy and procedure), falls risk assessment (refer to local policy and procedure), identification bracelet(s).
- Wellbeing: assess for mood, sleeping habits and outcome, coping strategies, reaction to admission, emotional state, support networks, reaction to admission and psychosocial assessments.
- Review the history of the patient recorded in the medical record, ask questions to add additional details to the history.

Focused assessment

A focused assessment is a detailed nursing assessment of a specific body system(s) related to the presenting problem or other current concern(s). The systems to be assessed will be determined by the patient's needs. This can involve one or more body systems, there are some systems that may not need to be examined, or it may be inappropriate to examine them, the nurse is required to use clinical judgement to decide on which elements of a focused assessment are appropriate for the patient.

Examination must always be carried out in a respectful and gentle manner. With practice the nurse will develop skills so as to identify any deviations from normal. The following four components (skills) will need to be developed:

- Inspection
- Auscultation
- Palpation
- Percussion

Inspection

This requires a visual examination, for example when examining the thorax note should be made of the shape of the chest, the presence of any skin abnormalities, any signs of the use of the accessory muscles of respiration, and the equal (or not) movement of both sides of the chest of the patient during respiration. Any abnormalities noticed on inspection can offer clues to altered pathology, these can then be investigated further using auscultation, palpation, and percussion if appropriate.

Auscultation

This is the term for using a stethoscope to listen to the sounds inside the body. Placing the stethoscope over the patient's bare skin, the nurse listens to the specific area of the body under examination, for example the abdomen (the gastrointestinal tract). There are no risks or side effects associated with auscultation.

Palpation

This concerns feeling by placing the finger over an artery to measure a patient's pulse, for example if an abnormality regarding pulse is detected, the nurse then plans care accordingly. Palpation on the abdominal wall, for example, can help to detect abdominal tenderness or the presence of abdominal masses (see Figure 7.1). The liver, kidneys, and spleen can also be palpated.

Percussion

This involves the skilled tapping of the fingers on different parts of the body, such as the abdomen. Percussion is used to listen for sounds related to the organs or body parts below the skin. During percussion, hollow sounds are heard and body parts filled with air (for example, the lungs) and much duller sounds above an organ, such as the liver or bodily fluids (for example, the urinary bladder). See Figure 7.2.

Underpinning all aspects of the assessment of a patient is the important issue of good record keeping. This is essential for the effective monitoring and interpretation of vital signs. It is an NMC requirement (NMC 2018) that nurses keep clear and accurate records relevant to their practice. Good record keeping is a key component to the provision of safe and effective care.

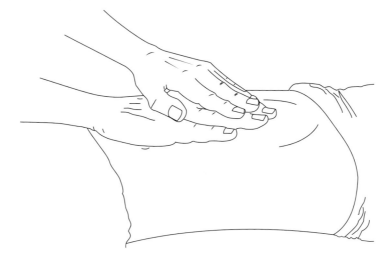

Figure 7.1   Palpation.

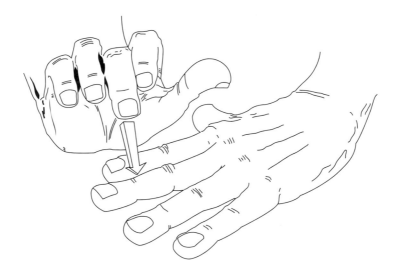

Figure 7.2   Percussion.

So far

Bringing together all of the skills associated with assessment enables the nurse, working with the patient to plan care interventions to meet needs.

Physical assessment requires a structured and coordinated approach as this allows the nurse to obtain a holistic assessment of the patient. Techniques such as observation/inspection, palpation, percussion, and auscultation are used to gather information. Clinical judgement is brought into play to decide on the degree of assessment needed.

Again, practice will enable the nurse to perfect the multitude of skills that are required to confidently assess the needs of the patient.

Take note

Respecting patients' dignity is a fundamental part of nursing care. At all times when obtaining a patent history or undertaking a physical examination it is essential that patient confidentiality is maintained and the patient's dignity is upheld.

All patients are entitled to have their dignity and privacy maintained throughout all stages of treatment.

Whenever possible the patient should always be given the option of having a chaperone present when an intimate examination is being performed.

Review

In your place of work what does your local policy and procedure say about the use of chaperones?
The General Medical Council (2013) suggest that a chaperone will:

- Be sensitive and respect the patient's dignity and confidentiality
- Reassure the patient if they show signs of distress or discomfort
- Be familiar with the procedures involved in a routine intimate examination
- Stay for the whole examination and be able to see what the doctor is doing, if practical
- Be prepared to raise concerns if they are concerned about the doctor's behaviour or actions.

Take note

Documenting the findings after assessing and examining a patent is a key facet of nursing care. The documented findings become an important reference document providing concise information about a patient's history and examination findings at the time of admission. It also outlines a plan for addressing the issues which prompted the hospitalisation/visit. The information should be presented in a logical manner featuring all data immediately relevant to the patient's condition. It is a means of communicating information to all those who are involved in the care of the patient. It is an important medical-legal document. At all times, local policy and procedure must be adhered to.

Planning care

Intended outcomes and goals are set which should be realistic and achievable and which can be short-term or long-term goals. Nursing diagnoses offer a focus for the planning and implementation of effective and evidence-based care. This process entails identification of nursing-sensitive patient outcomes and deciding on appropriate interventions (Alfaro-LeFevre 2014). When planning care and setting goals several factors and values have to be given consideration (throughout the process), these factors underpin patient-centred care:

- Every patient is the best expert in their own lives and should be actively involved in setting their own priorities and making decisions about how they want to be supported with their health
- Healthcare providers should build on a patient's strengths and capabilities and focus on doing with, as opposed to doing for
- The nurse has a key role in empowering patients by providing information and working with the patient to devise strategies that can be adopted to promote health and wellbeing
- Adopt a collaborative approach, whereby members of the multidisciplinary team work together with the patient, carers and others as they strive to deliver a holistic and individualised response to the patient's unique needs
- Nurses have to be empowered to apply their expertise and professional judgement as they plan flexible and appropriate solutions and bespoke service delivery to meet needs.

Goals should describe what it is that the patient hopes to achieve, goal setting provides the nurse with a clear focus about how they will work with the patient. A patient's goal shows the nurse the arrival point, working together with the patient and other health care providers to plan the roadmap that will be used to get there. Setting goals that are aligned with the patient's values and priorities can encourage them, when able, to take on responsibility and commit to making the changes that are needed to enhance their health and wellbeing.

So far

Another phase of the nursing process is planning care, this can only occur in an effective and patient-centred way if the nurse is skilled in assessment. It is evident that the nurse uses observation, measurement, and communication in order to holistically assess needs.

There are several tools that are available to help gather information and interpret findings.

Review

What types of assessment tools are you familiar with? Make a list of the tools you have seen in use in the care setting and describe the pros and cons with each of them.

Objectives and goals

There are many different terms covering goal setting, including goal planning, care planning, and action planning used by practitioners and researchers (Scobbie et al. 2009). An objective is a statement which explains a specific goal to be achieved, it should be something that can be measured by undertaking specific activities within a definite time frame. Writing goals that are patient-centred requires much practice and this will come in time. All nurses are accountable for their actions and omissions (NMC 2018), writing goals and setting objectives is one way in which this can be evidenced.

Objectives should be patient-focused and realistic, these state how the goals are to be achieved as well as when the outcomes should be evaluated. An outcome that is patient-focused will centre on the required results of care interventions – the impact of care provided on the patient. Outcomes and goals can be short- or long-term, enabling the nurse to identify the patient's health status and progress, if the patient's condition is stable, have they made an improvement or has the person deteriorated. Setting realistic outcomes and interventions requires the nurse to discriminate between those nursing diagnoses that are life-threatening or an immediate risk to the patient's safety and those that could be dealt with at a later stage (Grant-Frost et al. 2011). Identifying which nursing diagnoses/problems impact on other problems (for example, inability to swallow will contribute to a poor nutritional status) will lead to that problem being a higher priority. If the nurse, working with the patient addresses the issues with swallowing the patient's nutritional status will be improved.

By using the Specific, Measurable, Achievable, Realistic with a Timeframe (SMART) framework when writing objectives or this can help make them SMART. The objective or goal should state clearly:

- what is to be achieved (e.g. the specific skill or performance)
- how achievement will be measured (the standard or criteria that you will use to measure if the goal has been achieved)
- the timeframe that has been allocated for achievement (the time when the goal is to be accomplished)

Table 7.2 provides further detail of SMART approach. Table 7.3 lists some action verbs that can be used in goal setting.

Table 7.2 The specific, measurable, achievable, realistic with a timeframe (SMART) approach.

SMART Element	Meaning	Examples	Considerations
Specific	An objective or goal should relate to a specific skill or performance that needs to be achieved. Action verbs should be used to help measure your performance (see Box 7.3).	Must be clearly defined. 'I'm going to become fitter' this is not specific. 'I'm going to walk each day during my lunch hour, starting with 10 minutes and building this up by a couple of minutes when is becomes easy' is a very specific goal	What exactly needs to be achieved? What strategies have been identified? Is the objective or the goal clear and explicit? Has an 'action' verb been used?
Measurable	A measurable goal or objective has to make clear how the performance can be measured.	This demonstrates the progress towards the goal and if it has been achieved. 'Do some gardening' is not measurable – this could mean digging for 30 minutes or gently hoeing the border? 'I'm going to spend 30 minutes clearing the side border of weeds' is measurable, demonstrating time spent and what is to be achieved	How will it be known that the goal or outcome has been achieved? How can the changes or impact be measured?
Achievable	A goal or objective must be possible to achieve in terms of your role as a nursing student and the amount of time on placement.	Is the overall goal achievable? This is explored from the patient's viewpoint (asking about their confidence in achieving the goal) and also from the nurse's viewpoint, a goal to lose 20 kg might be achievable; however, consideration should also be given a realistic timeframe.	Can this goal or objective be achieved given the nurse's level of competence? Can this be achieved within the specified timeframe? Have limitations or constraints been considered?
Realistic	The goal or objective has to be realistic.	Goals have to be realistic. A 20 kg weight loss is achievable; however, this may not be realistic to state that this will occur in three weeks	Is this goal or objective achievable? Can the goal or objective be achieved by using the resources identified? Are the resources needed to achieve the goal or objective accessible?
Timeframe	A realistic timeframe to measure progress has to be included.	If a specific time has been set then goals are more likely to be achieved, in terms of time of day and in time for the task to be completed, a lunchtime (specific time of day) walk for 10 minutes (specific time of the task). These timeframes need to be thought of in terms of what fits in with the patient's usual daily routine so that they will eventually become fully incorporated into that routine	Is there a stated deadline for achieving the goal or objective? Is the timeframe realistic?

Source: Adapted Doran (1981), Furze (2015).

Table 7.3   Some measurable verbs.

• State	• Demonstrate
• Verbalise	• Perform
• Communicate	• Administer
• List	• Walk
• Describe	• Stand
• Identify	• Sit
• Name	• Lie
• Express	• Choose
	• Participate

For the goal to be SMART, all five parts must be interconnected and as such taken as a whole. A goal which is not being achieved may not be completely SMART or those interventions that have been put in place to achieve it may not be appropriate (Stonehouse 2018).

Review

When next working in a care area undertake an audit on a patient's care plan and determine if the care plan clearly identifies the patient's needs and if the goals that have been set have used the SMART approach.

Furze (2015) provides some tips for successful goal setting in the non-acute care setting. Goal setting is a key skill when supporting self-management of long-term conditions, appropriate goal setting can have significant effects on a person's physical and psychological functioning and quality of life. Table 7.4 offers some tips for goals setting.

Take note

Simple goal diaries available for patients to record their goal and success can be very helpful. Using diaries can help to:

• Accurately record the specific goal
• Encourage patients to engage with the activity
• Identify any problems that may be developing
• Reward success

There are a number of electronic devices available, for example activity trackers – these are akin to pedometers and may help people achieve their goals and record their success.

It is very important that the nurse, with the patient, monitors progress and offers feedback to the patient on their goal achievements, receiving positive feedback can help to encourage confidence and competence in relation to success, schedule regular appointments in the care process to discuss with the patient their goals. If the patient has been completing a goal diary or using an activity tracking device for example, these should be discussed as part of how the patient is progressing towards meeting their goals. Engaging patients in this way can reinforce success and can prevent the patient feeling isolated as they strive to achieve their goals and outcomes. If the patient is experiencing difficulties then work with them to devise ways of overcoming the difficulty, it may be that the goal that has been set needs to be re-set.

A goal needs to be measurable, functional, and have temporal element. An alternative to the SMART approach is a five-step approach that is described in Table 7.5.

Table 7.4 Tips for goal setting on the non-acute care setting.

Set goals that will take into account what it is the patient can do now	This is important when setting activity goals, the nurse should take into account what the patient can actually do now. Ask, for example, how long they can walk for on the flat. Take into account where the person will be going for a walk (is the route paved, is it hilly?). Then set the first week's goal at 80% of what the patient says they can do on a bad day; this way you are setting the first week's activity goal at a level that they should be able to easily achieve and this promotes success. Advise the patient that the goal should only be increased (a little) if they find it easy on three consecutive days
Set goals for fun things to do	Goals that include things that the patient enjoys might encourage them to see goals positively as opposed to a task that must be done. For example, a walking goal could include to go for a walk with the grandchildren
Ask if the patient would like their family involved in their goals	The family may or may not support the patient in achieving their goal. It is important to discuss this with the patient prior to involving the family. Bringing the family on board can help to prevent them unintentionally sabotaging the goals, for example saying, 'you are overdoing things – you should rest', when the patient is simply following the activity goal that you have set with them
Support the patient to write the goals down and to also make notes of their progress	This has two outcomes – it helps the patient to 'own' the goal, it also helps them to see that they are making progress, or can help them to see when they need to ask the nurse for more help
Break down complex goals	For example, maintaining a garden involves a variety of tasks, requiring different levels of ability. Gently hoeing well-dug ground is very light exercise, digging the ground to plant vegetable crops requires a different level of fitness. Even mowing the lawn will be different for a person with a ride-on mower compared to those with a manual mower. The nurse works with the patient to set small goals based on what they can do and that will build over the weeks towards achieving the overall goal.

Source: Adapted Furze (2015).

Table 7.5 An alternative approach to specific, measurable, achievable, realistic with a timeframe (SMART) goal setting – the five-step approach.

Component	Description
Who	A goal focuses on the patient receiving care. It follows therefore that 'who' is always the patient. Family members and significant others may be involved in goal setting and with the patient's care, but they are not the focus of the goal.
What	The 'what' of the goal is the activity that the patient performs. Activities described in goals relate to the desired outcomes of care, they should be observable and repeatable and have a definite beginning and end. Each goal focuses on an activity or activities with similar functional requirements. A general outcome of 'self-care', for example, has many components as each activity has different functional requirements, each activity requires a separate goal.
Under what conditions	The conditions under which the patient's achievement of the goal is measured is the next component…. The conditions often address the aspects of a goal that are unique to the patient. Conditions incorporate specific elements of a measure into the goal. This may include measures of distance, time to perform an activity, or other elements needed for performance of the activity.
How well	'How well' describes the amount of assistance needed, if any, from other people for the patient to perform the activity, or describes the number of successful attempts needed before considering that the patient has achieved the goal. 'How well' can also relate to a specific number of successful attempts of the activity out of a specific number of trials. This element provides a set criterion for consistency in performing the activity before considering a goal to have been achieved.
By when	The final component 'By when' is the target date for the patient to achieve the goal. It is usually the nurse who determines this time frame, basing it on evidence such as knowledge of the estimated tissue healing times, available research, personal experience and the past progress of the individual. The dates for achievement of goals may change as care advances.

Source: Adapted Randall and McEwen (2000).

So far

Producing patient-centred goals will require much practice, this is an important skill. Writing goals and setting objectives is one way in which the nurse may be judged on their actions or omissions.

Objectives should be patient-focused and realistic and state how the goals are to be achieved and also when outcomes should be evaluated. Outcomes and goals can be short- or long-term. Setting realistic outcomes and interventions requires the nurse to distinguish between those nursing diagnoses that are life-threatening or an immediate risk to the patient's safety and those that may be dealt with at a later stage.

Essential steps in goal setting require the use of a SMART approach to goal setting helping the patient and nurse reach outcomes set. Goals should be set in collaboration with the patient. A five stage approach to goal setting can also be used.

Writing goals or objectives

When writing goals or objectives it is important that they are written clearly and concisely and this means that the correct verbs are used. If goals have been badly planned and are unachievable then the nurse should not attempt to implement care activities. The following should be considered, have the wishes of the patient been taken into account when goals have been set? Have patients been equal partners during the planning process? Nurses must work openly and cooperatively with those who use health and social care services treating them and their families with respect, this means involving them in their care in an open supportive manner.

Using verbs that are vague (or woolly) should be avoided as these verbs are difficult to measure see Box 7.4

The verbs in Box 7.4 are about mental processes and it is difficult to provide evidence that can be measured with these kinds of verbs.

Once goals have been set using a SMART approach, the cyclical nursing process then continues. Interventions to achieve goals are identified and implemented. The final stage of the nursing process; evaluation then occurs to determine if the care delivered has been successful in achieving the goals and outcomes. If not, reassessment takes place and the goals may need to be changed or alternative interventions employed.

Review

Reflect on this, a patient with a wound.

Many of the goals that nurses write for those with wounds will frequently emphasise the wound and often neglect the individual with the wound. Often, for example, goals are pathophysiology oriented, 'decrease wound size by 75%' and 'prevent and control infection'.

It is vital that physiological issues are addressed and aiming to decrease wound size and to control and preventing infection are important. Such an approach, however, neglects to ensure that the patient (the person with the wound) is at the centre of all that is being done, in this instance this approach fails to address the whole picture of the patient and the limitations or disabilities that the wound may cause.

Patient-centred goals for patients with wounds should focus on those activities that are important to the patient, whilst at the same time considering the wound and methods to be used to promote wound healing.

Goals in this instance also need to address any functional activity that is important to the patient as well as incorporating issues regarding the wound to prevent infection. When providing care to those patients with wounds, the nurse is still required to measure and document wound size along with other aspects of injury and pathophysiologies, but there must also be a focus on the individual and any functional limitations and disabilities imposed by the wound.

Box 7.4 Some verbs to avoid

- Appreciate
- Improve
- Be aware of
- Know
- Understand
- Think
- Feel
- Realise

The goal is aimed at the nursing diagnosis and the expected outcomes are aimed at meeting the goal. Goals must be:

1. Patient-centred
2. Address only one response
3. Include observable and measurable factors
4. Need a target date
5. Use a measurable verb

It can be written like this:
Mrs Singh will state three ways to treat her hypoglycaemia by [DATE].
This goal:

1. Is patient-centred (it names Mrs Singh, she will…)
2. Addresses only one response (treat her hypoglycaemia)
3. Includes observable and measurable factors (it states three ways)
4. Had set a target date (by [DATE])
5. Used a measurable verb (will state).

It would be incorrect for the goal to say 'the patient will state 3 ways to treat hypoglycaemia and will know signs and symptoms of hypoglycaemia by [DATE]'

This is because this goal is addressing two responses, using the word 'know' is difficult to measure. In some situations, it would be very difficult to prove that the patient knows or understands something.

Review

Examine this goal for Mr Jakob Raheem, a gentleman who has a dry mouth, oliguria, loss of skin turgor and is dehydrated. Re-write the goal so that it contains all of the correct criteria that are required for care that is implemented is safe, patient centred way and is able to be evaluated.

Patient is dehydrated. Needs to have fluids encouraged so he looks better and is passing more urine by tomorrow.

So far

One of the most important reasons for writing patient-centred goals is that patients may be more likely to make the greatest gains when the goals set focus on activities that are meaningful to them and that will make a difference to their lives.

Often the best way to identify patient-centred goals is simply to ask the patient (if appropriate), 'What are your goals related to your condition'. In this case the patient is likely to respond with a focus on what they see as important to them. Their response can become the starting point for writing patient-centred measurable goals.

Review

Consider this case in a rehabilitation care setting:

Mr Johnson, who has a stable fracture of the right femoral neck and whose desired outcome is 'I want to go home and look after myself, I want to be able to garden again'.

How might you work with Mr Johnson to enable him to reach his desired outcome?

Think of these elements as you make your response:

- Who
- Will do what
- Under what conditions
- How well
- By when

The above is a variant on the SMART goal approach but can work equally as well

Conclusion

Nurses who adopt a patient-centred approach when assessing needs and formulating goals and outcomes can be confident in providing holistic care. When this approach is used the therapeutic nursing relationship will flourish and there will be a change in the way nurses and patients interact.

There are many skills associated with assessment and these will take time to perfect. The nurse is required to measure, communicate, and observe. These skills need to be practiced on a regular basis so as to achieve expertise, it can be helpful to obtain feedback from others on your assessing and goal setting performance. There are a number of assessment tools that are available in care areas. The use of assessment tools can offer a standardised approach to obtaining patient data, this can help to document change in a patient's condition over time and to evaluate clinical interventions and nursing care.

There is a need to obtain a patient history and to perform a physical examination. Once all of the data has been collected nursing diagnoses can be made and the ensuing formulation of patient-centred goals is required. Goal setting can be complex, they would usually be SMART.

References

Alfaro-LeFevre, R. (2014). *Applying Nursing Process: The Foundation for Clinical Reasoning*. Philadelphia: Lippincott.

Blainey, S. (2014). Consultation and clinical history taking. In: *Clinical Examination Skills for Healthcare Professionals* (ed. M. Ransom, H. Abbott and W. Braithwaite), 1–19. Keswick: M and K Publishing.

Cook, K. and Montgomery, H. (2010). Assessment. In: *Practices in Children's Nursing*, 3e (ed. E. Trigg and T.A. Mohammed), 67–80. London: Churchill Livingstone.

Doran, G.T. (1981). There's a S.M.A.R.T. way to write management's goals and objectives. *Management Review* 70 (11): 35–36.

Furze, G. (2015). Goal setting: a key skill for person-centred care. *Practice Nursing* 26 (5): 241–244.

General Medical Council (2013). Intimate examinations and chaperones. www.gmc-uk.org/-/media/documents/Maintaining_boundaries_Intimate_examinations_and_chaperones.pdf_58835231.pdf (accessed June 2018).

Grant-Frost, D., Hofland, J., Lister, S. et al. (2011). Assessment, discharge and end of life care. In: *The Royal Marsden Manual of Clinical Nursing Procedures*, 8e (ed. L. Dougherty and S. Lister), 21–78. Oxford: Wiley.

Le May, A. (2017). *Rapid Adult Nursing*. Oxford: Wiley.

National Health Service (2017). Re-ACT: the Respond to Ailing Children Tool. https://improvement.nhs.uk/resources/re-act-respond-ailing-children-tool (accessed May 2018).

National Health Service Improvement (2018). SBAR Communication Tool: Situation, Background, Assessment, Recommendation. https://improvement.nhs.uk/resources/sbar-communication-tool (accessed May 2018).

Nursing and Midwifery Council (2018). The Code. Professional Standards of Practice and Behaviour for Nurses, Midwives and Nursing Associates. https://www.nmc.org.uk/globalassets/sitedocuments/nmc-publications/nmc-code.pdf last accessed 8 May 2019.

Nursing and Midwifery Council (NMC) (2018). Future nurse: Standards of proficiency for registered nurses. www.nmc.org.uk/globalassets/sitedocuments/education-standards/future-nurse-proficiencies.pdf (accessed May 2018).

Randall, K.E. and McEwen, I.R. (2000). Writing patient-centered functional goals. *Physical Therapy* 80 (12): 1197–1203.

Royal College of Physicians (2017) National Early Warning Score 2. www.rcplondon.ac.uk/projects/outputs/national-early-warning-score-news-2 (accessed May 2018).

Scobbie, L., Wyke, S., and Dixon, D. (2009). Identifying and applying psychological theory to setting and achieving rehabilitation goals: development of a practice framework. *Clinical Rehabilitation* 23 (4): 321–333. https://doi: 10.1177/02692155 09102981.

Stonehouse, D. (2018). How SMART are your patient goals? *British Journal of Health Care Assistants* 12 (5): 233–235.

Weber, J.R. and Kelley, J.H. (2018). *Nursing Assessment in Health Care*. Philadelphia: Wolters Kluwer.

Chapter 8

Assessment tools

Aim

This chapter introduces the reader to the concept of assessment tools.

Learning outcomes

By the end of the chapter the reader will be able to:

1. Discuss the use of assessment tools in care areas
2. Provide an understanding of a number of terms associated with assessment tools such as reliability, validity, specificity, and sensitivity
3. Describe the value of using assessment tools when assessing needs
4. Outline the limitations associated with use of assessment tools

Introduction

Nursing assessment requires the nurse to gather information about a patient's physiological, psychological, sociological, and spiritual status. Assessment has been discussed in other chapters and in detail in Chapter 7 of this text. The appropriate use of assessment tools according to Lappin (2018) is to help the nurse ascertain a strongly balanced assessment that can lead to a robust plan of care that will meet the patient's individual needs.

Tools and instruments

There are many names given to assessment tools, the name often reflects the purpose of the tool, they can be called:

- Instruments
- Screening tools
- Screening instruments
- Risk assessment tools
- Risk assessment instruments
- Clinical algorithms

Most nurses will rely on tools or instruments to help them assess a patient's health status and how the patient is progressing (outcomes). They are used to help the nurse quantify things as concrete and to objectively measure phenomena such as the size of a pressure sore or to measure subjective

Fundamentals of Assessment and Care Planning for Nurses, First Edition. Ian Peate.
© 2020 John Wiley & Sons Ltd. Published 2020 by John Wiley & Sons Ltd.

concepts such as level of anxiety. The use of an assessment tool assists with measurement. There are many tools available, they are used in conjunction with the assessment process and also as a part of an appraisal of risk (Hill 2017) and can be handwritten or electronic. The risk assessment tools aims to predict a patient's level of risk of developing, for example, a pressure sore (Waterlow 2007) or the possibility that the patient's condition may change (for example, National Early Warning Score 2 (NEWS2)) (Royal College of Physicians 2017). If risk has been identified then appropriate interventions need to be put in place to mitigate the risk.

No instrument or tool that is in use in clinical practice is perfect, irrespective of how many years the tool has been in development or in use. There are a number of reasons why a tool may be imperfect, it can be a challenge to measure abstract concepts and errors may sit with the instrument itself, the person using the tool may lack confidence and competence, or how the tool is administered with the population being assessed. The aim, when using a tool, is to obtain the most accurate measurement possible and this is important as subsequent care interventions may be based on the outcomes of using the tool. It is important that the nurse is critical of the tool and ensures that the right tool is being used for the right purpose and the right population. It is equally important that the person who uses the tool knows how to use it and how to interpret and act on the results it provides.

With an increase in the number of risk assessment tools available in care areas, this can make the choice of an appropriate tool a challenge. The nurse needs to consider a number of issues prior to deciding on what tool to use (Fazel and Wolf 2018). The reliability, validity, sensitivity, and specificity of the instruments are important factors to consider when choosing an instrument (McNett et al. 2017).

So far

There are many tools available (and will continue to be made available) that can help nurses undertake an objective assessment of needs. Tools (or instruments as they are also known) help nurses assess a patient's status and how the patient is progressing (outcomes). It has to be acknowledged that there is no tool that is in use in clinical practice that is perfect, regardless of how many years the tool has been in use.

Take note

As the number of risk assessment tools that are available will continue to increase, beware that this can make choosing an appropriate tool a challenge.

Reliability

Glasper and Rees (2017) discuss the terms reliability and validity in the context of nursing and healthcare research. Reliability they suggest is the accuracy and consistency of a tool to measure data that is collected. The tool that has been chosen has to be chosen carefully, tools such as a pain tool (usually a named tool), for example the Faces Pain Scale – Revised (International Association of Pain 2014), has been demonstrated to be reliable when it comes to measuring pain. There are some specialist tools that require the user to be specifically trained in its use otherwise questions may arise about user reliability. Intra-rater reliability refers to the consistent use of the tool as it is used over and over again by the same person. Inter-rater reliability, however, also refers to the consistency of the tool or instrument when different people are using it. It can be difficult to assure inter-rater reliability as different people work in different ways and may be using the tool in different ways as they attempt to measure and assess. When an assessment tool is used that requires the nurse to consider concrete facts (objectivity) then inter-rater reliability should be good (high); however, when the nurse is asked for an opinion (subjectivity) related to assessment, then inter-rater reliability may not be so good and it is seen as having low inter-rater reliability.

Review

If you asked a group of people who have just watched a football match to tell you if they enjoyed the game, you are likely to get a number of responses. If you asked them the names of the two teams who played it is likely that 100% would give you the right answer. The enjoyment of the game will depend on each person's perspective and this would be subjective, the name of the teams playing is without doubt, so this is objective.

Inter-rater reliability is key in health and social care settings. There has to be inter-rater reliability, if this is not evident then each person using the tool to undertake assessment would provide a different response even if the patient's attributes had not altered, the response would not be based on a change in the patient's characteristics but, on how the tool is used by each nurse.

Not all assessment tools that are in use have high inter-rater reliability. Kelly (2005) undertook a study to determine inter-rater reliability when nurses used the Waterlow pressure ulcer risk assessment tool. There was much variance in inter-rater reliability in the sample tested. There may be consequences for patient care when inter-rater reliability is not reliable. In the incidence regarding the Waterlow pressure ulcer risk assessment tool those nurses tested could have underestimated the risk of a patient developing a pressure sore and failed to initiate evidence-based actions that could have alleviated risk or they may have overestimated and instigated precautions that were not needed which could have had a negative impact on the use of scarce human and material resources available.

Review

How do you think inter-rater reliability could be enhanced when using a popular assessment tool such as the Malnutrition Universal Screening Tool (MUST) (British Association for Parenteral and Enteral Nutrition 2018)?

Take note

Inter-rater reliability should be given serious consideration by the nurse when choosing any assessment tool as this can have serious implications for patient safety and quality of care.

Validity

Validity, according to Glasper and Rees (2017), is often discussed at the same time as reliability. Validity is associated with accuracy, whereas reliability is associated with precision (Jacobsen 2017). Take, for example, a dart thrower who hits the same spot on the dart board consistently this is reliable (precision). However, if the cluster is not on the bull's eye then the dart thrower lacks accuracy (validity).

The more abstract the concept being measured, for example anxiety, pain, resilience, the more difficult it will be to declare 100% the validity of the tool that sets out to measure anxiety, pain, resilience – it is rare for any tool to be 100% valid. Validity refers to the degree that the assessment tool (or the instrument) measures what it is intended to and performs as it is designed to perform. There are several statistical tests and measures that can be used to assess the validity of assessment tools which generally involve pilot testing.

Sensitivity and specificity

These terms are often used in research. An ideal screening tool would be 100% sensitive and 100% specific, that is, there would be no false positives and no false negatives. A tool that detects risk of pressure sore formation, for example, would be sensitive as the tool can predict the future, tools have to have

Table 8.1 Specificity and sensitivity.

Specificity	Sensitivity
The specificity of a test is the ability of the test to identify correctly the non-affected individuals.	The sensitivity of a test is the ability of the test to identify correctly the affected individuals.
Proportion of people testing negative amongst non-affected individuals	Proportion of people testing positive amongst affected individuals

a high level of sensitivity to be of any value. When tools are not sensitive to what they are measuring they can produce false negatives, false negative predictions can have serious implications for patient safety. See Table 8.1 for an overview of specificity and sensitivity in relation to predictive values.

It is important that nurses and other health care providers do not rely on the scores of tools, instruments, and scales alone when they are assessing an individual, they should consider other factors, such as the degree of impairment, length of episode, history of the condition, family history, other comorbid disorders, and specific circumstances relating to the patient.

So far

Assessment tools have to be reliable and valid. Tools that aim to predict or diagnose have to be sensitive and specific. When tools have been tested and they are used correctly with the right patient group then they are able to assist the nurse when making decisions about care provision and the allocation of human and material resources in an appropriate way.

Take note

Not all assessment tools are reliable. Nurses need to be aware of this and they must always know how to use a specific tool, as failure to understand the tool (and its limitations) could result in adverse patient outcomes.

Wound assessment tools

Greatrex-White and Moxey (2013) undertook an evaluatory research study to determine how well different wound assessment tools met the needs of nurses as they undertook general wound assessment and whether current tools are fit for purpose.

Caring for people with wounds can be challenging; there is a need for nurses and others to adopt a holistic and systematic approach to wound care. A key aspect of any holistic approach to care is to undertake initial and ongoing wound assessments. In doing this it provides baseline information against which progress can be monitored. It can enable goal setting and assist with the appropriate selection of dressings. If poor or inappropriate assessment is apparent, this can lead to inappropriate wound management along with poor patient outcomes. It is therefore essential that assessment is undertaken in alignment with the highest of standards: if assessment is not performed correctly, any wound care that follows will suffer and result in delayed healing and/or serious complications (Timmins 2009). Wound assessment is a key activity associated with good wound management, and must be seen as an integral element of wound care practice.

It is important for nurses to be able to accurately establish the current condition of a wound, evaluate whether the wound is improving or deteriorating and to make a decision upon the most suitable treatment. Nurses should consider a number of issues associated with wound assessment. Following the assessment of a wound, think about:

1. What stage is this wound at?
2. What do I want this wound to do next?
3. How can these objectives be achieved whilst at the same time preserving healthy tissue?

Clearly none of this can be left to chance, and the nurse must seek a way of ensuring that the assessment of a person with a wound is as objective as possible. Wound assessment tools can help to make the assessment in this case more objective. Benbow (2016) reiterates the point that wound classification tools are only effective when practitioners are confident in using the tools and understand the findings to determine an accurate diagnosis and the appropriate treatment. Without a universal approach and understanding, Watret (2005) emphasises that such tools in themselves can be a barrier to effective multidisciplinary working as well as best patient outcomes.

High-quality wound management will be ineffective if the nurse fails to consider the patient's risk and other contributing factors during the assessment, as well as their involvement in and approval of treatment planned. Consideration should be given to conditions, such as diabetes, cardiovascular disease, respiratory disease, anaemia, immune disorders, renal disorders, and obesity, as well as other systemic influences, for example ageing, smoking, ability to mobilise, nutrition, and stress. These factors are all important in ascertaining the development or occurrence of a wound and how, or whether, it heals (Benbow 2016).

It is important to determine if a wound is acute or chronic, the stage of healing, how it is healing, whether there are any obvious impediments to healing and how the patient is reacting to having a wound. Two challenges arise: the assessment of these parameters is mainly subjective; and accurate assessment relies on the knowledge, experience, and skill of the practitioner (Brown and Flanagan 2013; Benbow 2016). When a wound is first assessed it should be accurate and detailed in such a way as to afford a baseline for following assessments so these can be compared and measured against. The World Union of Wound Healing Societies (2004) offers a standardised, systematic, sequential approach to assessment to ensure that best practice enables accurate ongoing evaluation of wound progress, be this positive or negative.

Of wound assessment tools, Greatrex-White and Moxey (2013) conclude that there are several tools in existence which meet many of the needs of nurses as they undertake wound assessment. No tool, they note, has been identified which meets all the requirements of nurses.

Take note

Nurses have to be selective in the wound assessment tool that they use, as no one tool will meet all requirements.

So far

When a nurse purports to provide patients with wounds with holistic care, assessment must involve identifying, gathering, and interpreting information about the patient and wound to ensure that the diagnosis is accurate, the care provided is appropriate, and there is ongoing monitoring and prevention of complications.

A standardised, systematic approach to assessment should be adopted so as to assist the nurse in the accurate evaluation of the wound, with the overarching aim of ensuring optimal wound healing as well as positive patient outcomes.

Nutritional assessment tools

Mutrie and Hill (2018) emphasise the importance of nutritional support as it aims to provide patients with the nutrients required to meet their basal metabolic requirements. Assessment of the nutritional requirements of any patient will usually include multidisciplinary input from dieticians because of the patient's various requirements, as well as the potential complexity of their conditions.

The National Institute for Health and Care Excellence (NICE) (2017a) has provided guidelines to help nurses benchmark nutritional support for patients, recommending screening for malnutrition and risk of malnutrition in all hospital inpatients using a recognised tool, such as the MUST (British Association for Parenteral and Enteral Nutrition 2018). The MUST calculator is used in a variety of care settings it establishes nutritional risk by using objective measurements to obtain a score and a risk category or subjective criteria to estimate a risk category but not a score. Components of the tool include:

Table 8.2 The components of Malnutrition Universal Screening Tool (MUST) (British Association for Parenteral and Enteral Nutrition 2018).

Component	Description
Body mass index (BMI)	Clinical impression – thin, acceptable weight, overweight. Clear wasting (very thin) and obesity (very overweight) may also be recorded.
Unplanned weight loss	Clothes and/or jewellery have become loose/fitting (weight loss), dentures may be loose. History of a decline in food intake, a reduction in appetite or swallowing problems over three to six months and underlying disease or psychosocial/physical disabilities that are likely to cause weight loss.
Acute disease and effect	Acutely ill as well as no nutritional intake or possibility of no intake for more than five days. If the patient is currently affected by an acute pathophysiological or psychological condition and there has been no nutritional intake or possibility of no intake for more than five days, it is likely that they will be at nutritional risk. These patients would include those who are critically ill, those who have swallowing difficulties (e.g. after stroke), or head injuries or those undergoing gastrointestinal surgery.

Determine overall risk of malnutrition
The result of the estimated BMI category, any unplanned weight loss and acute disease effect, then allows the nurse to select the appropriate risk category.

Low	Medium	High

109

- The patient's body mass index (BMI)
- Percentage of unplanned weight loss
- Acute disease effect

(see Table 8.2).
When the components are brought together in a systematic way this can help to calculate risk of malnutrition.

Review

In the care area where you work or have worked, how is the need for nutritional support assessed? Who would be involved in the holistic assessment of a patient who may require nutritional support?

The MUST is a five-step screening tool to identify those adults who are malnourished, at risk of malnutrition (undernutrition), or obese (see Figure 8.1). The tool also provides management guidelines which can be used to help nurses develop a care plan. The tool can be used in hospitals, community, and other care settings and can be used by all care workers.

Review

How would you measure the height of patient who is unable to stand?

So far

Good nutrition is important for health, healing and recovery from illness and injury. There are a number of published nutritional screening/assessment tools that are available for use by nurses to screen or assess the nutritional status of patients and MUST is one of these tools. Many tools have not been subject to rigorous testing and the nurse is required to take this into account when undertaking a nutritional screen or assessment.

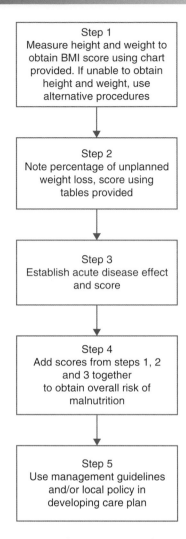

Figure 8.1 Malnutrition Universal Screening Tool (MUST): the five steps. Source: Adapted BAPEN 2018.

National Early Warning Score (NEWS) 2

The idea of using early warning scores (EWS) systems was introduced by the Department of Health in 2000 (DH 2000) this was due in part to the recommendations made in the comprehensive critical care report. The EWS, also known as 'track and trigger systems', according to Carberry and Clements (2014), is the calculation of an aggregate trigger score based on physiological abnormalities. It is intended to support objective decision making in order to help health care staff identify deteriorating patients.

Failing to identify or act on signs that a patient's condition is deteriorating will result in a serious patient safety issue. It can mean that an opportunity may be missed to provide the essential care to result in the best possible chance of survival. Royal College of Physicians (RCP) (2017) states that NEWS2 reliably detects deterioration in adults, triggering review, treatment, and the escalation of care.

NEWS2 is established on a simple scoring system where a score is allocated to six physiological measurements that are already taken in hospitals:

1. Respiratory rate
2. Oxygen saturations

3. Temperature
4. Systolic blood pressure
5. Pulse rate
6. Level of consciousness

This early warning system has been shown to be an extremely effective system for the detection of those patients who are at risk of clinical deterioration or death, the system when used correctly prompts a timely clinical response, aiming to improve patient outcomes. NEWS2 has been taken up by a number of hospitals around the world, to improve patient safety and to save lives (RCP 2017).

NEWS2 is a practical approach, with an emphasis on system-wide standardisation using physiological parameters that nurses and other staff are already routinely measuring in hospitals and in prehospital care. The findings are recorded on a standardised clinical chart, the NEWS2 chart. See Figure 8.2 showing the physiological parameters used.

NEWS2 is based on a simple combined scoring system whereby the nurse allocates a score to physiological measurements, when a patient presents to, or is being monitored in, hospital. Paper or electronic systems can be used to record the NEWS2 score.

A score is allocated to each parameter as they are measured, with the magnitude of the score reflecting how extremely the parameter varies from the norm. Scores range from 0 to 20, with a higher score representing further removal from normal physiology and a higher risk of morbidity. The score is then totalled and uplifted by two points for those patients requiring additional oxygen to maintain their recommended oxygen saturation (RCP 2017) – see Table 8.3 for scores and responses.

Using NEWS2

Nurses and other staff can use NEWS2 with all adults who are aged 16 or over (apart from pregnant women) and across all healthcare settings. The RCP (2017) recommend that the NEWS2 should be recorded during the initial prehospital and/or hospital assessment of a patient and

Physiological parameter	Score						
	3	2	1	0	1	2	3
Respiration rate (per minute)	≤8		9–11	12–20		21–24	≥25
SpO$_2$ Scale 1 (%)	≤91	92–93	94–95	≥96			
SpO$_2$ Scale 2 (%)	≤83	84–85	86–87	88–92 ≥93 on air	93–94 on oxygen	95–96 on oxygen	≥97 on oxygen
Air or oxygen?		Oxygen		Air			
Systolic blood pressure (mmHg)	≤90	91–100	101–110	111–219			≥220
Pulse (per minute)	≤40		41–50	51–90	91–110	111–130	≥131
Consciousness				Alert			CVPU
Temperature (°C)	≤35.0		35.1–36.0	36.1–38.0	38.1–39.0	≥39.1	

Figure 8.2 National Early Warning Score 2 (NEWS2) physiological parameters used. Source: Reproduced from: Royal College of Physicians. NEWS 2: Standardising the assessment of acute-illness severity in the NHS. Updated report of a working party. London: RCP (2017).

Table 8.3 National Early Warning Score 2 (NEWS2) early warning system scores and responses.

NEWS2 Score	Frequency of monitoring	Clinical response
0	Minimum 12 hourly	Continue routine NEWS monitoring with every set of observations
Total: 1–4	Minimum 4–6 hourly	• Inform registered nurse, who must assess the patient • Registered nurse to decide if increased frequency of monitoring and/or escalation of clinical care is required
Total: 5 or more or 3 in one parameter	Increase frequency to a minimum of 1 hourly	• Registered nurse to urgently inform the medical team caring for the patient • Urgent assessment by a clinician with core competencies to assess acutely ill patients • Clinical care in an environment with monitoring facilities
Total: 7 or more	Continuous monitoring of vital signs	• Registered nurse to immediately inform the medical team caring for the patient – this should be at least at specialist registrar level • Emergency assessment by a clinical team with critical care competencies, which also includes a practitioner/s with advanced airway skills • Consider transfer for clinical care to a level 2 or 3 care facility, i.e. higher dependency or intensive care unit

Source: Grant (2018), Merrifield (2017), RCP (2017).

during the patient's hospital stay, as part of the standard clinical observation chart across the NHS. The NEWS2 can also be used in prehospital assessment of the acutely ill patient by paramedics; this can help to improve the communication of acute-illness severity to the hospital receiving the patient.

NEWS2 is particularly valuable when a patient is transferred from one care setting to another, to ensure there is a clear understanding of the patient's clinical state, their risk of deterioration, and their prognosis. If the clinical team, in discussion with the patient (and if appropriate their family/carer), have made a decision that the routine recording of NEWS2 data is inappropriate, for example for those patients who are at the end of their life on an end-of-life care pathway, then this must be communicated and recorded in the patient's notes.

6Cs

End-of-life care

As patients become closer to their end of life, they become weaker. Inappropriate interventions, including measurement of vital signs and the routine recording of data for the NEWS2, should be discontinued. The decision to do this should only be done after discussion with the patient and their family/carer if appropriate, and the outcome of that decision should be recorded in the patient's notes.

Lim (2016) points out that the clinician should be able to recognise when the focus of care has to move from an aggressive life-sustaining approach to an approach that helps prepare and support the patient and their family members through a period of advancing, inevitable decline. Symptom management focuses on the goals to first and foremost provide comfort and let dignity take precedence.

Take note

Local policy and procedure must be followed at all times. This will include the methods required for reporting findings, documenting findings, and the actions taken or the reasons not to act on the NEWS2.

What do your local policies and procedure say about recording data related to NEWS2?

The nurse recording the physiological data for the NEWS2 must be appropriately trained to measure the physiological parameters accurately. The nurse must also understand the meaning of the NEWS2 as well as the response and policies in place for altering the frequency of monitoring and escalating clinical care.

When undertaking assessment, the nurse records the six NEWS2 physiological parameters, each one being allocated a score reflecting the degree of physiological disturbance. The NEWS2 should be used for continuous monitoring of a patient's wellbeing throughout their stay in hospital and not only for the initial assessment of severity of illness. Recording the NEWS2 on a regular basis provides the nurse with information trends in the patient's condition and their clinical response can be tracked, providing an early warning of any clinical deterioration and the necessity for more intensive treatment. The recording of the NEWS2 trends will also provide guidance about the patient's recovery. This can signal a reduction in the frequency and the intensity of clinical monitoring towards the patient's discharge.

The nurse must remember that clinical judgement should always be used, even if the NEWS2 score is normal, escalating deteriorating patients for review if they are concerned, even if the NEWS2 appears to be reassuring. As well as the recommended frequency of observations, review/escalation should be increased if there is any clinical concern that the patient appears to be more unwell than the recorded NEWS2 score.

Whilst accurate recording of the NEWS2 is important, reliable response and escalation is just as important. The frequency of observations and review/escalation is based upon the aggregate NEWS2 (according to local policy and procedure). However, this should be increased/escalated if the nurse is concerned that the patient is sicker than they appear.

So far

- Measure and record the score for each of the six physiological parameters.
- Aggregate the scores and add 2 for any use of supplemental oxygen to derive the final NEWS2 score.

Use the NEWS2 to define and record:

- If escalation of clinical care is needed and its urgency
- The competencies of the clinical review required
- The frequency of monitoring needed
- The most suitable clinical setting for continuing clinical care.

Review

In this NEWS2 chart, record Agnieszka Nowakowski's six NEWS2 physiological parameters.

Agnieszka (who prefers to be called Aggie) is a 73-year-old lady who is 22 hours post total gastrectomy and is being cared for in the surgical ward. The nurse assessing Aggie records the following:
Temperature: 38.1 °C

Oxygen saturations: 92%
Respiratory rate: 24 breaths per minute
Systolic blood pressure: 98 mmHg (98/50 mmHg)
Heart rate: 126 beats per minute
Level of consciousness: Disoriented
Aggie is receiving 60% humidified high flow supplemental oxygen via a face mask

114

NEWS key	FULL NAME		
0 1 2 3	DATE OF BIRTH		DATE OF ADMISSION

		DATE																			DATE
		TIME																			TIME
A+B Respirations Breaths/min	≥25	3																			≥25
	21–24	2																			21–24
	18–20																				18–20
	15–17																				15–17
	12–14																				12–14
	9–11	1																			9–11
	≤8	3																			≤8
A+B SpO$_2$ Scale 1 Oxygen saturation (%)	≥96																				≥96
	94–95	1																			94–95
	92–93	2																			92–93
	≤91	3																			≤91
SpO$_2$ Scale 2[†] Oxygen saturation (%) Use Scale 2 if target range is 88–92%, eg in hypercapnic respiratory failure	≥97 on O$_2$	3																			≥97 on O$_2$
	95–96 on O$_2$	2																			95–96 on O$_2$
	93–94 on O$_2$	1																			93–94 on O$_2$
	≥93 on air																				≥93 on air
	88–92																				88–92
[†]ONLY use Scale 2 under the direction of a qualified clinician	86–87	1																			86–87
	84–85	2																			84–85
	≤83%	3																			≤83%
Air or oxygen?	A=Air																				A=Air
	O$_2$ L/min	2																			O$_2$ L/min
	Device																				Device
C Blood pressure mmHg Score uses systolic BP only	≥220	3																			≥220
	201–219																				201–219
	181–200																				181–200
	161–180																				161–180
	141–160																				141–160
	121–140																				121–140
	111–120																				111–120
	101–110	1																			101–110
	91–100	2																			91–100
	81–90																				81–90
	71–80																				71–80
	61–70	3																			61–70
	51–60																				51–60
	≤50																				≤50
C Pulse Beats/min	≥131	3																			≥131
	121–130	2																			121–130
	111–120																				111–120
	101–110	1																			101–110
	91–100																				91–100
	81–90																				81–90
	71–80																				71–80
	61–70																				61–70
	51–60																				51–60
	41–50	1																			41–50
	31–40																				31–40
	≤30	3																			≤30
D Consciousness Score for NEW onset of confusion (no score if chronic)	Alert																				Alert
	Confusion																				Confusion
	V	3																			V
	P																				P
	U																				U
E Temperature °C	≥39.1°	2																			≥39.1°
	38.1–39.0°	1																			38.1–39.0°
	37.1–38.0°																				37.1–38.0°
	36.1–37.0°																				36.1–37.0°
	35.1–36.0°	1																			35.1–36.0°
	≤35.0°	3																			≤35.0°
NEWS TOTAL																					**TOTAL**
Monitoring frequency																					Monitoring
Escalation of care Y/N																					Escalation
Initials																					Initials

National Early Warning Score 2 (NEWS2) © Royal College of Physicians 2017

Source: Reproduced from: RCP. NEWS2: Standardising the assessment of acute-illness severity in the NHS. Updated report of a working party. London: RCP (2017).

Now, using the scores in Figure 8.2, aggregate the scores and add 2 for the use of supplemental oxygen and derive the NEWS2 score.

What is Aggie's NEWS2 score?

Having determined this, what are your next steps? Use Table 8.3 NEWS2 early warning system scores and responses to help you.

You are required to communicate your findings to a more senior member of the clinical team. Use the SBAR approach:

Component	Your response
Situation. The first step is stating the situation. What is the problem?	
Background. Provide information about the patient, the context.	
Assessment. What did you assess and what was the outcome of that assessment? What do you think the problem is, having assessed the patient?	
Recommendation. Provide a recommendation. What do you think needs to be done?	

Table 8.4   Parameters not included in National Early Warning Score 2 (NEWS2).

Parameters not included	Discussion
Age	Older age is associated with higher clinical risk. The relationship between age and the physiological response to acute illness is multifaceted. Chronological age is not always a good indicator of biological age.
Urine output	The monitoring of urine output is important in many clinical situations. Formal estimation of urine output, however, is not always available at first assessment, and measurement of urine output is not routinely required for the majority of those patients who are in hospital. It is recognised that urine output monitoring is important for some patients as is dictated by their clinical condition.
Pain	The symptom of pain must be recorded and responded to by the clinical team. Pain and/or its cause will generally, but not always, result in physiological disturbances that should be detected by the scoring system for the NEWS2. The symptom of pain should be routinely recorded and responded to; it should not form part of the aggregate score for the NEWS2.
Gender, ethnicity, and obesity	There is no evidence that these parameters have any significant influence.
Pregnancy	Physiological parameters and their response to illness are altered by pregnancy. Existing EWS systems and the NEWS2 may be less reliable in estimating acute-illness severity during pregnancy, the NEWS2 should not be used in pregnancy
Comorbidities including immunosuppression	For many comorbidities there are disease-specific scoring systems, the use of which is not precluded by the NEWS2. The NEWS2 was designed to be generic and should reflect the physiological concerns associated with various comorbidities.

Source: RCP (2017), Smith et al. (2008).

The parameters detailed in Table 8.4 have not been included as part of the scoring system for the NEWS2. This does not mean, however, that they are insignificant or unimportant or that they should not be recorded and considered as a part of the overall clinical assessment of the patient.

Cultural considerations

Ethnicity
There is no evidence that ethnicity has any significant influence on previously evaluated early warning systems. Whilst in the development stages the NEWS Development Group recommended that ethnicity should form no part of the weighting or scoring system for the NEWS2.

Patients not suitable for NEWS2

NHS England (2018) notes that NEWS2 should not be used in children (those under 16 years) or pregnant women. There are other scoring systems that NHS England and NHS Improvement are considering: Paediatric Early Warning Score (PEWS) and Modified Early Obstetric Warning Score (MEOWS).

NEWS2 should not be applied to the obstetric population. This is because the physiological changes that occur during pregnancy can render the existing NEWS2 unsuitable. Furthermore, the physiological response to acute illness in children can be modified as well as by pregnancy. Baseline physiological parameters are different in these two populations when they are compared with the non-pregnant adult population.

Track and trigger systems

NICE (2017b) note that a track and trigger system is a universal term for clinical tools that grade physiological observations and then trigger an escalation response. These systems have been designed to help nurses and other health care professionals to identify and respond to a deteriorating patient. A numerical score is attached to particular parameters to identify the meaning of a patient's vital signs. The parameter ranges are allocated scores that trigger an escalation response Examples of some track and trigger systems are identified in Table 8.5.

Grant (2018) discusses some limitations that are associated with the use of track and trigger systems. In the UK there are a number of track and trigger systems which are in use that have potential limitations. There is significant inconsistency between the various systems, with each of them having varying degrees of specificity and sensitivity.

The numerous track and trigger systems used across the NHS demonstrate significant variations in the parameters used and the scores that these are allocated. These variations bring concerns with regard to equity in practice, patient safety as well as the application of evidence-based practice (Quirke 2012).

Table 8.5 Some examples of track and trigger systems.

System	Description
EWS	Early Warning Score. There are different versions in use across the NHS, these systems are specific to each trust.
SEWS	Standardised Early Warning Score incorporates an escalation policy prompting more frequent observations and urgent medical assessment. The SEWS chart was designed to be visually striking and simple to complete.
MEWS	Modified Early Warning Score is a simple physiological score that may allow improvement in the quality and safety of management provided to patients. The key aim is to prevent delay in intervention or transfer of critically ill patients.
RRT	Rapid response trigger is based on the idea of early and rapid intervention, originally inspired by the management strategies of severe trauma, which included two key elements: the early detection of deterioration coupled to a rapid response.
NEWS 1	National Early Warning Score 1, launched in 2012, was a tool developed by the Royal College of Physicians which improves the detection and response to clinical deterioration in adults.
NEWS 2	National Early Warning Score 2, launched in 2017 is the early warning system for identifying acutely ill patients, including those with sepsis, in hospitals in England.

Source: Adapted Gardner-Thorpe et al. (2006), Grant (2018), Paterson et al. (2006), RCP (2017).

There is also significant variation in terms of the values that are identified as 'normal' parameters, for example Rhind and Greig (2002) suggest that the normal core temperature is 36–37°C, whereas Boore et al. (2016) uses 35.8–37.8°C as the normal value. A further limitation is that observations that could offer valuable information to identify deterioration may be missing from a track and trigger system.

Take note

Nurses need to be aware of the potential limitations when using any track and trigger system.

The RCP (2017) caution that the NEWS2 should be used as an objective data collecting tool that aids clinical decision making, it is not a barrier or alternative to proficient clinical judgement. It may be that in certain situations a nurse considers that the NEWS2 score underestimates their concern for the patient's clinical condition. When this occurs, concern must be escalated to a more senior clinical decision maker. In circumstances in which the nurse or healthcare professional feels the NEWS2 score might be overesti- mating the severity of the patient's clinical condition, they are also required to escalate decision making to a more senior decision maker to ascertain if escalation of care is justified or not.

Take note

Any track and trigger system (including NEWS2) should be used only as an objective tool that helps the nurse to collect data, which in turn assists with clinical decision making. They should not be seen as a barrier or an alternative to proficient clinical judgement.

Any track and trigger system can only work effectively if the nurse undertaking the routine measurements is appropriately trained in its use and response systems and staff are available to deliver the recommended urgency of response by a clinical team with an appropriate level of clinical competence. Grant (2018) concludes and reiterates that nurses should not rely solely on track and trigger systems (including NEWS2), but should use them to support their clinical judgement.

So far

Recognising and responding to patient deterioration depends on a whole-system approach and the revised NEWS2, published by the RCP in December 2017, reliably detects deterioration in adults. This triggers a review, treatment, and escalation of care where appropriate.

Conclusion

There are so many assessment tools available to nurses to assist them as they assess a patient's needs. The assessment tool, instrument rating scale aims to objectify data that may be seen as subjective, such as pain, anxiety, or the size of a wound. Choosing the right tool and questioning reliability, valid- ity, specificity, and sensitivity are important so as to ensure the most appropriate tool is used as well as the provision of safe, effective, and patient-centred care.

All tools have potential limitations (nutritional assessment tools, wound assessment tools, and track and trigger systems and others). In order to use any tool, instrument, or risk assessment tool the nurse needs to fully understand how to use the tool, apply it to clinical practice, act on the findings, and document the action taken or, if no actions were taken after assessment, the reason why.

It should be remembered that any tool is there to support clinical judgement. The tool is only as good as the nurse who is using it; the significance of clinical judgement must never be underestimated.

References

Benbow, M. (2016). Best practice in would assessment. *Nursing Standard* 30 (27): 40–47.
Boore, J., Cook, N., and Shepherd, A. (2016). *Essentials of Anatomy and Physiology for Nursing Practice*. London: Sage.

British Association for Parenteral and Enteral Nutrition (2018). 'MUST' Calculator. www.bapen.org.uk/screening-and-must/must-calculator (accessed June 2018).

Brown, A. and Flanagan, M. (2013). Assessing skin integrity. In: *Wound Healing and Skin Integrity: Principles and Practice* (ed. M. Flanagan), 52–65. Oxford: Wiley.

Carberry, M. and Clements, P. (2014). Early warning systems 1: how helpful are early warning scores? *Nursing Times* 110: 12–14.

Department of Health (2000). *Comprehensive Critical Care: A Review of Adult Critical Care Services*. London: Department of Health.

Fazel, S. and Wolf, A. (2018). Selecting a risk assessment tool to use in practice: A 10-point guide. *Evidence Based Mental Health*. http://ebmh.bmj.com/content/ebmental/21/2/41.full.pdf http://dx.doi.org/10.1136/eb-2017-102861.

Gardner-Thorpe, J., Love, N., Wrightson, J. et al. (2006). The value of Modified Early Warning Score (MEWS) in surgical in-patients: a prospective observational study. *Annals of the Royal College of Surgeons of England* 88 (6): 571–575.

Glasper, A. and Rees, C. (2017). *Nursing and Healthcare Research at a Glance*. Oxford: Wiley.

Grant, S. (2018). Limitations of track and trigger systems and the National Early Warning Score. Part 1: areas of contention. *British Journal of Nursing* 27 (11): 624–631.

Greatrex-White, S. and Moxey, H. (2013). Wound assessment tools and Nurses' needs: an evaluation study. *International Wound Journal* 12 (3): 293–301. https://doi.org/10.1111/iwj.1210.

Hill, R. (2017). Assessment, Planning, Implementation and Evaluation (APIE). In: *Essentials of Nursing of Practice* (ed. C. Delves-Yates), 197–210. London: Sage.

International Association of Pain (2014). Faces Pain Scale – revised home. www.iasp-pain.org/Education/Content.aspx?ItemNumber=1519 (accessed June 2018).

Jacobsen, K.H. (2017). *Introduction to Health Research Methods: A Practical Guide*, 2e. Burlington: Jones and Bartlett.

Kelly, J. (2005). Inter-rater reliability and Waterlow's pressure ulcer risk assessment tool. *Nursing Standard* 19 (32): 86–92.

Lappin, M. (2018). The nursing process. In: *Nursing Practice Knowledge and Care*, 2e (ed. I. Peate and K. Wild), 111–128. Oxford: Wiley.

Lim, R.B.L. (2016). End-of-life care in patients with advanced lung cancer. *Therapeutic Advances in Respiratory Disease* 10 (5): 455–465.

McNett, M., Shelly, A., and Olson, D.M. (2017). Sensitivity, specificity, and receiver operating characteristics: A primer for neuroscience nurses. *Journal of Neuroscience Nursing* 49 (2): 99–101. https://doi.org/10.1097/JNN.0000000000000267 (accessed June 2018).

Merrifield, N. (2017). Warning score system for patient deterioration due to be standard across NHS by 2019. *Nursing Times*. www.nursingtimes.net/news/hospital/trusts-told-to-use-same-nhs-warning-score-for-deterioration/7022531.article (accessed June 2018).

Mutrie, L. and Hill, B. (2018). Providing nutritional support for patients in critical care. *Nursing Standard* https://doi.org/10.7748/ns.2018.e10804.

National Institute for Health and Care Excellence (2017a). *Nutrition Support for Adults: Oral Nutrition Support, Enteral Tube Feeding and Parenteral Nutrition: Clinical Guideline No. 32*. London: NICE.

National Institute for Health and Care Excellence (2017b). Sepsis: Recognition, diagnosis and early management. www.nice.org.uk/guidance/ng51 (accessed June 2018).

NHS England (2018). National Early Warning Score (NEWS). www.england.nhs.uk/nationalearlywarningscore/#which-patient-groups-should-not-use-news (accessed June 2018).

Paterson, R., MacLeod, D.C., Thetford, D. et al. (2006). Prediction of in-hospital mortality and length of stay using an early warning scoring system: clinical audit. *Clinical Medicine* 6 (3): 281–284.

Quirke, M. (2012). The NEWS is bad for neurological patients. *British Journal of Neuroscience Nursing* 9 (2): 94–95.

Rhind, J. and Greig, J. (2002). *Anatomy and Physiology Applied to Health Professionals*, 7e. Edinburgh: Churchill Livingstone.

Royal College of Physicians (RCP) (2017). National Early Warning Score 2. www.rcplondon.ac.uk/projects/outputs/national-early-warning-score-news-2 (accessed June 2018).

Smith, G.B., Prytherch, D.R., Schmidt, P.E. et al. (2008). Should age be included as a component of track and trigger systems used to identify sick adult patients? *Resuscitation* 78: 109–115. https://doi.org/10.1016/j.resuscitation.2008.03.004.

Timmins, J. (2009). Can nurses' knowledge of wound care be improved by a systematic approach to wound management? In: *Applied Wound Management Part 3* (ed. Wounds UK), 14–17. Aberdeen: Wounds UK.

Waterlow, J. (2007). The Waterlow Assessment Tool. www.judy-waterlow.co.uk (accessed June 2018).

Watret, L. (2005). Wound bed preparation and the diabetic foot. *Diabetic Foot Journal* 8 (1): 18–26.

World Union of Wound Healing Societies (2004). Principles of Best Practice: Minimising pain at wound dressing-related procedures. A consensus document. London: MEP Ltd. www.woundsinternational.com/media/issues/79/files/content_39.pdf (accessed June 2018).

Chapter 9

Assessing the musculoskeletal system

Aim

This chapter introduces the reader to the assessment of the musculoskeletal system and the care required for people who experience musculoskeletal problems.

Learning outcomes

By the end of the chapter the reader will be able to:

1. Provide an overview of the musculoskeletal system
2. Discuss a number of conditions affecting the musculoskeletal system
3. Outline ways in which the nurse assesses the musculoskeletal system
4. Describe care planning related to the musculoskeletal system

Introduction

Kinesiology (also called body mechanics) is the study of the movement of body parts. The musculo-skeletal system (along with the nervous system) allows the body to move. The use of good body movement is important for the safety of both patient and nurse.

When the body is in a correct anatomical position or alignment (arrangement in a straight line, bringing a line into order) this is when it functions best. Correct, proper body movement is essential to prevent injuries. See Box 9.1 good posture and correct standing body alignment.

Movement of the whole of the body, or some parts of it, is required for many body activities such as breathing, eating and drinking, avoiding injury, and to reproduce. Body movement is mostly under conscious (voluntary) control (Waugh and Grant 2018). There are exceptions and these include protective movements that are carried out before the person is aware of them, for example reflex actions when a person reacts to the presence of a noxious substance or when a finger is removed very quickly from a very hot surface.

Musculoskeletal conditions affect the joints, bones, and muscles and include rarer autoimmune diseases and back pain. There are more years lived with musculoskeletal disability than any other long-term condition, these conditions therefore feature widely in all aspects of health and social care.

There are more than 200 musculoskeletal conditions which affect 1 in 4 of the adult population (many being young and of working age) which is around 9.6 million adults in the UK (House of Commons Hansard 2011). In England, musculoskeletal conditions account for around 30% of GP consultations (Margham 2011).

Fundamentals of Assessment and Care Planning for Nurses, First Edition. Ian Peate.
© 2020 John Wiley & Sons Ltd. Published 2020 by John Wiley & Sons Ltd.

Box 9.1 Correct standing body alignment

- Head up and eyes straight ahead
- Neck straight
- Chest out
- Back straight
- Arms relaxed and at the sides
- Abdominal muscles tucked in
- Knees slightly flexed
- Feet straight and toes forward

Source: Williams (2018)

Musculoskeletal conditions have an enormous impact on the quality of life of millions of people in the UK with 10.8 million days lost as a consequence of musculoskeletal conditions (House of Commons Hansard 2011). They are also associated with a large number of comorbidities, these include diabetes, depression, and obesity (Arthritis Research UK 2013).

Of all surgical interventions in the NHS, musculoskeletal conditions account for over 25%, with a prediction that this is set to rise significantly over the next 10 years (Arthritis Research UK 2013). Musculoskeletal conditions account for a considerable amount of NHS spending each year, it also brings with it much personal and emotional distress for patients and their families.

This chapter considers assessment of the musculoskeletal system. An overview of the system is provided in order to offer context. Sometimes the skeletal and muscular systems are treated as two separate entities. It is also sometimes called the locomotor system. The three key components of the musculoskeletal system are:

1. Bones
2. Joints
3. Muscles

The characteristics of these three key components are discussed along with an overview of the assessment that is needed to allow the nurse to make a nursing diagnosis (or diagnoses), plan care, implement that care, and to evaluate nursing interventions.

Review

Before the nurse can undertake a confident and competent assessment of the musculoskeletal system there is a need to have an understanding of the anatomy and physiology of this system as well as understanding the range of motions of the joints.

Bones

Bones provide the scaffold or the framework for the body. The skeleton is made up of 206 bones at birth, there are around 300 bones and cartilage elements in the human body. As the baby develops, some of the bones combine to form larger, stronger bones. The skeleton is divided up into two parts, the axial skeleton, the central core of the body (offering protection), and the appendicular skeleton, this forms the extremities of the arms and legs (offering support as well as flexibility). The bones of the axial skeleton (there are 80 of these) function as a hard-shell offering protection to the internal organs: for example, the cranium protects the brain and the ribs provide protection to the heart.

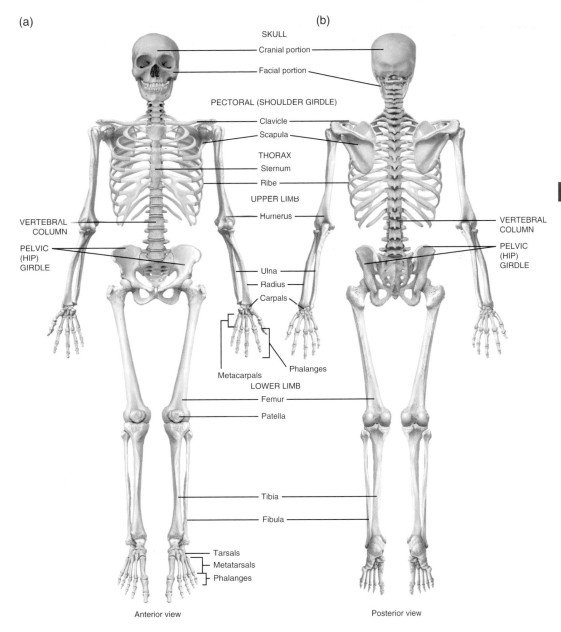

(a)

SKULL
Cranial portion
Facial portion

PECTORAL (SHOULDER GIRDLE)
Clavicle
Scapula

THORAX
Sternum
Ribe

UPPER LIMB
Humerus

VERTEBRAL
COLUMN

PELVIC
(HIP)
GIRDLE

Ulna
Radius
Carpals

Phalanges
Metacarpals
LOWER LIMB
Femur
Patella

Tibia

Fibula

Tarsals
Metatarsals
Phalanges

Anterior view

(b)

VERTEBRAL
COLUMN

PELVIC
(HIP)
GIRDLE

Posterior view

Figure 9.1   The human skeleton.

The bones of the appendicular skeleton (comprising 126) offer support and flexibility at the joints, they anchor the muscles that move the limbs (see Figure 9.1).

Bone is the most rigid of the connective tissues and is made of bone cells that are surrounded by a very hard matrix that contains calcium and a large number of collagen fibres. Bones provide protection, support, and muscle attachment. The functions of the skeletal system are:

- To support the body
- Facilitate movement
- Protect internal organs
- Produce blood cells (known as haemopoiesis)
- Store and release minerals and fat

The formation of bone

Bone formation is known also as ossification or osteogenesis. The skeleton is a structure of living tissue growing, repairing, and renewing itself. Bones are active and complex organs that have a number of important functions, some of these functions are required to maintain homeostasis. It is during development of the foetus that bone formation commences, continuing throughout childhood and adolescence as the skeleton grows. Bone remodelling, however, is a lifelong process that consists of the breaking down of old bone (resorption) and the formation of new bone (ossification). This is key to shaping the skeleton and to the repair of bone fractures.

There are three cell types present in bone, osteoblasts, osteocytes, and osteoclasts. These cells are responsible for the production, maintenance, and resorption of bone (respectively) (see Table 9.1).

Bone remodelling is the process in which matrix is resorbed on one surface of a bone and then deposited on another, primarily occurring during bone growth. In adult life, however, bone undergoes remodelling, in which resorption of old or damaged bone takes place on the same surface, where osteoblasts lay new bone to replace that which is resorbed (McCance and Heuther 2018).

Osteoclasts, large cells which dissolve the bone, come from the bone marrow and are related to white blood cells. Osteoblasts are the cells that form new bone. They also come from the bone marrow, functioning in order to build bone, producing new bone called osteoid.

The 206 bones making up the adult skeleton are divided into five categories, classified according to their shapes:

1. Long bones
2. Short bones
3. Flat bones
4. Irregular bones
5. Sesamoid bones

See Table 9.2.

Joints

Joints are also called articulations they provide flexibility of the skeleton; without joints, there would be no movement. Joints are a place where two or more bones meet, moving in relation to each other and attached to each other by ligaments. There are a number of different types of joints:

- Synovial (including ball and socket and hinge joints)
- Fibrous (joints between the teeth and between the maxilla and mandible)
- Cartilaginous (joints between the vertebrae and at the symphysis pubis)

Synovial joints are the most common type of articulation, appearing where there is a small gap between the bones. This gap allows a free range of movement and space for the synovial fluid to lubricate the joint, for example the joint at the knee (see Figure 9.2).

Fibrous joints occur where bones are very tightly joined, providing little or no movement between the bones – there is no movement between the structures of the skull, for example.

Table 9.1 Cells present in the bone.

Osteoblasts	Bone-forming cells located near the surface of bones, responsible for making osteoid, consisting mainly of collagen. Osteoblasts secrete alkaline phosphatase to create sites for calcium and phosphate deposition. This allows crystals of bone mineral to grow at these sites. The osteoid becomes mineralised, forming bone.
Osteocytes	Osteocytes are osteoblasts no longer on the surface of the bone, instead they are found in lacunae between the lamellae in bone. Their main role is homeostasis, maintaining the correct oxygen and mineral levels in the bone.
Osteoclasts	Multinucleated cells responsible for bone resorption. They travel to specific sites on the surface of bone, secreting acid phosphatase, which unfixes the calcium in mineralised bone to break it down.

Table 9.2 Bone shapes.

Type of bone	Description
Long bones	Cylindrical in shape, these bones are longer than they are wide. The name describes the shape of a bone, not its size. Long bones are found in the arms (they have a shaft and two extremities): • Humerus • Ulna • Radius In the legs: • Femur (the longest bone in the body) • Tibia • Fibula Also found in the fingers and toes are metatarsals and phalanges. These bones act as levers – when they contract, the muscles move.
Short bones	These bones are cube-like; they are roughly equal in length, width, and thickness; they have no shaft and no extremity. Located only in the carpals of the wrists and the tarsals of the ankles. They offer stability and support; they also have some limited motion.
Flat bones	Flat bones vary in size and shape and not all are flat. They have the common feature of being very thin in one direction and can also provide large areas of attachment for muscles. The function of flat bones is to protect internal organs, such as the brain, heart, and pelvic organs. Flat bones include: • Frontal • Parietal • Occipital • Ribs • Sternum • Bones of the pelvis (ilium, ischium, and pubis)
Irregular bones	These vary in shape and structure, they do not fit the pattern of the long, short, flat, or sesamoid bones. Examples are the vertebrae (protecting the spinal cord from compressive forces), sacrum, and coccyx, as well as the sphenoid, ethmoid, and zygomatic bones of the skull.
Sesamoid bones	These bones are small, round bones that are shaped like a sesame seed. These bones form in tendons, where there is much pressure generated in a joint. These bones protect tendons, helping them overcome compressive forces. Sesamoid bones can be found on joints throughout the body, including the patella in the knee and the pisiform bone found in the wrist.

123

Cartilaginous joints are formed where bone meets cartilage or where there is a layer of cartilage between two bones, such as the intervertebral joints between the vertebral bodies. These joints provide a small amount of flexibility as a result of the gel-like consistency of cartilage.

Skeletal muscles

Skeletal muscle is connected to bones by tendons which allow the muscle to pull on bone. A tendon is a band of connective tissue and when a muscle contracts, it pulls the bone, causing movement. Skeletal muscle also contributes to the maintenance of homeostasis as it generates heat. This type of muscle is made up of groups of muscle fibres in an organised arrangement. Small muscles may only be comprised of a few bundles of fibres. However, the major muscles in the body, such as the gluteus maximus (forming the bulk of the buttock), is made up of hundreds of bundles.

The brain controls movement of skeletal muscle. All muscle fibres have a nerve ending, receiving impulses from the brain that then stimulates the muscle, resulting in the filaments of myosin sliding over the actin filaments. This results in the muscle shortening in length. See Figure 9.3, a diagrammatic representation of a skeletal muscle fibre.

Skeletal muscle is richly supplied by blood vessels for nourishment, delivery of oxygen as well as the removal of waste.

The musculoskeletal system has a number of other important functions including haematopoiesis and as a repository centre.

The bone has a responsibility to produce red and white blood cells in a process that is called haematopoiesis. Red bone marrow is situated in the hollow space inside of bones (the medullary cavity).

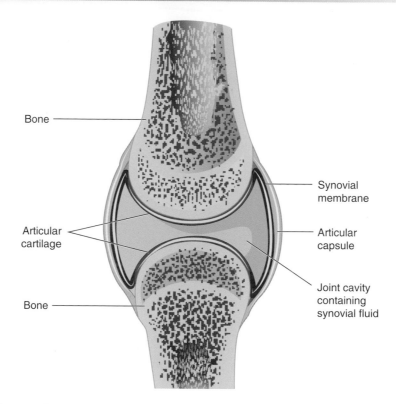

Figure 9.2   A synovial joint.

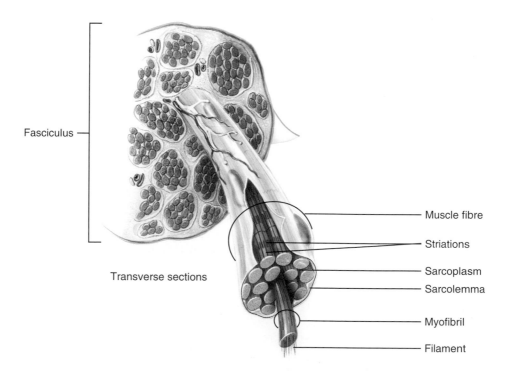

Figure 9.3   Skeletal muscle fibre.

Children have more red bone marrow than adults; this is due to a child's constant growth and development. The amount of red bone marrow tails off at the end of puberty and is replaced by yellow bone marrow.

Storage

The skeletal system also acts as a storage centre, storing a number of types of essential substances needed for growth and repair of the body. The skeletal system's cell matrix acts as a calcium bank, storing and releasing calcium ions into the blood steam as required. Appropriate levels of calcium ions in the blood are crucial for the efficient function of the nervous and muscular systems. Bone cells also release osteocalcin, a hormone that helps in the regulation of blood sugar and fat deposition. The yellow bone marrow located inside the hollow long bones is used to store energy in the form of lipids. Red bone marrow stores some iron in the form of ferritin and uses this iron to produce haemoglobin that is present in red blood cells.

125

Anatomical terms

See Table 9.3 – angular movements possible at the joints.

Review

Why is it important for the nurse to have an understanding of the anatomical terms related to joint movement?

Assessing needs

Everything that we do depends on an intact musculoskeletal system – all of the activities of living are dependent on the musculoskeletal system. How extensive an assessment is performed will depend largely on each patient's problems and needs.

Musculoskeletal problems are common in every age group, impacting on individuals, families, and communities. Primary problems can result from congenital, developmental, infectious, cancer (abnormal tissue growth), traumatic, or degenerative disorders of the system. Secondary problems can arise from disorders of other body systems. The aim of a complete musculoskeletal assessment is to detect risk factors, potential problems, or musculoskeletal dysfunction early and then to plan appropriate interventions, these can include teaching health promotion and disease prevention and implementing treatment measures. The nurse has a significant role to play in assisting patients in the prevention of pain and dysfunction.

The health history

The data collection phase begins by obtaining a detailed and accurate health history. Engaging with the patient to seek of what exactly the patient means by certain subjective complaints, including the location, character, and the onset of any symptoms. It is only the patient who can provide data concerning pain, stiffness, ability to move, and how their activities of living have been affected.

The history provides the subjective data that will then direct the physical examination (see Chapter 7). If time is an issue and you are unable to perform a complete health history, perform a focused history on the motor-musculoskeletal system.

Biographical data

A review of the biographical data may identify those at risk for musculoskeletal problems. Take into account the patient's age, sex, ethnicity, and occupation and consider these as possible risk factors. Women, for example, are at a higher risk than men for osteoporosis and rheumatoid arthritis, an occupation that requires heavy lifting can increase the risk for injury to bones, muscles, joints, and supporting structures, the risk for degenerative joint disease (for example, osteoarthritis) increases with age.

Table 9.3 Angular movements possible at joints.

Term	Description	Image
Flexion	Bending of a body part at a joint so that the angle between the bones is decreased	
Extension	Straightening of a body part at a joint so that the angle between the bones is increased	
Dorsiflexion	Upward movement of the foot so the feet point upwards	
Plantar flexion	Downward movement of the foot so that feet face downwards towards the ground	

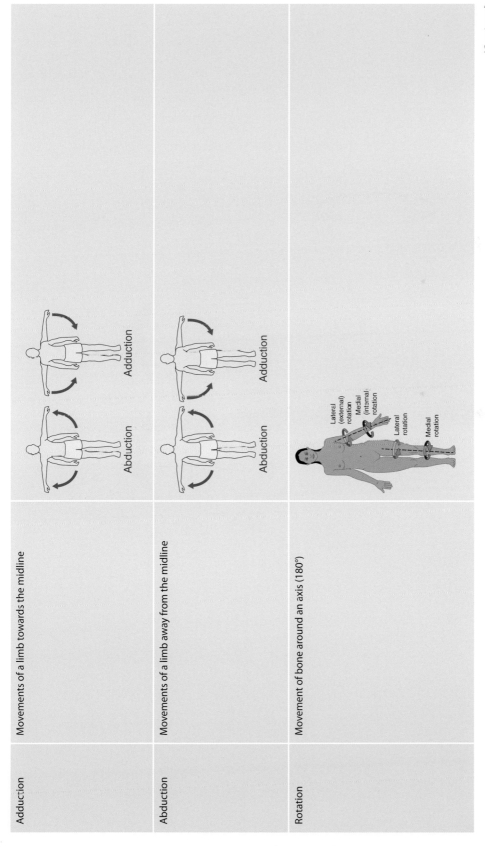

Adduction	Movements of a limb towards the midline	
Abduction	Movements of a limb away from the midline	
Rotation	Movement of bone around an axis (180°)	

Abduction   Adduction

Abduction   Adduction

Lateral (external) rotation
Medial (internal) rotation
Lateral rotation
Medial rotation

(Continued)

Table 9.3 (Continued)

Term	Description	Image
Circumduction	A circular movement of a joint (360°)	
Supination	Turning the hand so that the palm is facing upwards	Supination Pronation

Pronation	Turning the hand so that the palm is facing downwards	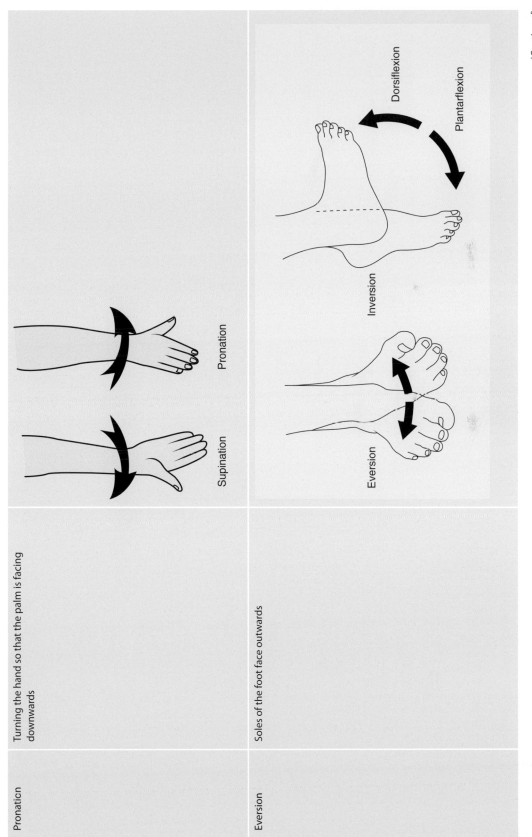
Eversion	Soles of the foot face outwards	

Supination   Pronation

Eversion   Inversion

Dorsiflexion

Plantarflexion

129

(Continued)

Table 9.3 (Continued)

Term	Description	Image
Inversion	Soles of the foot face inwards	

Dorsiflexion

Plantarflexion

Inversion

Eversion

Current health status

Begin the assessment with questions about the patient's current health status. Key symptoms to give specific consideration to, in order of importance, are pain, weakness, and stiffness.

Pain

This can be caused by bone, muscle, or joint problems. Bone pain is not usually associated with movement unless there is a fracture, but muscle pain is. Current or recent illness may cause muscle aches. Bone pain is deep, dull, and throbbing; muscle pain takes the form of cramping or soreness. In rheumatoid arthritis, joint pain and stiffness are worse in the morning. In osteoarthritis, the joints are stiff after rest and pain exacerbated towards the end of the day. In order to evaluate the nature of pain that the patient is experiencing the mnemonic SOCRATES can be helpful:

Site – Where is the pain? Or the maximal site of the pain.
Onset – When did the pain start, and was it sudden or gradual? Include also whether it is progressive or regressive.
Character – What is the pain like? An ache? Stabbing?
Radiation – Does the pain radiate anywhere?
Associations – Any other signs or symptoms associated with the pain?
Time course – Does the pain follow any pattern?
Exacerbating/Relieving factors – Does anything change the pain?
Severity – How bad is the pain?

Weakness

Muscle weakness associated with certain diseases travels from muscle to muscle or to groups of muscles. Ask the patient if the weakness interferes with their ability to perform the activities of living. Weakness of the upper extremities, for example, often presents itself as difficulty when lifting objects or combing hair. Weakness of the lower extremities presents as difficulty with walking and crossing the knees. Patients with myasthenia gravis, for example, have difficulty with diplopia, swallowing, and chewing, along with generalised muscle weakness.

Stiffness

This is a common musculoskeletal complaint. It is important to determine if the stiffness is worse at any particular time of the day. For example, patients with rheumatoid arthritis are stiff on arising because of the period of joint rest that occurs during sleep.

So far

Effective communication skills are required to collect meaningful data in order to obtain a detailed and accurate health history. The nurse actively engages with the patient so as to seek clarity as to what exactly the patient means by certain subjective complaints, where in the body the issue manifests, and the type and onset of symptoms. If the patient is unable to provide the health history secondary sources should be sought, such as family, carers, and other health and social care professionals.

Balance and coordination problems

Patients who have problems with balance and coordination may also have a neurological problem. These problems often manifest as gait problems or difficulty in performing the activities of living. The patient may complain of falling or losing balance or may have ataxia (irregular and uncoordinated voluntary movements). Gait problems are associated with a number of disorders for example:

- Parkinson's disease
- Multiple sclerosis
- Herniated disc
- Stroke

131

- Brain tumour
- Inner ear problems, medications
- Exposure to chemical toxins

Other related symptoms

Musculoskeletal diseases may produce multiple symptoms such as acute rheumatic fever, gout, and autoimmune inflammatory diseases may cause pyrexia and joint pain. Bowel and bladder dysfunction, for example, may suggest a herniated disc.

Past health history

When the past health history has been completed, compare this with the patient's present musculoskeletal status or uncover risk factors that might predispose the patient to musculoskeletal disorders (see Table 9.4).

Cultural considerations

Black males have the densest bones, with a relatively low incidence of osteoporosis. White people tend to have a higher bone density than Chinese people.

Source: Hochberg (2007).

Table 9.4   Some risk factors that might predispose the patient to musculoskeletal disorders.

Factor	Ask about	Discussion
Childhood illnesses	History of juvenile rheumatoid arthritis Cerebral palsy, muscular dystrophy	Symptoms related to childhood illnesses may be seen in adulthood
Surgery	Any surgery regarding bone, muscle, joints, other supporting structures. What type and when?	May explain physical findings
Serious injury	Any past injuries to bone, muscle, joints, other supporting structures. What type and when? What was the treatment? Any residual effects?	Could explain physical findings Past trauma may impact on a person's range of movement
Serious/chronic illness	Any other medical problems? Recent problems including infection	A range of other problems can result in musculoskeletal issues. TB can affect bones and joints; some sexual acquired infections may cause problems with joints. Diabetes may lead to muscle atrophy and joint problems
Allergies	Do you have any allergies, allergic to dairy products, lactose intolerance	Those with an allergy or lactose intolerance may have a reduced calcium intake as they avoid dairy products
Medications	What type, what for, prescribed or over-the-counter? Women: are you receiving oestrogen replacement therapy?	Some medications can affect the musculoskeletal system – diuretics, for example, can cause muscle cramps, benzodiazepines can cause ataxia and the use of corticosteroids can result in, for example, muscle weakness, myopathy, pathological fractures. Women who begin menopause early are at a greater risk for osteoporosis
Recent travel	Where to? What for? Any exposure to infectious or contagious disease?	Travel may bring with it exposure to risk factors that could impact on the musculoskeletal system

Family history

Obtaining the family history may help the nurse to identify predisposing or causative factors for musculoskeletal problems. After undertaking an assessment of the current and past musculoskeletal health status, move on to investigate possible familial tendencies towards problems. For example, is there a family history of gout, arthritis, or osteoporosis? Risk increases when there is a family history for these conditions.

Review of systems

When the nurse undertakes a review of systems this allows an assessment of the interrelationship of the musculoskeletal system to every other system. Often, when doing this, the nurse can uncover important facts that the patient may have failed to mention previously. Numbness, tingling, and loss of sensation may be associated with neurological issues, a herniated disc. Sickle cell anaemia can cause joint pain.

133

Psychosocial profile

The psychosocial profile may uncover patterns in the patient's life that could affect the musculoskeletal system and puts the person at risk for musculoskeletal disorders. When the person undertakes activities to promote the health of musculoskeletal system this helps the nurse with the patient identify health promotion and preventative activities. Understanding what patient's hobbies or recreation activities can identify activities that may put the patient at a higher risk of musculoskeletal injury. Repetitive strain injury can result from knitting, playing football, playing tennis, or working at a computer and using other electronic hand-held devices. Knowing where the patient lives, if they have stairs to climb, or if they live with anyone assists with the important activity of discharge planning.

See Table 9.5 outlines some social factors that are related to musculoskeletal conditions.

So far

A detailed assessment requires the nurses to obtain subjective information about the past history, family history, a review of the systems is required permitting the nurse to understand the interrelationship of the musculoskeletal system to every other system. The patient's psychosocial profile has the potential to uncover patterns in the patient's life that might impact on the musculoskeletal system, putting the patient at risk of musculoskeletal disorders.

Table 9.5   Some social factors related to musculoskeletal conditions.

Alcohol	Trauma Gout Myopathy Rhabdomyolysis Neuropathy
Smoking	Lung cancer with bony metastases Hypertrophic pulmonary osteoarthropathy Rheumatoid arthritis
Drug misuse	Trauma Hepatitis B and C HIV
Diet	Vitamin deficiencies, vitamin D (rickets, osteomalacia), vitamin C (scurvy) Anorexia nervosa (osteoporosis) Obesity (osteoarthritis, diabetes mellitus, Charcot joint)

Source: Gibson and Huntley (2013).

The physical assessment

Once the subjective data has been gathered, objective data is gathered by undertaking a physical assessment (see also Chapter 7). Once again, how extensive the physical assessment is will depend on each patient's individual needs and problems. Sometimes, because the musculoskeletal systems and the central nervous systems are interrelated they may be assessed at the same time.

Take note

The nurse may need assistance in undertaking the physical assessment. The patient may need support before, during, or after the assessment.

The nurse should keep all relevant history findings in mind as the physical examination is carried out. Findings from the physical examination and history taking provide the nurse with the complete assessment picture. Data is analysed, the nursing diagnosis(es) is formulated and a plan of care developed. Because a musculoskeletal problem might be present it is essential that the nurse understands normal musculoskeletal function prior to establishing any abnormal findings.

Method

Data on the patient's posture, gait, coordination, balance, movement and bone structure, muscle strength, joint mobility, and their ability to perform the activities of living is revealed as the nurse performs a physical assessment of the musculoskeletal system.

Inspection, palpation, and percussion are used to assess the musculoskeletal system. A systematic approach is required as the nurse works from head to toe, making a comparison of one side with the other. Inspect and palpate each joint and muscle; then assess range of motion and test muscle strength, if the patient is unable to perform an active range of movements then the nurse should gently perform a passive range of motion. Inspection and palpation are performed simultaneously during the physical assessment.

Take note

Prior to undertaking, and upon completion of any physical examination, the nurse must adhere to local policy and procedure regarding hand washing.

Undertaking a general survey

Before examining specific areas, observe the patient from head to toe, noting general appearance and signs of musculoskeletal problems. Assess vital signs and be alert to signs of pain or discomfort as the patient performs a range of movement. If there are any signs or symptoms of pain associated with movement, the nurse should never force a joint.

Take note

The nurse should never force a joint when undertaking physical assessment.

Physical examination

Perform a head-to-toe physical assessment looking for changes in every system that might indicate a musculoskeletal problem. As the musculoskeletal system is about locomotion (movement) it is essential that the nurse looks at how the patient moves (or does not move).

6Cs

The patient's dignity should be preserved at all times. The examination room should be warm, the examination conducted in private and the presence of a chaperone should be offered in line with local policy and procedure.

Carrying out a musculoskeletal physical assessment

Once the head-to-toe examination is completed the nurse should focus on the specifics of the examination:

- Assess posture, gait, and cerebellar function
- Measure limbs
- Assess joints and test joint movement
- Assess muscle strength and ROM
- Perform additional tests to assess for wrist, spine, hip, and knee problems, if necessary

Williams (2018) suggests that when assessing the standing patient's body alignment, the nurse should begin by noting the head position in relation to the rest of the body:

- Is the head centred and erect?
- Are the shoulders and hips parallel?
- Are the knees and ankles slightly flexed and parallel to the hips and shoulders?
- Do the arms hang comfortably at the side of the patient?
- Are the feet slightly apart, providing a base of support?

During the assessment, also observe for any muscle weakness or paralysis, and check symmetry (meaning equality in size, form, and arrangement of parts on the opposite sides of a plane; a mirror image) of extremities.

When the patient is sitting observe for symmetry. Establish whether the patient's head is erect and centred over the shoulders. Are the buttocks in the same plane as the shoulders and are the thighs aligned with the shoulders? The patient's weight should be distributed evenly over the buttocks and thighs. The knees should be flexed at around 90°, with the feet resting comfortably on the floor. Offer a footstool if the feet do not reach the floor. The arms should lie comfortably in the lap or be supported by the armrests of the chair.

When assessing the lying patient, assess carefully for alignment and correct position. Patients often lie on their back when in bed. Support the head with one pillow preventing hyperflexion of the neck. The vertebral column should be centred and in alignment, without observable curves. The mattress should support the body in this position.

Finally, assess the patient's ability to walk and to change position independently. Observe the patient walking if appropriate and note:

- Is the head centred over the vertebral column?
- Is the gait even and unlaboured?
- Is the patient balanced?
- Is there any weakness or favouring of one side?

This will determine the patient's ability to ambulate independently or determine the type of assistance needed. Assess cerebellar function, this includes balance, coordination, and accuracy of movements.

Take note

Prior to undertaking a physical assessment, the nurse must seek consent from the patient; to do otherwise could contravene common law and the Code of Conduct (NMC 2018).

Balance

To assess balance, observe the patient's gait. If there are any gait problems, proceed no further. If there are no gait problems and the patient is able, ask the patient to tandem (heel-to-toe) walk, heel-and-toe walk, hop in place and do a deep knee bend, and perform the Romberg test.

Ask the patient to stand with feet together and eyes open, then close the eyes. If cerebellar function is intact, the patient will be able to maintain balance with minimal swaying with eyes closed. This is called the Romberg test. Remember, balance problems may also occur with inner ear disorders.

Coordination

When assessing coordination, note the patient's dominant side – this side is usually more coordinated. To test upper extremity coordination, ask the patient to perform rapid alternating movements by patting the thigh with one hand, alternating between the supinate and the pronate hand position. Perform finger-thumb opposition to further test hand coordination. To test lower extremity coordination, ask the patient to perform rhythmic toe tapping and then run the heel of one foot down the shin of the opposite leg. Each side has to be tested separately so findings can be compared.

Accuracy of movements

Point-to-point localisation is used to assess accuracy of movements. The patient should touch the finger to the nose with the eyes open, then closed.

Taking limb measurements

Limb measurements include both length and circumference. Measure arm lengths from the acromion process to the tip of the middle finger. Measure leg lengths from the anterior superior iliac crest crossing over the knee to the medial malleolus. This is known as true leg length. An apparent leg length measurement is measured from a nonfixed point, the umbilicus, to the medial malleolus.

Limb circumference reflects actual muscle size or muscle mass. Measure circumference on forearms, upper arms, thighs, and calves. Note the patient's dominant side, which can normally be up to 1 cm larger than the non-dominant side. Accurate circumference measurement requires the nurse to determine the midpoint of the extremity being assessed. If the upper arm circumference is being measured, measure the distance from the acromion process to the olecranon process, use the midpoint to determine circumference; then repeat for the opposite arm.

Assessing joints and muscles

Inspect the size, shape, colour and symmetry of each joint, noting masses, deformities, and muscle atrophy. Compare muscle and joint findings bilaterally and palpate for oedema, heat, tenderness, pain, nodules, crepitus, and stability. Test active range of movement and gentle passive range of movement. If there are any changes in articular cartilage, scarring of the joint capsule, and muscle contractures these will all limit motion. It is important to determine the types of motion the patient can no longer perform, particularly associated with the activities of living.

Take note

When testing passive range of movement, the nurse should always be gentle when performing this activity being aware of the patient's verbal and non-verbal communication.

Table 9.6   The Oxford Scale.

Grade	Description	Category/interpretation
0/5	No contraction	Paralysis
1/5	Visible/palpable muscle contraction but no movement (flicker of movement)	Severe weakness
2/5	Movement with gravity eliminated (gravity counterbalance)	Poor range of motion
3/5	Movement against gravity only (through full range actively against gravity)	Average weakness
4/5	Movement against gravity with some resistance (through full range actively against some resistance)	Slight weakness
5/5	Movement against gravity with full resistance (through full range actively against strong resistance)	Normal

Review

In this table, provide examples of the type synovial joint.

Type of synovial joint	Example
Ball and socket	
Hinge	
Condyloid	
Gliding	
Pivot	
Saddle	

Test muscle strength by requesting the patient to put each joint through a range of motions whilst applying gentle resistance to the part being moved. Document muscle strength using a scale for muscle strength, for example the Oxford Scale (Porter 2013). The Oxford Scale is commonly used by physiotherapists to manually assess muscle strength, muscle strength is graded 0 to 5 (see Table 9.6).

So far

The physical examination requires the nurse to assess the musculoskeletal system paying attention to the range of movement, tone, and strength. The nurse may require assistance to position the person throughout the examination.

Additional tests

The nurse can perform a range of additional specific tests to assess for wrist, spinal, hip, and knee problems.

Take note

When the assessment has been undertaken, the nurse must explain to the patient the next steps in the process. It is essential that the nurse documents findings according to local policy and procedure (NMC 2018).

Abnormal findings

When a thorough assessment has been undertaken, the nurse can then identify any abnormalities. See Table 9.7 for some common abnormal musculoskeletal findings.

Table 9.7   Some abnormal musculoskeletal findings.

Findings (signs and symptoms)	Likely cause
Pain radiating through a limb Movement exacerbates pain Crepitus felt and heard Deformity of the limb Erythema and oedema Impaired circulation Paraesthesia	Fracture
Aching, shooting tingling pain that radiates down the leg, behind the thigh and knee Pain maybe felt in the lower leg Pain exacerbated by activity and relieved by rest Difficulty moving from a sitting position to a standing position Limping	Sciatica
Painful aching in the legs when walking Pain may range from mild to severe, usually relived when legs are rested Both legs are often affected at the same time; however, pain may be worse in one leg Numbness Spasms Loss of peripheral pulses Pallor or cyanosis Diminished sensation Oedema Ulceration Shiny skin on the legs Hair loss on legs and feet	Arterial occlusion (insufficiency)
Pain and stiffness in the joints of the hand Symptoms can come and go in episodes Pain exacerbated by increased activity levels and even the weather In some cases, the symptoms can be continuous On palpation joints may be tender Pain and stiffness increase when the joints have not been moved for a whilst Joints appear slightly larger or more 'knobbly' than usual Crepitus Range of movement in the joints decreased Weakness and muscle wasting	Osteoarthritis
Lower back pain Numbness or tingling in shoulders, back, arms, hands, legs or feet (sensory changes) this is usually unilateral Neck pain Problems bending or straightening the back Muscle weakness Pain in the buttocks, hips, or legs if the disc is sciatic nerve (sciatica) Diminished reflexes	Herniated disc (slipped disc)
Acute onset of severe pain in any joint Pain may develop in the night or the early hours of the morning Pain in big toe, or fingers, wrists, elbows or knees Skin over the affected joint is red, hot, oedematous, shiny, and skin may peel Pyrexia may be a sign Rigors may be present if pyrexial	Gout

Maurice Samuda (Father)

Maurice attended the GP and was seen by the practice nurse Tisha. Maurice complained of a three-month history of lower back pain and more recently pain in the right leg. Maurice had avoided coming to the practice due to 'issues' at home with the family.

Maurice could not recall a single event relating to the onset of his back pain. In the weeks prior to developing back pain he had been helping others at his work to move office. He has been spending more time in his shed lately fixing up old motor bikes. The pain began in his lower back quite centrally and with time has started radiating straight down the back of his right thigh and into his calf, it stops at the ankle (Figure 9.4).

Maurice tells the nurse that the pain is worse in the morning. He feels stiff and crooked in the morning and is sometimes unable to get out of bed without assistance from his wife. He sometimes requires help to shower and dress.

The pain is getting worse waking him in the night every two to three hours with severe buttock and posterior thigh pain. The right leg feels 'heavy'. He denies experiencing any pins and needles or numbness.

Lying down and sitting down, being still or getting cold seems to aggravate his back and leg pain (indeed Tisha notices that Maurice is shifting a lot in the chair during the assessment).

Pain levels increase within 30 minutes of each sustained posture and take up to two hours to ease, he relives this mainly by walking. There was no position or movement that completely reduced Maurice's leg pain. Maurice was asked to rate his pain and his pain was recorded as 9 out of 10, with 10 being the worst possible pain imaginable.

Maurice is a full-time civil servant; however, he has been taking more time off work due to worsening pain.

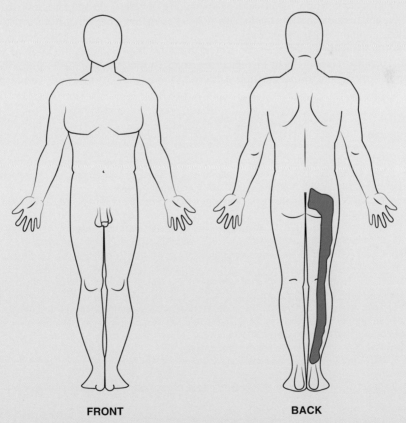

FRONT   **BACK**

Figure 9.4   Maurice's subjective assessment of pain distribution.

Maurice expressed his concerns regarding his pain and the lack of improvement, he was puzzled about the cause of his problem.

Tisha performed a musculoskeletal assessment. Following objective and subjective assessment, her primary hypothesis for the source of symptoms was a lumbar disc herniation with associated radiculopathy.

Consider, in a holistic manner, the case of Maurice and his lumbar disc herniation-associated radiculopathy.

What type of pain assessment tool might Tisha have used in order to obtain an objective score related to pain severity?

What other tests and investigations might be needed in order to make a definitive diagnosis?

Choose one of Maurice's problems (identified during assessment) and write a care plan to help allevi-ate the issue that you have chosen (revise Chapters 5 and 6).

Conclusion

The musculoskeletal system is responsible for movement of the human body, without the musculo-skeletal system breathing would cease and other life-supporting systems would fail. This chapter provided insight on how to undertake a thorough musculoskeletal assessment, including a health history and physical examination.

It is essential that the nurse has insight and understanding of the musculoskeletal system prior to undertaking the assessment. The musculoskeletal system has a major impact on a person's wellbeing and their ability to function. The physical examination of the musculoskeletal system uses inspection, palpation, and percussion. The examination includes assessment of gait, posture, cerebellar function, limb measurement, joints, and muscles.

When the assessment has been completed the nurse then analyses the findings so actual and potential health problems can be identified, a nursing diagnosis can be made, and a plan of care can be written. To complete the nursing process the nurse must evaluate the care given, and this requires reassessment.

References

Arthritis Research UK (2013). *Musculoskeletal Health: A Public Health Approach*. Chesterfield: Arthritis Research UK.

Gibson, J. and Huntley, J. (2013). The musculoskeletal system. In: *Macleod's Clinical Examination*, 13e (ed. G. Douglas, F. Nicol and C. Robertson), 315–354. Edinburgh: Elsevier.

Hochberg, M.C. (2007). Racial differences in bone strength. *Transactions of the American Clinical and Climatological Association* 18: 305–315.

House of Commons Hansard (2011). Musculoskeletal diseases 530. https://hansard.parliament.uk/Commons/2011-07-04/debates/11070442000002/MusculoskeletalDiseases (accessed June 2018).

Margham, T. (2011). Musculoskeletal disorders: time for joint action in primary care. *British Journal of General Practice* 61 (592): 657–685.

McCance, K.L. and Heuther, S.E. (2018). *Pathophysiology: The Biologic Basis for Disease in Adults and Children*, 8e. St Louis: Mosby.

Nursing and Midwifery Council (2018). The Code. Professional Standards of Practice and Behaviour for Nurses, Midwives and Nursing Associates. https://www.nmc.org.uk/globalassets/sitedocuments/nmc-publications/nmc-code.pdf last accessed 8 May 2019.

Porter, S. (2013). *Tidy's Physiotherapy*. Edinburgh: Elsevier.

Waugh, A. and Grant, A. (2018). *Ross and Wilson's Anatomy and Physiology in Illness and in Health*, 13e. Edinburgh: Elsevier.

Williams, P. (2018). *de Wit's Fundamentals Concepts and Skills for Nursing*, 5e. St Louis: Elsevier.

Chapter 10

Assessing the circulatory system

Aim

This chapter introduces the reader to the assessment of the circulatory system and the care required for people who experience circulatory problems.

Learning outcomes

By the end of the chapter the reader will be able to:

1. Provide a brief overview of the circulatory system
2. Discuss a number of conditions affecting the circulatory system
3. Outline ways in which the nurse assesses the circulatory system
4. Describe care planning related to the circulatory system

Introduction

Assessment of the circulatory system is one of the most important areas of the nurse's daily patient assessment (the cardiac system is discussed in Chapter 11). This chapter provides insight and understanding regarding the circulatory system so that the nurse is able to undertake a competent and confident assessment in order to come to a nursing diagnosis, plan care, implement that plan of care, and undertake an evaluation of nursing interventions.

The chapter provides a foundation of relevant anatomical and physiological concepts required to assist the nurse to perform a competent and confident nursing assessment. One of the most powerful tools that the nurse should use is the power of observation. If you detect something that is abnormal, even a slight deviation from the norm, further assess that area, and report your findings.

When undertaking the assessment, the nurse should be as objective as possible and make known any uncertainty and investigate further. There are many tools available to assist the nurse in making an objective assessment: observation, communication, inspection, and palpation are all key. Report your findings as clearly as possible, documentation of findings according to local policy and procedure is essential as it permits other members of the multidisciplinary team to provide continuity of care. Good documentation is also key for effective, safe, and patient-centred nursing care (NMC 2018).

Fundamentals of Assessment and Care Planning for Nurses, First Edition. Ian Peate.
© 2020 John Wiley & Sons Ltd. Published 2020 by John Wiley & Sons Ltd.

The circulatory system

The circulatory system is a complex system that distributes nutrients, gases, and electrolytes as well as removing the waste products of metabolism and other substances. The circulatory system, according to Nair (2017) includes the heart, the blood, the blood vessels, and the lymphatic system. The blood vessels transport blood throughout the body. Blood contains formed elements and a fluid portion called plasma.

The blood vessels form a network that enables blood to flow from the heart to all living cells and then back again to the heart. The blood has many functions, and these include the transportation of nutrients, respiratory gases such as oxygen and carbon dioxide, nutrients, metabolic waste such as urea and uric acid, hormones, electrolytes, and antibodies. As the blood circulates throughout the body, cells are continually removing nutrients, hormones, electrolytes, oxygen, and other substances as well as excreting unwanted waste into the blood.

A network of blood vessels leading away from and returning to the heart transports blood through a network of blood vessels. The main types of blood vessels include:

- Arteries
- Arterioles
- Capillaries
- Venules
- Veins

One other important aspect of the circulatory system is the lymphatic system. This system drains lymph. The lymphatic system is made up of the lymph vessels, lymph nodes, and lymph glands, for example the spleen and the thymus gland. See Figure 10.1, for the arterial and venous systems.

Blood

The blood contains formed elements such as red blood cells (erythrocytes), leukocytes (white blood cells) and platelets. Plasma is the fluid portion of blood containing various forms of proteins and other soluble molecules. When centrifuged, the content of the blood sample accounts for 45% of the blood and plasma makes up 55% of the total blood volume.

Normally, more than 99% of the formed elements are cells named for their red colour (red blood cells). White blood cells (pale in appearance) and platelets comprise less than 1% of the formed elements. Between the plasma and erythrocytes is the buffy coat, consisting of white blood cells and platelets (see Figure 10.2). The percentage of the formed elements comprises the haematocrit or packed cell volume. Haematocrit is a blood test measuring the percentage of red blood cells in whole blood. The volume of blood is constant unless a person has physiological problems, for example haemorrhage.

The properties of blood

The average adult has a blood volume of approximately 5 L, which comprises around 7–9% of the body's weight, men have 5–6 L and women 4–5 L. As blood is thicker and denser than water, it flows much slower due to the red blood cells and plasma proteins, such as albumin and fibrinogen.

Plasma proteins, including albumin, fibrinogen, prothrombin, and the gamma globulins, make up around 8% of the blood plasma in the body. These proteins help maintain water balance and they also affect osmotic pressure, increase blood viscosity, and help to maintain blood pressure.

Blood has a high viscosity which offers resistance to blood flow. The red blood cells and proteins contribute to the viscosity of the blood, and this ranges from 3.5 to 5.5 compared with 1.000 to water (Nair 2017). Viscosity relates to the stickiness of blood, the normal viscosity of blood is low, permitting it to flow smoothly. However, the more red blood cells and plasma proteins in blood, the higher the viscosity and the slower the flow of blood. Normal blood varies in viscosity as it flows through the blood vessels, but the viscosity decreases when it arrives at the capillaries. The specific gravity (density) of blood is 1.045–1.065 compared with 1.000 for water, and the pH of blood ranges from 7.35 to 7.45 (Nair 2017).

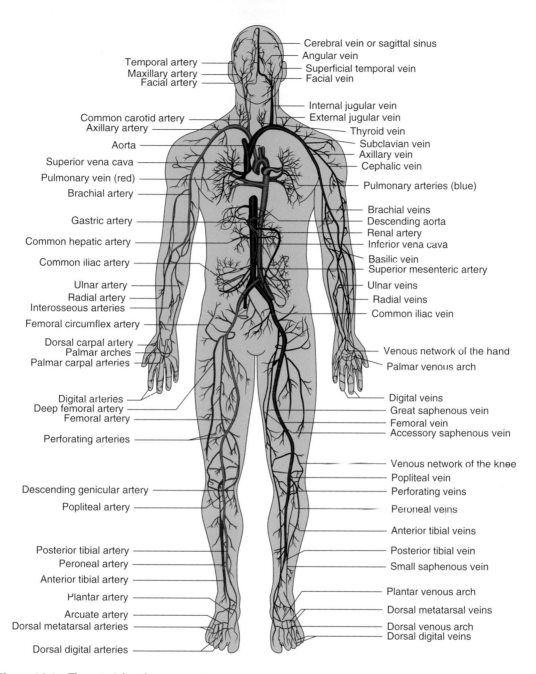

Figure 10.1   The arterial and venous systems.

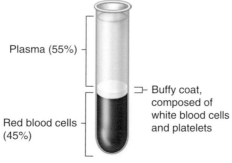

Appearance of centrifuged blood

Figure 10.2   The appearance of centrifuged blood.

The functions of blood

The blood has a number of functions which include:

- The blood acts as a transport mechanism whereby all nourishment and respiratory gases are transported into and out of the cells.
- Blood helps to maintain the body temperature and does this by distributing the heat produced by the chemical activity of the cells evenly, throughout the body (it helps to maintain body temperature).
- The pH of the blood pH is maintained by the excretion or reabsorption of hydrogen ions and bicarbonate ions.
- When blood reaches the kidneys, excess fluid is excreted or reabsorbed to maintain fluid balance which helps to regulate fluid balance.
- Removal of waste products. The blood removes all waste products from the tissues and cells, waste products are transported to the appropriate organs for excretion such as lungs, kidneys, intestine, skin, and so on.
- By the mechanism of clotting, loss of blood cells and body fluids are prevented, the blood plays a part in blood clotting.
- The blood aids in the defence of the body against the invasion of micro-organisms and their toxins.

Formation of blood cells

Red blood cells and the majority of white blood cells and platelets are manufactured in the bone marrow. The red blood and white blood cells and the platelets are the formed elements of blood (see Figure 10.3). The bone marrow is the soft fatty substance that is found in bone cavities. Within the bone marrow, all blood cells originate from a single type of unspecialised cell that is called a stem cell.

When a stem cell divides, it first becomes an immature red blood cell, white blood cell, or platelet-producing cell. The immature cell then divides, matures further, and ultimately becomes a mature red blood cell, white blood cell, or platelet.

Review

What is the local policy and procedure where you work as regards blood transfusion?

How would you reassure a patient who has been prescribed a blood transfusion that the transfusion they are to receive is safe?

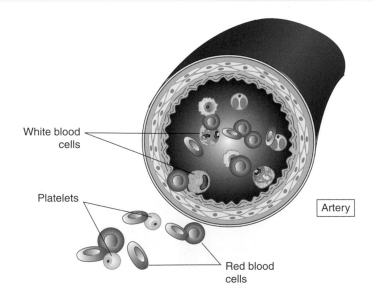

White blood cells

Platelets

Artery

Red blood cells

Figure 10.3   The formed elements of blood.

The blood cells

Red blood cells (also called erythrocytes) are the most abundant blood cells. They are biconcave discs (see Figure 10.4), containing the oxygen-carrying protein haemoglobin. The biconcave shape is maintained by a network of proteins called spectrin which allows the red blood cells to change shape as they are conveyed through the blood vessel. There are approximately 4 million to 5.5 million red blood cells in each cubic millimetre of blood.

The key function of haemoglobin in the red blood cell is to transport oxygen and carbon dioxide. As the blood flows through the capillaries in the tissues, carbon dioxide is picked up by the haemo-globin and oxygen is released. The blood reaches the lungs, carbon dioxide is released, and oxygen is picked up by the haemoglobin molecules. Apart from transporting oxygen and carbon dioxide, the haemoglobin plays an important role in maintaining blood pressure and blood flow. Haemoglobin is made up of a protein called globin bound to the iron-containing pigments called haem. There are around 250 million haemoglobin molecules in one red blood cell; as such one red blood cell trans-ports 1 billion molecules of oxygen. At the capillary end the haemoglobin releases the oxygen mol-ecule into the interstitial fluid, which is then transported into the cells.

Without a nucleus and other organelles, the red blood cell is unable to create new structures to replace the ones damaged. The breakdown (haemolysis) of the red blood cell is carried out by mac-rophages in the spleen; liver and the bone marrow (see Figure 10.5). The globin is broken down into amino acids and reused for protein synthesis. Iron is separated from haem and is stored in muscles and the liver and reused in the bone marrow to manufacture new red blood cells.

145

The transportation of respiratory gases

The chief responsibility of red blood cells is to transport oxygen from the lungs to the tissues. The oxygen in the alveoli (air sac) of the lungs combines with iron molecules in the haemoglobin to form oxyhaemoglobin. This is then transported by the blood to the tissues. As the oxygen level in the red blood cell increases it becomes bright red and when the level of oxygen content drops, the colour changes to dark bluish-red.

In addition to transporting oxygen from the lungs to the body tissues, red blood cells transport carbon dioxide from the tissues to the lungs.

The white blood cells

These cells are also called leukocytes, with approximately 5000–10 000 white blood cells in every cubic millimetre of blood. The number may increase in infections to approximately 25 000 per cubic millimetre of blood. An increase in white blood cells is leukocytosis, and an abnormally low level of white blood cell is leukopenia. White blood cells, unlike red blood cells have nuclei and are able to move out of blood vessel walls into the tissues.

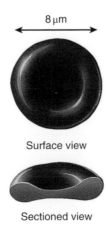

8 μm

Surface view

Sectioned view

RBC shape

Figure 10.4   Red blood cell.

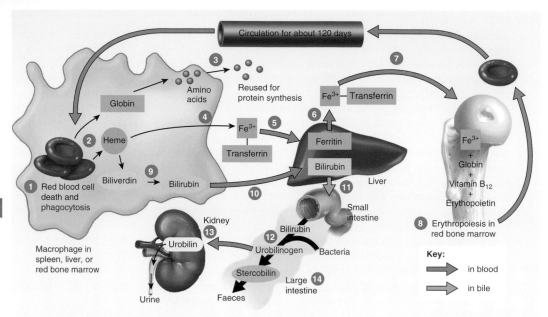

Figure 10.5   The destruction of a red blood cell.

White blood cells produce a continuous supply of energy, unlike the red blood cells. They are able to synthesise proteins, and thus their life span can be from a few days to years. The two main types of white blood cells are:

- granulocytes (containing granules in the cytoplasm)
  - neutrophils
  - eosinophils
  - basophils

- agranulocytes (containing a few granules in the cytoplasm)
  - monocytes
  - lymphocytes.

Review

What do you understand by the term 'protective isolation'?

Platelets

These are small blood cells produced in the bone marrow, approximately 2–4 μm in diameter but having no nucleus, the life span is approximately five to nine days. Old and dead platelets are removed by macrophages in the spleen and the Kupffer cells in the liver. The surface of platelets contains proteins and glycoproteins allowing them to adhere to other proteins such as collagen in the connective tissues.

These cells play a vital role in blood loss by the formation of platelet plugs, sealing the holes in the blood vessels and releasing chemicals to aid blood clotting. If the platelet number is low, excessive bleeding may occur; however, if the number increases, blood clots (thrombosis) can form, leading to cerebrovascular accident, deep vein thrombosis, heart attack, or pulmonary embolism. Haemostasis is a sequence of responses that can stop bleeding and prevent haemorrhage from smaller blood vessels. Haemostasis plays an important part in maintaining homeostasis, it consists of three main components: vasoconstriction, platelet aggregation, and coagulation.

Blood groups

The red blood cells define an individual's blood group. On the surface of the red cells there are markers called antigens. Apart from identical twins, each person has different antigens. These antigens are the key to identifying blood types and must be matched in transfusions to avoid serious complications. ABO system is the system used for defining blood groups. If a person has blood group A, then they have A antigens covering their red cells. Group B has B antigens on their red blood cell, whilst group O has neither antigen and group AB has both antigens (Tortora and Derrickson 2014).

The ABO system also covers antibodies in the plasma that are the body's natural defence against foreign antigens. If, for example, blood group A has anti-B in their plasma, B has anti-A, and so on, however, group AB has no antibodies and group O has both (see Figure 10.6).

Factor D is another factor that has to be considered is the rhesus factor (Rh) system. Rh antigens can be present in each of the blood groups. Not everyone has the Rh antigen on the red blood cell; however, if a person has Rh antigen on their red blood cells then they are Rh positive and if they do not have the Rh antigen then they are Rh negative. A person with blood group A and Rh positive is known as A+, whilst if the Rh is negative they are A−. The same applies for B, AB, and O.

147

Take note

- Transfusion is very safe in the UK, with a very low risk of bacterial or viral infection
- Correct patient identification and adherence to basic procedures are key to safer practice
- Acute transfusion reactions are the leading cause of major morbidity
- Transfusion-associated circulatory overload is a serious complication
- Local policy and procedure need to be adhered to at all times

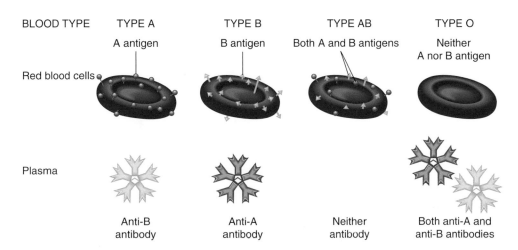

Figure 10.6   The ABO blood group system.

The blood vessels

Blood vessels are part of the circulatory system transporting blood throughout the body. There are three major types of blood vessels:

1. Arteries, carrying blood away from the heart
2. Capillaries, which enable the actual exchange of water, nutrients, and chemicals between the blood and the tissues
3. Veins, carrying blood from the capillaries back towards the heart

See Figure 10.7.

All arteries apart from the pulmonary and umbilical arteries, carry oxygenated blood, most veins carry deoxygenated blood from the tissues back to the heart; exceptions are the pulmonary and umbilical veins – both carry oxygenated blood. The structure of the arteries and veins can be seen in Figure 10.8.

The capillaries form the microcirculatory system. At this point nutrients, gases, water, and electrolytes are exchanged between the blood and tissue fluid. Capillaries are tiny, very thin-walled vessels acting as a bridge between arteries and veins. The thin walls of the capillaries allow oxygen and nutrients to pass from the blood into tissue fluid and allow waste products to pass from tissue fluid into the blood.

The differences between arteries and veins are outlined in Table 10.1 and Figure 10.9.

The capillaries

These are tiny blood vessels, approximately 5–20 μm in diameter. There are networks of capillaries in most of the organs and tissues. The capillary walls are only one cell thick, allowing exchange of material between the contents of the capillary and surrounding tissue fluid. The single layer of cells (the endothelium) is so thin that molecules such as oxygen, water, and lipids can pass through them by diffusion, entering tissues. Waste products such as carbon dioxide and urea can diffuse back into the blood to be carried away for removal. Capillaries are so small the red blood cells need to change shape so as to pass through them in single file.

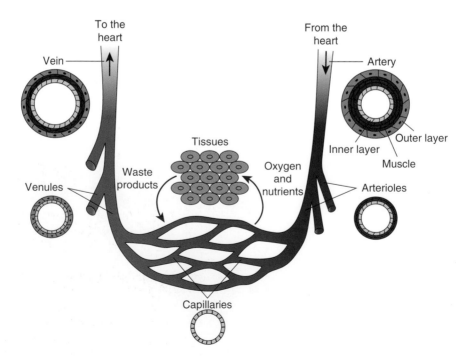

Figure 10.7   The blood vessels.

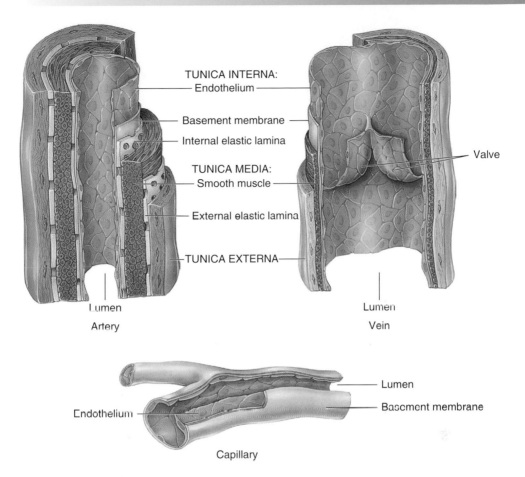

TUNICA INTERNA:
Endothelium

Basement membrane

Internal elastic lamina

TUNICA MEDIA:
Smooth muscle

External elastic lamina

TUNICA EXTERNA

Valve

Lumen   Lumen
Artery   Vein

Lumen

Basement membrane

Endothelium

Capillary

Figure 10.8   The structure of arteries, veins, and capillaries.

Table 10.1   Differences between arteries and veins.

Arteries	Veins
Transport blood away from the heart	Transport blood to the heart
Carry oxygenated blood, apart from the pulmonary and umbilical arteries	Carry deoxygenated blood, apart from the pulmonary and umbilical veins
Have a narrow lumen	Have a wide lumen
Have more elastic tissue	Have less elastic tissue
Do not have valves	Have valves
Transport blood under pressure	Transport blood under low pressure

Blood pressure

This is the pressure exerted by blood within the blood vessel. The pressure is at its greatest near the heart and decreases as the blood moves further from the heart. There are three factors that regulate blood pressure, these are:

- Neuronal regulation – through the autonomic nervous system
- Hormonal regulation – adrenaline, noradrenaline, renin, and others
- Autoregulation – through the renin-angiotensin system.

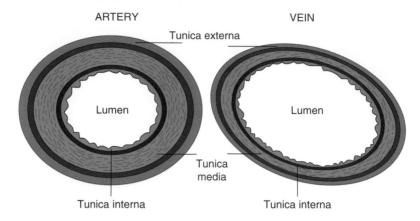

ARTERY   VEIN

Tunica externa

Lumen   Lumen

Tunica
media

Tunica interna   Tunica interna

Figure 10.9   Artery and vein.

There are a number of factors that affect blood pressure, including:

- Cardiac output, the volume of blood pumped out by the heart in one minute
- Circulating volume, the volume of circulating blood perfusing tissues
- Peripheral resistance, the resistance provided by the blood vessels
- Blood viscosity, the measure of the resistance of blood flow, resistance is provided by plasma proteins and other substances in the blood
- Hydrostatic pressure, the pressure exerted by the blood on the vessel wall

The lymphatic system

This component of the circulatory system transports lymph (see Figure 10.10). The lymphatic system begins with very small, closed-end vessels called lymphatic capillaries, which are in contact with the surrounding tissues and the interstitial fluid. The lymphatic system consists of:

- Lymph
- Lymph vessels
- Lymph nodes
- Lymphatic organs, for example spleen and thymus

The body contains around 1–2 L of lymph, forming approximately 1–3% of body weight. Lymph transports plasma proteins, bacteria, fat from the small intestine and damaged tissues to the lymph nodes for destruction. The lymph contains lymphocytes and macrophages, playing an important role in the immune system. Lymph nodes are bean-shaped organs located along the lymphatic vessels, found in the largest concentrations in the neck, axillae, thorax, abdomen, and groin.

So far

The circulatory system is an extensive network of organs and vessels that is responsible for the flow of blood, nutrients, hormones, oxygen, and other gases to and from cells. The body would not be able to fight disease or maintain a stable internal environment, such as temperature regulation and maintenance of pH (homeostasis).

Assessing needs

The nurse must be able to demonstrate proficiency in their ability to assess the circulatory system. This can take time and confidence grows with practice. An up-to-date evidence-based approach to care needs has to be applied to the assessment, planning, and implementation of care to ensure the

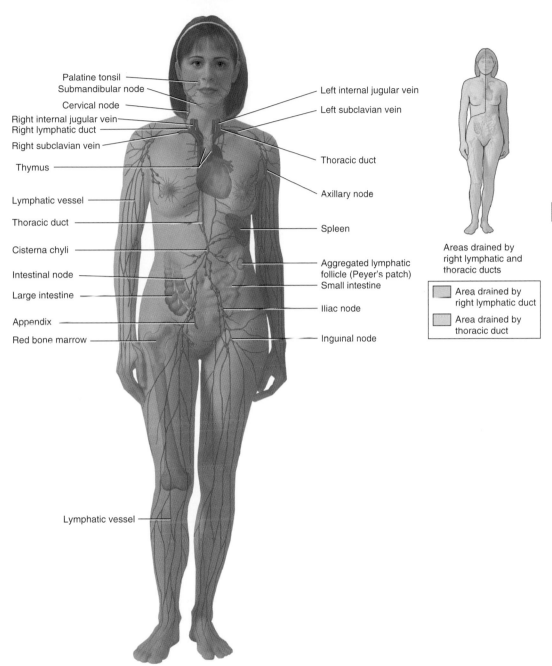

Palatine tonsil
Submandibular node
Cervical node
Right internal jugular vein
Right lymphatic duct
Right subclavian vein
Thymus
Lymphatic vessel
Thoracic duct
Cisterna chyli
Intestinal node
Large intestine
Appendix
Red bone marrow

Left internal jugular vein
Left subclavian vein
Thoracic duct
Axillary node
Spleen
Aggregated lymphatic
follicle (Peyer's patch)
Small intestine
Iliac node
Inguinal node

Lymphatic vessel

Anterior view of principal components of lymphatic system

Areas drained by
right lymphatic and
thoracic ducts

	Area drained by right lymphatic duct
	Area drained by thoracic duct

151

Figure 10.10   The lymphatic system.

best possible outcome. The focus here will be on obtaining a health history and the skills required to inspect, palpate, and auscultate as the nurse strives to assess needs in a holistic way, make a nursing diagnosis, plan care that is patient-centred, implement care, and evaluate interventions.

When providing care to patients with a cardiovascular disorder it is key that the nurse is sensitive to the physical as well as the psychological effects such a condition can create. For many patients, particularly those who have been first diagnosed with a cardiovascular condition, they may show evidence of anxiety and potential fear. There can often be a real fear of death (impending or otherwise) and the patient can be concerned about their future life as regards their ability to work, being a family member, and making a meaningful contribution to society. When people are anxious or/ and afraid they can exhibit this in a number of ways, and it is essential to understand the responses being made.

The health history

Taking a patient history requires the nurse to establish a rapport with the patient and their family and this is undertaken by using effective verbal and non-verbal communication skills. The nurse has to consider, for example:

- Symptoms experienced (elicit the patient's presenting complaint)
- Past and current medical history
- Medication history (remember to note any known allergies)
- Lifestyle factors (for example, smoking, obesity, diet, physical activity, occupation)
- The individual's overall health status
- Family and social history, (does the person have any carer input?) Include alcohol consumption, recreational drug use. Ask about the patient's living situation: Where do they live? Who do they live with?
- Emotional health and well being
- Assess the ability to perform the activities of living
- The patient's perception (their ideas, concerns, and expectations)

History taking should be undertaken using a systematic approach as this can help to avoid inadvertently missing any key information. Throughout the whole process the nurse has to ensure that they undertake documentation in a clear and thorough way adhering to local policy and procedure and any professional requirements. Prior to undertaking the examination, the nurse must ensure they have gained consent as to do otherwise will be in contravention of the Code NMC 2018.

So far

A careful and detailed clinical assessment is essential as the nurse assesses the likely cause and severity of symptoms, requests appropriate investigations and makes referrals.

Physical examination
Inspection, palpation, and auscultation

Examining an individual's arms and legs has the potential to reveal venous or arterial abnormalities. Arms can be examined when the nurse is assessing the patient's vital signs and legs examined when supine (on the back), veins have to be assessed when the person is standing up. The absence of hair or slow hair growth on the arms and legs may indicate arterial insufficiency (diminished arterial blood flow to those areas).

Inspection

The skill of observation is an important skill that the nurse uses throughout the assessment process. As with any assessment, a general survey (general observations) is undertaken whereby the nurse notes if arms are equal in length and if the legs are symmetrical. Make note of the person's skin colour, pay attention to any scars, lesions, clubbing of the digits (an important manifestation sometimes associated with chronic cardiopulmonary disease, characterised by a painless enlargement of the terminal phalanges of the fingers and toes, with widening and deepening of the nail bed), and any oedema of the extremities.

Cultural considerations

Cyanosis

This is a bluish discoloration of the skin that is caused by a relative decrease in oxygen saturation within the capillaries of the skin. Cyanosis, when present in fingers, toes, and ear lobes, i.e. peripheral cyanosis, is usually related to circulatory problems, such as heart failure. Central cyanosis is present when the patient's more central regions are affected, e.g. the tongue and lips, and the trunk. This is related to a lack of oxygenation of arterial blood through the pulmonary system.

Skin colour can reflect a patient's overall health and is an important part of the assessment process, it may, for example, indicate hypoxia. However, the exact nature of such colour changes, such as pallor, cyanosis, and redness, will vary with the patient's natural skin colour. This may present a challenge in providing clinically competent and culturally sensitive care.

Most skin care guidelines will apply primarily to those patients with light skin, yet nurses must bear in mind that they offer healthcare to diverse populations many from various ethnic backgrounds and with various skin colours.

153

Source: Sommers (2011).

The blood vessels in the neck (the carotid artery, the internal jugular) must be assessed, and this requires the nurse to observe these vessels. Pulsation is visible when pressure in the internal jugular vein is elevated.

Jugular venous pressure

Jugular venous pressure offers an indirect evaluation of central venous pressure. The internal jugular vein is connected to the right atrium, there are no intervening valves and because of this it acts as a column for the blood in the right atrium. The jugular venous pressure consists of waveforms and abnormalities that can assist in the diagnosis of certain conditions (Kumar and Clarke 2014). Jugular venous pressure, however, can be difficult to assess and the nurse may have to access other diagnostic methods to assist. See Table 10.2 for the carotid artery and internal jugular vein.

Assessing jugular venous pressure, this is the pressure in the jugular veins which can be seen as a pulsating column in the neck (jugular vein distension), and is used to estimate whether cardiac filling pressures are high. When evaluating jugular venous pressure the patient should be asked to lie on his/her back (the nurse may need assistance to help the patient into this position) and the head of the bed should be elevated to 45°. Ask the patient to turn their head slightly left, away from the examiner. The observation of waveform pulsation is noted. Gauge the level of the jugular venous pressure by using a ruler. Measure and record the height; this is usually less than 4 cm (Jevon and Cunnington 2007). See Box 10.1 for the procedure.

Table 10.2 The carotid artery and internal jugular vein.

The carotid artery	Has a brisk localised pulsation, rapid outward movement Carotid pulsation does not decrease when the patient is upright, inhales, or when this artery is palpated Determine if carotid pulsations are bounding or weak
The internal jugular vein	The internal jugular vein provides a softer more undulating pulsation Rapid inward movement While there is no decrease in carotid artery pulsation, the internal jugular vein changes in response to position, breathing, and palpation Inspect the jugular veins as this can provide valuable information regarding the blood volume and pressure on the right side of the heart (jugular vein distension)

Box 10.1 Measuring jugular venous pressure

- Wash hands
- Explain the procedure to the patient.
- Ensure there is adequate lighting.
- Stand to the patient's right.
- Ensure privacy and maintain the patient's dignity, expose the upper chest.
- Remove restrictive clothing from around the patient's neck and chest.
- Position the patient at an angle of 45°, leaving one pillow under the head.
- Request the patient turns their head to the left.
- Observe the level of the jugular venous pulsations just above the clavicle.
- Measure the vertical distance (cm) between the sternal angle (manubrio sternal joint) and the highest visible level of jugular vein pulsation (see Figure 10.11).
- The normal distance is less than 4 cm; add 5 cm because the right atrium is situated 5 cm below the sternal angle.
- Shine a bright light directly onto the patient's neck if it is difficult to see the jugular venous pulsation,
- If there is still difficulty seeing jugular venous pulsation and uncertainty whether the pulsation is venous or arterial, gentle compression on the right upper quadrant of the abdomen increases venous pressure briefly, which produces a more prominent internal jugular vein. After a few seconds (even with continued abdominal pressure) venous pulsation usually returns to normal; if it remains elevated, this is suggestive of right-sided heart failure
- Document the findings of whether the jugular venous pulsation is visible and, if so, whether it is normal or elevated.
- Assist the patient to a comfortable position.
- Wash hands.

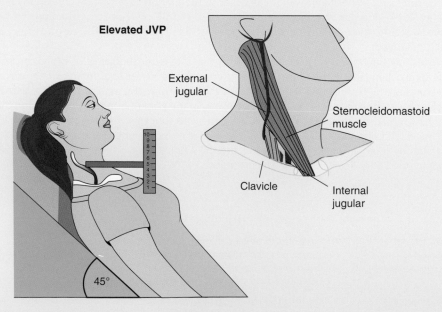

Figure 10.11 Measuring jugular venous pressure.

Source: Jevon and Cunnington (2007) and Roper (2014).

Take note

Only those staff who have been trained, supervised, and deemed competent to undertake the measurement of jugular venous pressure should do so. At all times, local policy and procedure should be adhered to.

So far

Inspection (observation, applying a clinical eye) is a skill that the nurse must continually develop; it is a key skill that is used throughout the assessment process.

Observing jugular venous pressure requires much skill. Jugular venous pressure offers an indirect evaluation of central venous pressure.

155

Palpation

Assess the skin temperature, texture, and turgor. Check capillary refill. This is done by assessing the nail beds on the fingers or toes. Capillary refill time should be no more than three seconds. The capillary nail refill test is also known as the nail blanch test.

Capillary refill time

Capillary refill time is a quick and simple test that requires minimal equipment or time to perform and can be measured in any care setting. If there is a prolonged capillary refill time the nurse should consider this as a 'red flag', it may identify those at an increased risk of significant morbidity or mortality (see Box 10.2). Brady et al. (2015) note that a slower capillary refill time could indicate fluid deficit and a faster one fluid overload. A delayed capillary refill time according to Dutton et al. (2012) is consistent with poor cardiac output.

Box 10.2 Measurement of capillary nail bed refill

- Wash hands.
- Explain the procedure to the patient, there will be minor pressure to the bed of the nail, this should not cause discomfort.
- Hold the hand to the level of the heart (if using the toenail bed, ensure that the leg is horizontal).
- Use the finger as the preferred measurement site (toes may also be used).
- If possible, measure at room temperature (between 20 and 25 °C).
- Allow time for skin temperature to acclimatise if the patient has been moved recently from a warmer or colder environment.
- Using gentle but moderate pressure, press for five seconds.
- Count the seconds it takes for the finger to regain its original colour.
- Normal capillary refill is two seconds or less, an abnormality has occurred if this is three seconds or more
- Record measurements using the actual number of seconds, for example capillary refill time '4 seconds' or '2 seconds or less' as opposed to using terms such as 'prolonged' or mathematical symbols such as +, ++, +++.
- If needed, assist the patient to a comfortable position.
- Wash hands.

Remove coloured nail polish before this test. Pressure is applied to the nail bed until it turns white, indicating that the blood has been forced from the tissue (this is called blanching). Once the tissue has blanched, pressure is removed, whilst the patient holds their hand above their heart, the nurse measures the time it takes for blood to return to the tissue. Return of blood is indicated as the nail turns back to a pink colour.

Pulse

Taking a pulse is a fundamental aspect associated with the role of the nurse, the nurse is required to take the pulse – palpate the pulse. The most common site for assessing the pulse (the heartbeat) is at the wrist, where the radial artery can be felt pulsating. Table 10.3 lists the sites of the peripheral pulses.

During each heartbeat the arteries stretch and relax momentarily. This is the pulse, and it should have a regular and consistent rhythm. The pulse originates in the aorta and spreads as a 'pulse wave', travelling through all the arteries. The farther away from the heart the artery is located, the fainter the

Table 10.3   Peripheral pulses.

Pulse/artery	Technique	Comments
Radial artery	Radial side of the wrist Use the tips of the index and middle fingers	Assess rate, rhythm, and volume
Brachial artery	Medial border of humerus at elbow medial to biceps tendon (on the elbow's side). Use the index and middle of left hand.	Assess rate, rhythm, and volume Can assess the character of the pulse The pulse used when taking blood pressure measurements
Carotid artery	The carotid pulse is located by placing the second and third finger gently on the patient's trachea, locate the Adam's apple or cricoid cartilage. Move fingers laterally (sideways) approximately 4–5 cm to the sternomastoid muscle mass. Pushing medially, you should locate the carotid artery.	Best for pulse character. To detect carotid stenosis. Also used during emergency situations such as cardiac arrest Never palpate both carotid arteries simultaneously
Femoral artery	With the patient lying flat and undressed, (ensure dignity is preserved) place finger directly above pubic ramus and midway between pubic tubercle and anterior superior iliac spine (this is the area between the hips and groin) Draw an imaginary line from the hip bone to the pubic bone. This should be just above the natural crease in the body where the lower abdomen meets the thigh.	This pulse is the most easily felt pulse To assess cardiac output To assess peripheral vascular disease
Popliteal artery	This pulse is located in the knee in the back of the leg deep within the popliteal fossa Gently palpate against posterior distal femur with knee slightly flexed	This site is used mainly to assess peripheral vascular disease The popliteal pulse may be difficult to palpate because the artery lies deep to other structures.
Dorsalis pedis	Place fingers just lateral (towards the side) to the extensor tendon of the great toe, move fingers more laterally if needed With the fingers in position the nurse may linger on the site Varying pressure may assist in picking up a weak pulsation	This site is used mainly to assess peripheral vascular disease

Source: Rhoads and Wiggins Petersen (2018).

pulse. When the blood reaches the capillaries, there is no longer a pulse. Pulses cannot be felt in those veins that return blood to the heart.

The pulse is a pressure wave in the wall of the artery. If an artery wall is gently palpated at a pulse point, the pulse of pressure in the arterial wall can be felt as blood is squeezed along with each contraction of the heart. The pulse occurs with each heartbeat; the frequency, or rate, at which it is felt indicates the rate at which the heart is beating.

Take note

Pressing too hard when taking a pulse may cause discomfort and could also obliterate the pulse.

The strength (or amplitude) of the pulse will depend on the volume of blood that is squeezed out of the heart with each beat, this is known as the stroke volume. The strength of the pulse is also influenced by the extent of elasticity of the artery wall. There are scoring systems and scales available that allocate a score of the amplitude of the pulse; however, the nurse should be cautious in using such tools, paying attention to reliability and validity of any tool used.

As a person ages, the arteries become stiffer (arteriosclerosis) and the extent to which they can stretch with each pulse reduces (Lowry and Ashelford 2015). Boore et al. (2016) suggest that the normal value associated with a pulse ranges between 60 and 100 beats per minute. They note that in a very fit and healthy person this is 40–60 beats per minute.

Usually the pulse is easy to palpate, but in patients with a weak or unstable pulse they should be assessed further. A weak pulse can indicate reduced cardiac output and may progress to deterioration. Pulses should be assessed on each side and should be equal and strong.

The rhythm of the pulses should be regular and consistent. An unstable or irregular pulse can indicate irregular contractions of the heart and should be referred to a senior clinician. A patient with a strong, bounding pulse may have high blood pressure. The nurse is assessing the patient's pulse for the rate, rhythm, and volume. The pulse is counted for one full minute. The peripheral pulses can be felt at various sites. See Table 10.3 and Figure 10.12.

Take note

The nurse must never palpate both carotid arteries simultaneously.

6Cs

When assessing the patient's pulse (for example, the femoral pulse), the role of the nurse is to ensure that the patient's dignity is preserved, only exposing the least aspect of the patient's body that is required to perform the procedure.

Determining which pulse will need to be examined will depend on individual patient circumstances and whether there are specific clinical reasons for examining a specific pulse or there may be a need to systematically examine all arterial pulses. Traditionally it is the radial pulse that is assessed first. However, routinely following this with examination of the larger brachial and carotid arteries to feel the nature of the wall and particularly the character of the pulse can also be advantageous.

It should be remembered that there are specific reasons to examine all the pulses at different sites undertaken as part of a complete and systematic cardiovascular examination.

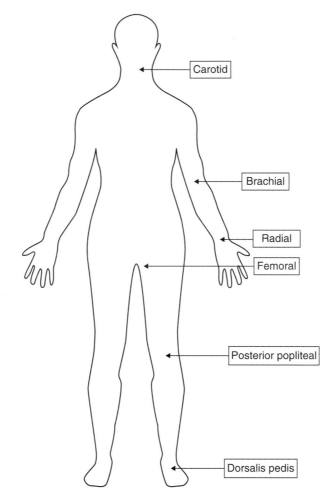

Figure 10.12   The peripheral pulses.

Take note

When taking the pulse it must be documented in the patient's notes what site has been used to obtain the pulse as this provides consistency and more accurate ways of comparing previous results.

Increases in pulse rate (tachycardia) could, for example, suggest hyperthyroidism, anxiety, infection, or anaemia. A slowing of the pulse rate (bradycardia) may be seen in heart block, hypothyroidism, or associated with the use of certain drugs (e.g. digoxin, propranolol). Irregularities in the pulse are suggestive of the presence of premature beats and a pulse that is completely irregular implies the presence of atrial fibrillation. Diminished or absent pulses in the various arteries that are examined could be indicative of impaired blood flow due to a number of conditions.

A systematic examination of the pulse provides the nurse with a great deal of information, and remains an essential part of nursing practice. Any abnormalities noted must be reported and acted upon. The results obtained through the measurement of the pulse may lead the nurse to undertake further examination of the rest of the cardiovascular system.

So far

Palpation requires the nurse to touch the patient with different parts of the hand.

Capillary refill time is a quick and simple test that can monitor flow of blood to the tissues.

Examination of the pulse provides the nurse with numerous clues to the presence of systemic diseases. In contemporary health care there are a number of tests that have been developed to assist in the work-up of systemic illness; however, examination of the pulse is still an important aspect of patient assessment.

Review

What do you think are the advantages of using automatic vital sign devices?

Can you think of the advantages associated with manually taking a patient's pulse compared with using an automated electronic device?

Oedema

Oedema is an abnormal collection of fluid in the tissues which can collect in either the interstitial or intracellular spaces and can be observed and palpated. Oedema can be generalised, postural, or localised (Douglas and Bevan 2014) and is often associated with venous problems. There are several causes of oedema. Interstitial oedema can lead to swelling, and this can cut off blood supply, leading to intracellular oedema. Intracellular oedema can lead to cellular damage, which will stimulate the release of mediators and the inflammatory response

The tissue fluid is mobile and can be moved by finger pressure. The nurse assesses peripheral oedema by pressing fingers gently but firmly for five seconds on the lowest part of the body where fluid may accumulate. This is usually the ankles (oedema may also form at the sacrum and abdomen). When finger pressure is released, an indentation or pit is left and is evaluated on a scale of +1 (minimal) to +4 (severe). Oedema does not become evident until interstitial volume has increased by 2.5–3 l (Porth 2015). The nurse should consider right-sided heart failure, fluid/electrolyte imbalance, low albumin levels, venous obstruction, kidney disease, and sepsis if peripheral oedema is present.

There are scales available that can assist with the grading of pitting oedema. Oedema grading generally depends on the depth and duration of the indention.

It is sometimes very difficult to differentiate between peripheral arterial and venous conditions. When the patient is experiencing a number of systemic and chronic medical problems, fatigue, and when oedema is present in the extremities, the likelihood is that the patient is experiencing problems associated with their venous system. When the symptoms include numbness, tingling, and/or sensory and/or motor changes, then this might indicate an arterial problem. Whatever the case, the nurse has to assess the patient very carefully, keeping in mind the immediate nursing measures that have to be taken.

So far

There are several causes of oedema. Assessment of peripheral oedema occurs by pressing fingers gently but firmly for five seconds on the lowest part of the body where fluid may accumulate. When finger pressure is released an indentation or pit is left and is evaluated. There are scales available that can assist with the grading of pitting oedema.

Auscultation
Bruits

Auscultation is used for assessing vascular sounds and the nurse uses the diaphragm of the stethoscope to do this. After the artery has been palpated, auscultation for a bruit should be performed. The noise of turbulent blood flow (bruit) may also be heard as a murmur, hum, or abnormal sound when a stethoscope is placed over areas of turbulence in arteries that are still pulsating. Bruits are detected by auscultation over the large and medium-sized arteries (such as the carotid, brachial, femoral, abdominal aorta) with the diaphragm of the stethoscope using light to moderate pressure.

Excessive pressure may produce, intensify, or prevent a bruit from being detected by indenting the vessel wall or occluding blood flow in the artery. Listen over the artery after palpation of the artery has occurred to prevent overlooking a significant lesion. The nurse may detect a 'thrill' or palpable vibratory sensation over a vessel in which a loud bruit is audible. The thrill indicates marked turbulence in local blood flow suggesting significant vascular pathology, for example arteriosclerotic plaque formation. If a thrill is noted during examination of the pulses, it should be recorded and reported in line with local policy and procedure.

So far

A bruit, a whoosh, or a blowing sound detected when the diaphragm of the stethoscope is placed over a large artery may indicate important vascular pathology such as atherosclerosis. Detection of a bruit may lead to a referral for further detailed examination and investigations such as a colour duplex ultrasound, CT angiography, or MR angiography.

Arterial and venous insufficiency
Peripheral arterial deficiency

Peripheral arterial deficiency (also called peripheral vascular disease) occurs when there is narrowing or occlusion of the peripheral arteries, affecting the blood supply to the lower limbs (NICE 2012). Pulses may be absent or decreased in those with arterial insufficiency. The skin can be cool to touch, pale, and shiny, and there may be loss of hair with pain in the legs or feet. The patient may experience a number of symptoms including calf pain on exercise (intermittent claudication), pain whilst at rest (critical limb ischaemia), skin ulceration, and gangrene.

Patients diagnosed as having peripheral arterial disease, including those who are asymptomatic, have an increased risk of mortality, myocardial infarction, and stroke. Acute limb ischaemia manifests as a sudden decrease in arterial perfusion in the limb, as a result of thrombotic or embolic causes. There may be ulceration that typically occurs around the toes, the foot often turns deep red when in the dependent position. Upper extremity limb arterial disease can also exist. Clinical features may include pulse deficit, arm pain, pallor, paraesthesia, coldness, as well as unequal arm pressures.

Chronic venous insufficiency

This is a common cause of leg pain and swelling, it is often associated with varicose veins. Patients complain of skin changes (pigmentation, eczema, and ulceration) and pain, tightness, aching, and itching. It occurs when the valves of the veins are not functioning properly and the circulation of blood in the leg veins is impaired. Chronic venous insufficiency can be caused by damaged valves in the veins or vein blockage. Ulcers can occur, particularly around the ankles. Pulses are present but because of the oedema they may be difficult to palpate. When the foot is in a dependent position, it can become cyanotic. It is common for skin discoloration to occur including hyperpigmentation.

Varicose veins are tortuous, dilated, superficial leg veins (Wright and Fitridge 2013), enlarged and swollen veins that are normally found in the legs and ankles (see Figure 10.13). They are often associated with an itching sensation or pain. The symptoms are usually worse when the patient has been standing for a long time and may be eased by resting and elevating the legs.

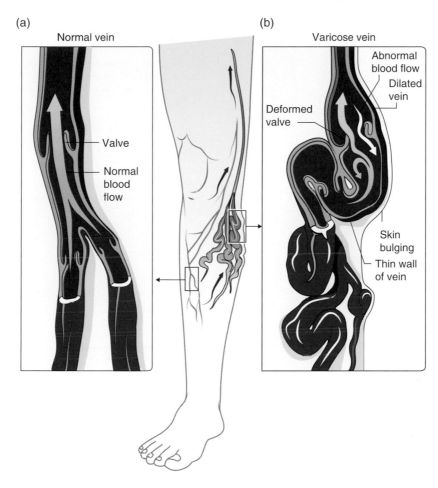

(a) Normal vein

Valve

Normal blood flow

(b) Varicose vein

Abnormal blood flow

Dilated vein

Deformed valve

Skin bulging

Thin wall of vein

Figure 10.13   Varicose veins.

Varicose veins can be caused by the failure of the valves inside the veins of the legs, leading to 'backward flow' and pooling of the blood in the veins. Alternatively, they may be caused by small clots in the veins that reduce the flow of blood back to the heart and act as a 'dam', thus trapping blood in the vein.

There are known risk factors for varicose veins, including: obesity, female sex, family history of varicose veins, or having a job that requires long periods of standing.

The diagnosis of varicose veins involves inspecting the legs. In significant cases, there may be a need for an ultrasound scan of the veins. The treatment for varicose veins will depend on the severity of the condition. The most common form of treatment is self-care, including losing weight, elevating the legs when resting, and avoiding long periods of standing. Compression stockings can be required in more severe cases. Patients should be encouraged to remove the stockings at night and to inspect the legs whilst washing. If dry skin becomes a problem, then emollient creams may help (these can be bought over-the-counter). NICE (2013) have issued guidance on varicose veins, diagnosis, and management.

For those cases where the symptoms are severe, the patient is referred to a surgeon, who will discuss surgical possibilities with the patient. There are two main treatment options for varicose veins; either the veins can be sealed using various techniques or they can be surgically removed.

Classifications using the CEAP grading system provides a method of classifying varicose veins, providing information on the clinical severity, aetiology, anatomical location, and pathophysiology of varicose veins (see Table 10.4). The CEAP classification system is:

C = Clinical and is the part used most frequently
E = Etiological (aetiological)

Table 10.4   CEAP classification system.

Clinical classification	
	C0 – no visible or palpable signs of venous disease C1 – telangiectasies or reticular veins C2 – varicose veins C3 – oedema C4a – pigmentation or eczema C4b – lipodermatosclerosis C5 – healed venous ulcer C6 – active venous ulcer S – symptomatic, including ache, pain, tightness, skin irritation, heaviness, and muscle cramps, and other complaints attributable to venous dysfunction A – asymptomatic
Etiology (aetiological) classification	
	Ec – congenital Ep – primary Es – secondary En – no venous cause identified
Anatomical classification	
	As – superficial veins Ap – perforating veins Ad – deep veins An – no venous location identified
Pathophysiological	
	Pr – reflux Po – obstruction Pr,o – reflux and obstruction Pn – no venous pathophysiology identifiable

A = Anatomical
P = Pathophysiological

The most commonly used component of the classification is C, this is often used without the other components. As a patient with venous insufficiency moves from C0 through to C5/6, this would indicate that they are developing progressive signs of chronic venous insufficiency. A patient at a level of C4 or above is considered to have chronic venous insufficiency.

The nurse must be aware that there is no universally accepted classification of chronic venous disease, and of those classifications that exist (for example, CEAP), few have been based on objective measurements of abnormal venous pressure/flow. The CEAP classification system was presented by the American Venous Forum in 1995. It was developed to provide a comprehensive, objective classification that could be promoted worldwide. The classification system was updated in 2004 (Eklöf et al. 2004). Vowden and Vowden (2013) stated that the CEAP classification system is now the internationally recognised descriptive grading system for classifying patients with lower limb venous disease.

So far

Peripheral vascular disease includes disorders that alter the natural flow of blood through the arteries and the veins outside the brain and heart; the peripheral circulation.

Peripheral vascular disease is a condition in which in which narrowed blood vessels (outside the heart) cannot deliver enough oxygen and nutrients to the body. If left untreated, this may result in chronic wounds on the limbs and increases the risk of heart attack or stroke.

CEAP classification system provides a method of classifying varicose veins, providing information on the clinical severity, aetiology, anatomical location, and pathophysiology of varicose veins.

Shahine Samuda (Mother)

After Shahine had her first child she first began experiencing aching in her legs, she did not seek any advice regarding this and just thought this was a normal occurrence.

Eighteen months ago, she went to see her GP. She was complaining of a 'heavy, aching feeling' in her legs (the left one is much worse than the right), she had been experiencing this for a number of years. At that point, she felt the aching and the pain in the left leg were significant enough to prompt a GP visit.

Shahine used to smoke, but she attended a smoking cessation clinic held at the GP surgery by the practice nurse and has been a non-smoker for the last five years. She is a part-time ward clerk; her job requires her to constantly walk and stand. Shahine has no significant medical history. She has three children, she was taking the contraceptive pill but she has not used this for the last four years. Shahine informs the GP that things at home have not been as good as they could be, her children are 'acting up' and she is having 'marital problems'.

When she first visited the GP, the GP suggested to Shahine that she lose some weight, wear compression stockings (removing them at night), avoid standing for long periods of time, and rest her legs as often as she can. If her legs became dry and itchy, she was advised to go to the chemist, buy and apply an emollient cream. She was encouraged to inspect both legs whilst washing and to report any changes in colour or the development of any lesions to the practice nurse or GP.

Now at this return visit to the GP she reports that her symptoms in her left leg have become much worse, with significant leg ache, heaviness, fatigue, itching, burning, and swelling. She tells the GP that even putting her feet up now is not doing the trick. Her symptoms have started to significantly limit her performance of the activities of living as well as impairing her work performance, despite her wearing compression stockings.

At the GP practice a physical examination was undertaken. Shahine was asked to stand in the first instance. The GP confirmed that the swelling noted is a number of varicose veins in the left leg, as she gently pressed over the area, the vein emptied and then refilled. The accuracy of physical examination is improved with the aid of a hand-held Doppler instrument, allowing the GP to listen to the blood flow.

Shahine's observations

Temperature: 36.7°C (tympanic)
Blood pressure: 194/98 mm/Hg
Respiration rate: 18 breaths per minute
Pulses (pulses on both side compared left side only described):

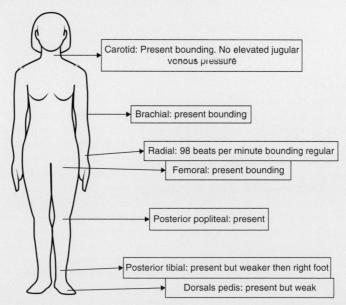

Carotid: Present bounding. No elevated jugular venous pressure

Brachial: present bounding

Radial: 98 beats per minute bounding regular

Femoral: present bounding

Posterior popliteal: present

Posterior tibial: present but weaker then right foot

Dorsals pedis: present but weak

Height: 160 m
Weight: 82 kg
BMI: 32

CEAP:

- C: C2/C3
- E: Es
- A: Ap
- P: Pr,o

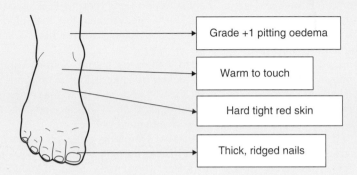

Grade +1 pitting oedema

Warm to touch

Hard tight red skin

Thick, ridged nails

Left foot

A referral was made to a specialist who would be able to make a more accurate and detailed test by using a duplex ultrasound examination. This provides an ultrasound image of the vein to detect any blockage caused by blood clots and to determine whether the vein valves are working correctly. Measurement of the venous function of the leg can be obtained with other tests such as plethysmography.

After the assessment and the examination, Shahine was thanked for attending the practice, and the GP explained the plan of care. Shahine was advised to exercise, to elevate her feet to avoid causing any damage to the skin on her lower limbs, and to attend a secondary care centre (a walk in centre, emergency department) if there is any bleeding. She may be offered surgical intervention (NICE 2013).

How might Shahine's quality of life be affected given the problems she is experiencing?

Conclusion

The circulatory system has been discussed in this chapter. This system, whilst being discussed as an entity in its own right, as is the case in all body systems, is interrelated with all other systems.

Understanding the anatomy and physiology associated with this complex and integrated system is an absolute key requisite as the nurse will meet numerous patients with issues related to the circulatory system. As the nurse undertakes a detailed assessment of needs, the skills of inspection, palpation, and auscultation are required as a diagnosis is made, goals are set with the patient, the care plan is implemented, and evaluation of efforts undertaken come to the fore.

There are a number of tools available to assist nurses in considering needs in a more objective manner, and some tools have been discussed here. It has to be remembered, however, that the nurse must choose the most appropriate tool as well as giving consideration to the reliability and validity of those tools.

References

Boore, J., Cook, N., and Shepherd, A. (2016). *Essentials of Anatomy and Physiology for Nursing Practice*. London: Sage.

Brady, G., Davies, M., McHugh, H. et al. (2015). Nutrition, fluid balance and blood transfusion. In: *The Royal Marsden Manual of Clinical Nursing Procedures*, 9e (ed. L. Dougherty and S. Lister), 253–329. Oxford: Wiley.

164

Douglas, G. and Bevan, J. (2014). The general examination. In: *Macleod's Clinical Examination*, 13e (ed. G. Douglas, F. Neil and C. Robertson), 41–62. Edinburgh: Elsevier.

Dutton, H., Elliot, S., and Sargent, A. (2012). The patient with acute cardiovascular problems. In: *Acute Nursing Care: Recognising and Responding to Medical Emergencies* (ed. I. Peate and H. Dutton), 107–162. Harlow: Pearson.

Eklöf, B., Rutherford, R.B., Bergan, J.J. et al. (2004). Revision of the CEAP classification for chronic venous disorders: consensus statement. *Journal of Vascular Surgery* 30 (2): 103–106.

Jevon, P. and Cunnington, A. (2007). Cardiovascular examination – part one of a four-part series – measuring jugular venous pressure. *Nursing Times* 103 (25): 28.

Kumar, P. and Clarke, M. (2014). *Kumar and Clarke's Clinical Medicine*, 8e. Edinburgh: Elsevier.

Lowry, M. and Ashelford, S. (2015). Assessing the pulse rate in adult patients. *Nursing Times* 111 (36/37): 18–20.

Nair, M. (2017). Circulatory system. In: *Fundamentals of Anatomy and Physiology for Nursing and Health Care Students*, 2e (ed. I. Peate and M. Nair), 185–222. Oxford: Wiley.

National Institute for Health and Care Excellence (2012). Peripheral arterial disease: Diagnosis and management. www.nice.org.uk/guidance/cg147/resources/peripheral-arterial-disease-diagnosis-and-management-pdf-35109575873989 (accessed June 2018).

National Institute for Health and Care Excellence (2013). Varicose veins: Diagnosis and management. www.nice.org.uk/guidance/cg168/resources/varicose-veins-diagnosis-and-management-pdf-35109698485957 (accessed July 2018).

Nursing and Midwifery Council (2018). The Code. Professional Standards of Practice and Behaviour for Nurses, Midwives and Nursing Associates. https://www.nmc.org.uk/globalassets/sitedocuments/nmc-publications/nmc-code.pdf last accessed 8 May 2019.

Porth, C.M. (2015). *Essentials of Pathophysiology. Concepts of Altered Health States*, 4e. Philadelphia: Wolters Kluwer.

Rhoads, J. and Wiggins Petersen, S. (2018). *Advanced Health Assessment and Diagnostic Reasoning*, 3e. Burlington: Nelson Bartlett.

Roper, T.A. (2014). *Clinical Skills*, 2e. Oxford: Oxford University Press.

Sommers, M.S. (2011). Color awareness: a must for patient assessment. *American Nurse Today* 6 (1): 6.

Tortora, G.J. and Derrickson, B.H. (2014). *Principles of Anatomy and Physiology*, 14e. New Jersey: Wiley.

Vowden, P. and Vowden, K. (2013). Are we fully implementing guidelines and working within a multidisciplinary team when managing venous leg ulceration? *Wounds UK* 9 (2): 19–21.

Wright, N. and Fitridge, R. (2013). Varicose veins – Natural history, assessment and management. *Australian Family Physician* 42 (6): 380–384.

165

Chapter 11

Assessing the cardiac system

Aim

This chapter introduces the reader to the assessment of the cardiac system and the care required for people who experience problems associated with the cardiac system.

Learning outcomes

By the end of the chapter the reader will be able to:

1. Provide a brief overview of the cardiac system
2. Discuss a number of conditions affecting the cardiac system
3. Outline ways in which the nurse assesses the cardiac system
4. Describe care planning related to the cardiac system

Introduction

The cardiac system (a part of the cardiovascular system) is composed of the heart and closed system of vessels that include the arteries, veins, and capillaries. Assessment of the circulatory system has been discussed in Chapter 10. The heart continuously pumps blood throughout the vessels, working in partnership with a number of other body systems in order to keep us alive. This system never works in isolation and is dependent on other systems to function effectively.

This chapter provides a brief overview of the cardiac system. Nurses must have an understanding of this system so that the care they deliver adheres to local, national, and international standards. The skills required to work in a patient-centred manner demand that the nurse is able to communicate effectively, use an evidence base to support any decisions made, and to develop psychomotor skills to perform hands-on safe and effective care.

When providing care the appropriate use of psychomotor skills requires coordination between thought and understanding and physical movements. These skills are seen through how the body moves, how the skills are performed with dexterity, coordination, care, compassion, strength, speed, and accuracy. It takes time, confidence and competence to develop psychomotor skills that are required to assess the complex needs of people who have issues associated with the cardiovascular system. This chapter provides the reader with a fundamental introduction to the assessment of the cardiac system.

The heart is the muscular pump that provides the pressure necessary to propel the blood throughout the body. It must continue its cycle of contraction and relaxation; otherwise blood will

Fundamentals of Assessment and Care Planning for Nurses, First Edition. Ian Peate.
© 2020 John Wiley & Sons Ltd. Published 2020 by John Wiley & Sons Ltd.

stop flowing and the cells in the body will be unable to obtain nutrients from food sources and remove waste such as carbon dioxide and other products. A healthy and efficient heart is essential for cellular function. This chapter will include a discussion of the structure and functions of the heart, the conducting system, and the blood flow through the heart.

Review

List the psychomotor skills that might be required to undertake an assessment of the cardiac system. You already use some of these skills on your list; what other skills do you need to develop to a proficient level so you can assess a person safely and effectively?

The cardiac system

The cardiac system, working as part of the cardiovascular system, is seen as a closed transport system required to deliver oxygen and nutrients to the various parts of the body as well as transporting waste products for excretion. If there is any disorder of this system (mechanically or electrically) this will lead to disruption of this conveyance mechanism, which could also, in some cases, result in the system's complete failure. Each component part of the cardiac system (see Figure 11.1) is vital to the continuing health of the system as a whole.

The heart

This is a relatively small but very muscular organ, resting on the diaphragm close to the midline of the thoracic cavity in the mediastinum (the space in the middle of the thorax between the right and left lungs). It lies more to the left than to the right side of the chest, and the base of the heart is over its apex (Figure 11.2). It is about the size of the owner's closed fist and is approximately 12 cm long and 9 cm wide. In men, it weighs approximately 250–390 g and in women it is 200–275 g (Tortora and Derrickson 2014).

Structures of the heart

The heart is composed of specialised cardiac muscle and is surrounded by the pericardium. The pericardium is divided into parietal and visceral pericardium. The parietal pericardium, which is the outer layer, is a fibrous sac. The inner layer, the visceral pericardium, is a serous membrane, close to the

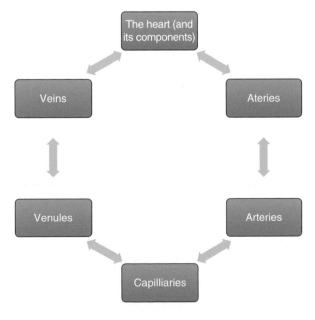

Figure 11.1   The cardiovascular (cardiac) system.

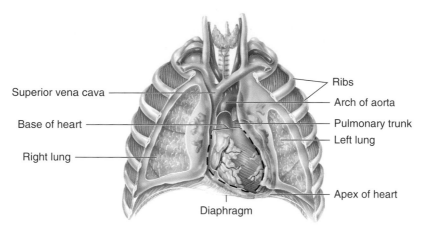

Superior vena cava

Base of heart

Right lung

Ribs

Arch of aorta

Pulmonary trunk

Left lung

Apex of heart

Diaphragm

Figure 11.2   Location of the heart.

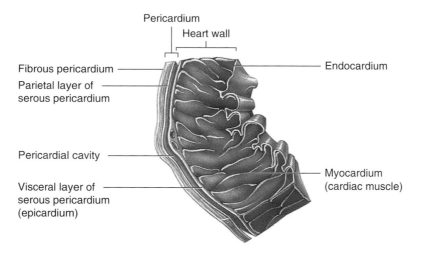

Pericardium

Heart wall

Fibrous pericardium

Parietal layer of
serous pericardium

Pericardial cavity

Visceral layer of
serous pericardium
(epicardium)

Endocardium

Myocardium
(cardiac muscle)

Figure 11.3   The heart wall.

heart (Figure 11.3). The two layers are separated by a thin film of serous fluid, permitting the heart to move freely. The cardiac muscle is called the myocardium, found only in the heart. The fibres of the myocardium branch and join with each other. Cardiac muscle cells are known as myocytes (see Figure 11.4). The endocardium lines the chambers and valves of the heart. It is a thin, smooth, and shiny membrane, allowing the smooth flow of blood (Waugh and Grant 2018). The heart therefore can be described as having three layers:

- The pericardium – the outer layer
- The myocardium – the middle layer
- The endocardium – the inner layer

The chambers of the heart

The heart is divided into two sides, right and left, separated by a muscle called the septum. The septum ensures that the oxygen-rich blood from the left side of the heart does not mix with the oxygen-depleted blood on the right side (Tortora and Derrickson 2014). Each side of the heart is divided into two chambers. The upper chambers are known as the atria (the right and left atrium) and the lower chambers are the ventricles (the right and left ventricle) (see Figure 11.5). The walls of the atria are much thinner than the walls of the ventricles.

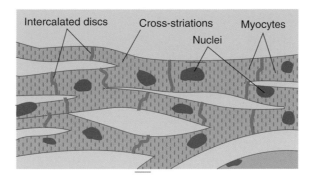

Figure 11.4 Cardiac muscle cells.

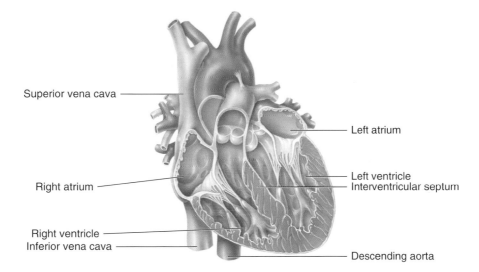

Figure 11.5 The chambers of the heart.

Valves of the heart

The valves between the atria and the ventricles are called the atrioventricular valves (AVs). The right AV is known as the tricuspid valve as it has three cusps, the left has two cusps and is also known as the bicuspid (mitral) valve (McCance and Heuther 2018). These valves will only allow the flow of blood from the atria to the ventricles, preventing the blood from flowing in the opposite direction. The pulmonary valve is situated between the right ventricle and the arteries supplying the lungs (the pulmonary arteries), preventing the backwards flow of blood into the right ventricle from the pulmonary arteries. The aortic valve is located between the left ventricle and the aorta, preventing the backwards flow of blood into the left ventricle from the systemic circulation.

Vessels of the heart

Blood flows in and out of the heart via a number of large vessels. The right atrium receives venous blood through the superior and inferior venae cavae. Oxygen-depleted blood from the right ventricle is transported to the lungs by the pulmonary artery. The pulmonary veins return oxygen-rich blood from the lungs to the left atrium. The aorta transports oxygenated blood from the left ventricle to the whole body (McCance and Heuther 2018). The heart has its own blood supply and this is delivered by the coronary arteries. The coronary veins return oxygen-depleted blood from the heart tissue to the right atrium (see Figure 11.6, the vessels of the heart). Table 11.1 provides a summary of the vessels and their functions.

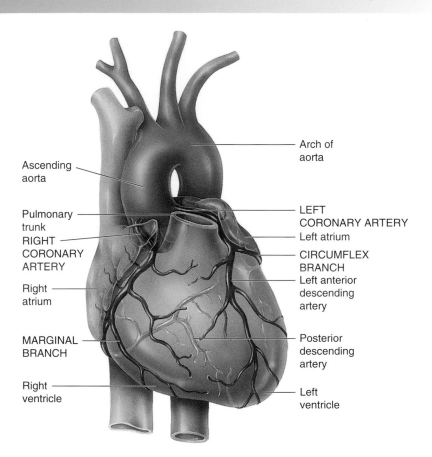

Figure 11.6   The vessels of the heart.

Table 11.1   Summary of the vessels and their functions.

Vessel	Function
Superior vena cava	Returns oxygen-depleted blood to the right atrium from the thoracic organs, head, neck, and both arms
Inferior vena cava	Returns oxygen-depleted blood to the right atrium from the rest of the body
Pulmonary artery (divides into the right and left pulmonary artery)	Takes oxygen-depleted blood from the right ventricle to the lungs
Pulmonary veins (two from the right lung and two from the left lung)	Returns oxygen-rich blood from the lungs to the left atrium
Aorta	Takes oxygen-rich blood from the left ventricle to the whole body
Coronary arteries	Takes oxygen-rich blood to the heart tissues
Coronary veins	Returns oxygen-depleted blood from the heart tissues to the right atrium via the coronary sinus

Blood flow through the heart

The right atrium receives oxygen-depleted blood via the superior and inferior venae cavae and the coronary sinus. The right atrium then empties the blood into the right ventricle via the tricuspid valve. By opening the pulmonary artery, the right ventricle pumps the blood to the lungs via the pulmonary arteries (right and left) and by opening the pulmonary semilunar valve. In the lungs, carbon dioxide is exchanged for oxygen molecules. Blood returning to the lungs has a higher content of carbon dioxide, which diffuses out of the lung capillaries into the alveolar sac and is disposed of during expiration. During inspiration, oxygen diffuses from the alveolar sac into the lung capillaries attaching itself to the haemoglobin molecules in the red blood cells. The oxygen-rich red blood cells are transported in the blood to the left atrium by four sets of pulmonary veins. The short circulation from the right ventricle to the lungs and from the lungs to the left atrium is called the pulmonary circulation (Marieb and Hoehn 2016).

From the left atrium, blood is then pumped into the left ventricle via the bicuspid (mitral) valve. From the left ventricle, the blood is then pumped to the rest of the body via the aorta through the aortic semilunar valve (see Figure 11.7). The aorta and its branches transport the oxygen-rich blood to all parts of the body. The blood is then returned to the right atrium via the venae cavae. This loop is called the systemic circulation (Marieb and Hoehn 2016).

Conducting systems of the heart

The heart has its own built-in regulatory mechanism producing a coordinated myocardial contraction of the four chambers, achieved by the cardiac conducting system (see Figure 11.8), which is composed of the:

1. Sinoatrial (SA) node
2. AV node
3. AV (bundle of His)
4. Right and left bundle branches
5. Purkinje fibres.

The SA node

The SA node is located in the right atrium, just below the opening of the superior vena cava. It is also called the pacemaker, as it initiates impulses much faster than other groups of neuromuscular cells (Waugh and Grant 2018). Impulses from the SA node trigger the atria to contract.

The AV node

The AV node is situated at the base of the right atrium. This is the last region of the atria to be stimulated, thereby allowing time for the atria to empty the blood into the ventricles prior to the ventricles starting to contract again. This ensures that the blood flows in one direction only.

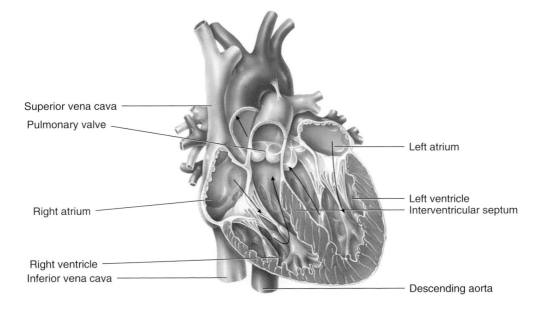

Figure 11.7   Flow of blood through the heart.

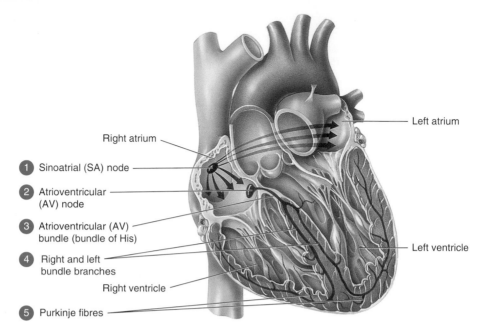

Left atrium

Right atrium

1 Sinoatrial (SA) node

2 Atrioventricular
(AV) node

3 Atrioventricular (AV)
bundle (bundle of His)

4 Right and left
bundle branches

Right ventricle

5 Purkinje fibres

Left ventricle

Figure 11.8   Conduction system of the heart.

Bundle of his

This is a set of fibres that originate from the AV node.

Right and left bundle branches

From the bundle of His, the nerve fibres split into the right and left bundle branches.

Purkinje fibres

These are tiny nerve fibres that innervate the right and left ventricular myocardial cells.

Nerve supply of the heart

The pumping action of the heart is regular and rhythmic. Cardiac muscle has the intrinsic ability of automatic rhythmic contraction that is independent of its nerve supply. However, the rate of contraction is influenced by the nerve supply to the heart.

The nerve supply originates from the cardioregulatory centre located in the medulla oblongata which is situated in the brainstem (see Figure 11.9). These nerves are a branch of the autonomic nervous system and are called the sympathetic and parasympathetic nerves (Waugh and Grant 2018).

The sympathetic nerve causes an increase in the heart rate; innervating the SA node, AV node and the myocardium of the atria and ventricles. The parasympathetic (vagus) nerve slows down the heart rate supplying the SA and AV nodes and the atria muscles. Factors affecting heart rate include (Waugh and Grant 2018):

- Hormones such as epinephrine, steroids
- Stress
- Age
- Drugs, for example propranolol, dopamine
- Body temperature
- Autonomic nervous system
- Circulating volume of blood
- Electrolyte imbalance
- Oxygen and carbon dioxide levels in the blood.

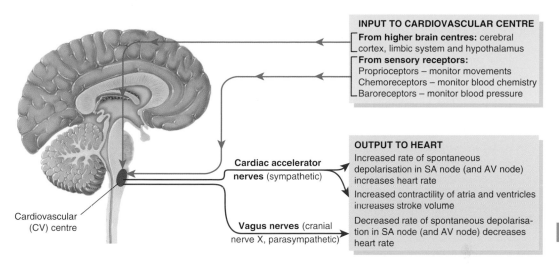

INPUT TO CARDIOVASCULAR CENTRE

⌈ **From higher brain centres:** cerebral
⌊ cortex, limbic system and hypothalamus
⌈ **From sensory receptors:**
   Proprioceptors – monitor movements
   Chemoreceptors – monitor blood chemistry
⌊ Baroreceptors – monitor blood pressure

OUTPUT TO HEART

Increased rate of spontaneous
depolarisation in SA node (and AV node)
increases heart rate

Increased contractility of atria and ventricles
increases stroke volume

Decreased rate of spontaneous depolarisation in SA node (and AV node) decreases
heart rate

**Cardiac accelerator
nerves** (sympathetic)

Cardiovascular
(CV) centre

Vagus nerves (cranial
nerve X, parasympathetic)

173

Figure 11.9   The cardio regulatory centre.

The cardiac cycle

The cardiac cycle is the cyclical contraction (systole) and relaxation (diastole) of the two syncytia (two atria and the two ventricles). Each cycle is initiated by the spontaneous generation of an action potential located in the SA node.

During diastole (which normally lasts around 0.4 second), blood enters the relaxed atria, flowing passively into the ventricles. The atria contract fractionally before the ventricles and complete ventricular filling. As the ventricles begin to contract, ventricular pressure increases and for a short time (this is the isometric phase) all four valves are closed with the volume of blood in the ventricles remaining constant. Increasing pressure finally forces the pulmonary and aortic valves to open and blood is ejected into the pulmonary artery and aorta. When the ventricles stop contracting, the pressure within them falls below that in the major blood vessels, the aortic and pulmonary valves close and the cycle begins again with diastole.

The normal heart rate is approximately 70 beats per minute in the resting adult, with each cardiac cycle lasting approximately 0.8 second. With each ventricular contraction, 65–75% of the blood in the ventricle at the end of diastole is ejected. This is usually a volume of 70–80 mL of blood and is known as the stroke volume.

Cardiac output is the volume of blood that is ejected from one ventricle in one minute. Whilst cardiac output is a traditional measure of cardiac function, it differs markedly with body size. A more useful measure is the cardiac index. This is the cardiac output per minute per metre squared of the body surface area. Usually this is about $3.2 \, l/m^2$. The primary factors that determine cardiac output are:

- Preload – the amount of tension on the ventricular muscle fibres before they contract, determined primarily by the end-diastolic volume (EDV)
- Afterload – the resistance against which the heart must pump. It is determined by blood pressure in the aorta, resistance in the peripheral vessels, the size of the aortic valve opening, left ventricular size, contractility of the heart, and the heart rate.

Within physiological limits, the volume of blood pumped out by a ventricle is the same as that entering the atrium on the same side of the heart, that is, cardiac output matches venous return. This principle is referred to as the Frank–Starling law of the heart. This means that the heart is able to adapt to changing loads of inflowing blood from the systemic and pulmonary circulations. Within limits, cardiac muscle fibres contract more forcibly the more they are stretched when contraction begins. When venous return increases beyond a certain limit, the myocardium will begin to fail. This regulation of the heart, responding to the amount of blood to be pumped, is known as intrinsic regulation.

Assessing needs

A careful and detailed clinical assessment is essential in order to assess the probable cause and severity of symptoms, to request appropriate investigations and referral, to avoid needless investigations and to assess an individual's risk of cardiac disease.

How the history is taken and information gathered in different health care settings is variable and will depend on, for example, the patient's presenting symptoms, patient concerns, the past medical, psychological, and social history. However, the general framework for history taking is discussed in Chapter 7 of this text. This framework may need to be amended depending on the care setting (in a general practice, an acute care ward, emergency department) and the nature of the patient encounter (an emergency situation or a pre-planned consultation). Many health care providers have protocols and procedures in place for taking a patient history, if this is the case, then local policy and procedure must be followed.

The history provides subjective information about the presenting symptoms, previous patterns of health and illness and the patient's ability to perform the activities of living. A family history, together with risk factor identification and social and psychological background, enriches the history-gathering activity. An in-depth physical examination is also needed that will provide additional objective data.

Explaining to the patient how the history taking is to progress, what it will entail, and how long it may take can help to develop rapport and even alleviate anxiety. The assessment of the cardiovascular system could be considered as one of the most important aspects of patient assessment. Throughout the whole assessment process the nurse must always be observant for even a slight deviation from the norm, if something is abnormal and uncovered then this warrants further investigation, any finding or concerns must be acted upon and reported.

Take note

Always explain to the person why you are doing what you are doing, you must seek permission from the patient to undertake the assessment. In doing this the nurse is gaining consent and also going someway to alleviating stress and anxiety.

When meeting the patient (in their own home, a cubicle, behind screens, in the consultation room), introduce yourself and explain that you will be carrying out an interview and a physical examination. Try to make the patient (and family) relax as much as possible, the patient will probably be very anxious. Remember not to rush the patient give them time, rushing the patient can make them even more anxious. Provide time for them to answer questions and do not interrupt when the patient is trying to answer, let them finish prior to asking the next question.

6Cs

'Hello my name is…'

The 'Hello my name is'…campaign is focused on reminding staff to introduce themselves to patients properly. A confident and clear introduction is the first step to providing compassionate care and is often all it takes to put patients at ease and help them feel relaxed whilst using health and social care services.

The key aim during the assessment phase is to be as objective as possible. When the nurse is unsure, then further investigation is needed. The use of validated tools along with inspection, palpation, and auscultation gives more credence to findings and subsequent care delivery. The nurse must act on and report findings as clearly as possible, adhering to local policy and procedure. Clearly documenting and communicating findings is essential for the treatment of the patient and the nursing care they are to receive.

Due to the nature of the person's condition the person may be so unwell that they cannot give a history (or only a partial history). The nurse may need to seek a secondary source to provide data.

Chief complaint and history of present condition

Prior to undertaking the assessment, access and read any pertinent patient-related data that has already been recorded about the patient, for example notes from any previous admissions. This can help to set the screen and contextualise.

Chief complaint and history of present condition is the story of the illness. Determining what it was that contributed to the patient coming to the health provider (hospital, GP practice, walk-in clinic) will provide information about the history of the present illness. Seek information concerning the present symptoms along with other recent symptoms relevant to this present illness. Obtain the following information specifically related to the cardiac system:

- Chest, jaw pain
- Pain in the extremities (pain radiating to the arms, leg pain or cramps)
- Irregular heart rate or palpitations
- Shortness of breath on exertion when lying down (orthopnoea) or at night (paroxysmal nocturnal dyspnoea)
- Cough
- Cyanosis
- Pallor
- Weakness
- Fatigue
- Unexplained weight changes
- Peripheral oedema
- Dizziness
- Headaches
- Hypo- or hypertension

Family history

Seek information from the patient regarding family history. Ask the age of any living relatives and include here relationships and health of immediate relatives. Ask the patient about hypertension, coronary heart disease, stroke, diabetes, hyperlipidaemia, congenital heart disease, and any early deaths (before the age of 60) in the family.

Cultural considerations

In the UK smoking rates vary noticeably between ethnic groups. In 2004, 40% of Bangladeshi men smoked, compared to 21% of Black African and Chinese men.

Source: British Heart Foundation (2012).

Obtaining a family history provides a useful tool to identify those who may have, or be at risk of developing an illness that has a genetic component. Asking a patient about their family history can also provide further information that may allow a diagnosis to be made.

The patient's reaction to an illness in the family may influence a response to personal medical problems. A family history of hypertension and myocardial infarction would be included with the history of present illness of a patient with new-onset chest pain. Time limitations may preclude a detailed inquiry into the health of each family member, the nurse should use discretion if the family is very large.

Lifestyle

Gather details about the current family unit, and the nature of the patient's work (to determine physical exertion and stress). How does the patient relax, do they have any hobbies? Enquire about exercise, note type, duration, and how often this is undertaken.

Ask about tobacco use and type, age when started, and age when stopped (if at all). How much does the patient smoke? Have there been any efforts to attempt to stop smoking? Does the patient drink alcohol, what type and what age did they start, how much is consumed (in units) and how often? Is the patient using any recreational drugs? How much? How often which type?

Calculate the patient's body mass index (BMI) to determine obesity or overweight. Ask about diet, is this healthy or unhealthy?

Take note

Body mass index

BMI is a measurement of a person's leanness or corpulence based on height and weight and is intended to quantify tissue mass. Although BMI has limitations in that it is an estimate that cannot take body composition into account, it can be used as a general indicator of a healthy body weight that is based on a person's height. The value obtained from the calculation of BMI is widely used to categorise whether a person is underweight, normal weight, overweight, or obese, depending on what range the value falls between.

Past medical history

A detailed exploration of the patient's past medical history helps in identifying any prior diseases or significant lifestyle factors:

- Ask about any raised blood pressure, heart problems, fainting, dizziness, or collapses.
- Take note if there have been any heart attacks, any history of angina and any cardiac procedures or operations (note type and date of intervention and outcome).
- Previous levels of lipids if ever checked or known.
- Enquire whether there is any history of rheumatic fever or heart problems as a child.
- Note any other operations or illnesses, particularly history of myocardial infarction, hyperlipidaemia, hypertension, stroke, diabetes mellitus.

The physical examination

Physical examination is the process of evaluating objective anatomical findings as the nurse uses observation, palpation, percussion, and auscultation. The information obtained has to be thoughtfully integrated with the patient's history and pathophysiology. This unique situation allows the patient and the nurse to understand that the aim of the interaction is diagnostic and therapeutic.

6Cs

As the environment affects the quality of the physical examination, it is important to arrange for quiet and privacy, the nurse should remember that in a ward area curtains are not soundproof and your conversation can be easily overheard.

The patient's dignity must be preserved at all times. Only expose those parts of the body being examined. The aim is to make the patient feel comfortable and safe.

Table 11.2 Common manifestations of cardiovascular problems.

System	Manifestation	Associated possible disorder
General	Fatigue, weight loss, weight gain, disturbed sleep pattern	Coronary heart disease, infective endocarditis, congestive heart failure, valvular disease
Skin	Pyrexia, rigours Skin change in colour/pigmentation, hair loss, oedema Clammy skin Malar flush – redness around the cheeks	Infective endocarditis, pericarditis Peripheral vascular disease, deep vein thrombosis Myocardial infarction Mitral stenosis
Eyes	Visual disturbance (blurred/double), decreased visual acuity, vertigo, headache	Hypertension
Respiratory	Persistent cough (productive or non-productive), pain associated with respiration, dyspnoea, orthopnoea, crackles, or wheeze on auscultation	Congestive heart failure, endocarditis, valvular disease
Gastrointestinal	Nausea, vomiting, anorexia Hepatomegaly Splenomegaly	Congestive heart failure Myocardial infarction Congestive heart failure
Musculoskeletal	Arthralgia Jaw pain, back pain	Infective endocarditis Myocardial infarction

Source: Adapted Rhoads and Wiggins Petersen (2018).

A number of cardiovascular diseases and disorders have manifestations in systems other than the cardiovascular system. The nurse must undertake a complete review of other systems whenever possible. However, due to time constraints and other issues the nurse may need to undertake a focused systems review. The information gained from examining other systems can have a significant impact on decisions the nurse makes.

Undertake a general survey, observe the patient as you meet them, note build, (overweight, obesity, wasting), are they short of breath (at rest on exertion), does the patient have difficulty in talking?

Look at the patient. Look at the person's face and determine: is the patient pale (pallor), are there any signs of jaundice? Inspect the person's lips and skin: is there any cyanosis? Is there xanthelasma (fatty lumps forming near the inner corners of the upper and lower eyelids, often due to high cholesterol levels)? Is the patient sweaty, do they feel clammy? See Table 11.2 for a list of common manifestations of cardiovascular problems.

A focused, systematic review of the systems along with the physical assessment will lead to prompt diagnosis and subsequent treatment. A careful assessment can allow the nurse to identify the cause, anatomical, and physiological components of a specific cardiovascular disorder, as well as to determine overall cardiac function.

The blood pressure

Blood pressure is an important guide to cardiovascular risk and provides the nurse with essential information on the patient's haemodynamic status. The blood pressure varies constantly in response to the environment, excitement, and stress.

Take note

'White coat hypertension' (white coat syndrome) is a phenomenon in which patients exhibit a blood pressure level above the normal range when in a clinical setting, but they do not exhibit it in other settings. This can have an impact on the blood pressure reading.

Usually the blood pressure is measured in the brachial artery, using a cuff around the upper arm. A large cuff must be used for those people who are obese; using a small cuff will result in the blood pressure being overestimated. In some instances (often in the intensive care unit) the blood pressure is measured using an invasive device such as an indwelling intra-arterial catheter connected to a pressure sensor.

In those patients complaining of chest pain, or if ever the radial pulses seem asymmetrical, the pressure should be measured in both arms, as a difference between the two could indicate aortic dissection. The blood pressure is measured in mmHg and recorded as systolic/diastolic.

Take note

The nurse should also record how the blood pressure reading was taken, for example BP 142/80 mmHg left arm, standing.

So far

The nurse has to obtain a full history using effective communication skills in order to gather as much information as possible ensuring the physical and psychological needs of the patient are being met. History taking is accompanied by a physical examination.

Chest examination

Inspection of jugular venous pressure has been discussed in Chapter 10. There are several techniques that can be used to examine the chest, and not all are discussed here. The nurse needs to identify the cardiovascular landmarks, understanding and locating these can help with detailing the findings.

Explain to the patient what you are about to do and why. You may need help as you assess the chest. Chest wall inspection can reveal scars that could indicate previous cardiac surgery or pacemaker implantation. Look to see if there are any chest wall deformities such as funnel chest. Take note to determine if the chest moves equally (symmetry); inequality of expansion is often the result of respiratory disease. Take note of the respiratory rate, rhythm, and depth.

Ask the patient to breathe out, and using both palms of your hands, rest them lightly on the side walls of the chest with thumbs meeting in the middle then ask the patient to breathe in. Assess the expansion of the chest on full inspiration by noting how far the your thumbs move apart.

Observe and palpate the trachea as you detect any deviation to the left or right (take note of any thyroid swelling).

Palpate and percuss to find any areas of dullness (fluid or lung collapse). Do this by palpating with the flat hand over the 5th intercostal space to feel the maximum impulse (apex of the heart) and note its position; the apex is better defined by the light use of two fingers (noting the rib space and its position relative to an imaginary line dropped from the middle of the clavicle). The nurse must be skilled and competent in performing this skill.

Take note

In order to develop the skills of chest examination watch a more experienced colleague perform the examination. With permission from the patient, practise these important skills.

Cardiac auscultation

Auscultation of the heart is an important skill for the nurse to master, it can take time to perform this skill competently. Learning the correct technique for auscultation is essential in order to distinguish the normal from the abnormal. All cardiac areas must be auscultated, and this has to be done in a structured and methodical fashion.

Take note

Using a stethoscope for auscultation

A simple stethoscope consists of a diaphragm or an open bell-shaped structure which is applied to the body, connected by rubber or plastic tubes to shaped earpieces for the examiner.

Prior to using a stethoscope, explain to the patient what you about to do and seek their consent.

The nurse can use the stethoscope during auscultation to assess breath and heart sounds.

Hold the diaphragm of the stethoscope firmly against the patient's skin to listen for high-pitched sounds.

Hold the bell of the stethoscope lightly against the patient's skin to listen for low-pitched sounds.

The nurse should never attempt to auscultate over clothing, i.e. a gown, a bra, a vest.

It may be helpful to close the eyes during auscultation to aid concentration.

Note the intensity and location of auscultation and document according to local policy.

Infection prevention and control principles also apply when using a stethoscope.

Source: O'Neill (2003).

179

Cardiac auscultation can identify abnormalities of blood flow through the valves in the heart. The blood that flows through the heart and the closing of the heart valves produce sounds that can be heard when a stethoscope is placed on key areas of the chest wall (see Figure 11.10). The clearest of the sounds are S1 (the first heart sound heard), caused by the closure of the mitral and tricuspid valve, heralding the onset of systole, and S2 (second heart sound), generated by the aortic and pulmonary valves closing, marking the beginning of diastole. Damaged and leaky valves will cause turbulent flow and produce murmurs that can be heard in the quiet time between systole and diastole (Jones et al. 2010).

The patient should be seated and leaning forward in order to auscultate heart sounds. If the heart signs are faint, ask the patient to lie on their left side, as this brings the heart nearer to the chest wall. When auscultating for heart sounds the nurse should place the stethoscope over the four sites illustrated in Figure 11.10, following the numbered sequence. The auscultation sites are denoted by the names of the heart valves. These sites are located along the pathway that the blood takes as it flows through the chambers of the heart and the valves.

By comprehensively assessing cardiovascular status and identifying problems early, the nurse can put in place appropriate interventions and if required escalate care in a timely manner to help prevent further deterioration, or to arrange for the patient to be transferred to a more appropriate care area.

Take note

Learning the skills of chest auscultation can take time and much practice. It is essential that you are proficient in all areas when performing this important skill. Having perfected the skill, the nurse needs to make sense of the findings and apply these to the care of the patient.

Electrocardiogram

An electrocardiogram (ECG) is a recording of the heart's electrical activity. It has two approaches. The 12-lead ECG provides a definitive diagnosis as it measures electrical activity from a three-dimensional perspective. The information that the 12-lead ECG provides can serve as a basis for which other diagnostic tests may be required (for example, echocardiogram).

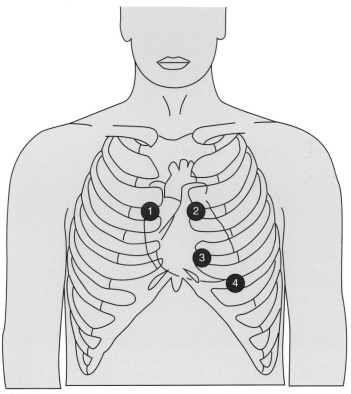

1 Aortic area - second intercostal space, right sternal border

2 Pulmonic area - second intercostal space, left sternal border

3 Tricuspid area -fourth (or fifth) intercostal space, left sternal border

4 Mitral area or apex - fifth intercostal space, left midclavicular line

Figure 11.10   Cardiac auscultation points.

A 12-lead ECG should be recorded at the earliest opportunity and will almost immediately show the tell-tale signs of cardiac dysfunction such as ischaemia and infarction. The 12-lead ECG is one of the essential criteria for diagnosing acute coronary syndromes. The ECG provides a quick and non-invasive approach to acquiring data to determine information about the heart's electro physiology (Marieb and Hoehn 2016). The 2-lead ECG is a basic monitoring technique that provides a less-detailed view of the basic heart rhythm and is used as a continual process (real time), this approach only shows the activity of the heart from one viewpoint at a time. Prior to recording a 12-lead ECG:

- Explain procedure to patient
- Seek consent to proceed
- Check that each electrode is attached and correctly placed
- Ask the patient to lie still and not speak whilst the recording is made
- Adhere to local policy and procedure
- Follow guidance issued by the National Institute of Health and Care Excellence (2010)

To record a 12-lead ECG, six electrodes are placed across the front of the chest on the left side. These electrodes provide a series of views of the left ventricle as observed from the right side of the heart around to the left side (see Figure 11.11).

Four electrodes are placed on the limbs, these electrodes can be placed either on the extremities (the ankles and wrists) or on the torso (upper chest and lower abdomen). It is important that these electrodes are placed symmetrically (see Figure 11.12).

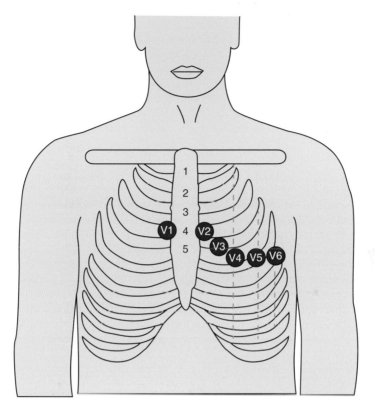

Figure 11.11   Lead placement.

There are 12 views of the heart obtained from the 12 electrodes: six are views of the heart from the sides, top, and bottom (on the vertical plane); six are views of the anterior surface of the left ventricle (on the horizontal plane). See Figure 11.13; this is a normal ECG.

When the ECG has been printed, the nurse should check, prior to detaching the cables, that the tracing is free from artefact. Artefact is the name given to disturbances in rhythm monitoring caused by movement of the electrodes, which can be caused by any electrical activity, for example shivering and the presence of nearby electrical equipment. If required, replace the electrodes and repeat the tracing. The nurse must write the date, time, and patient identity on the printout (there are some machines that automatically do this). Remember to record any clinical information, for example recent chest pain, and any medications that may have been administered. The nurse must be trained and deemed competent prior to carrying out this procedure.

Take note

When performing an ECG:
- The ECG machine should be checked, charged, and ready for use.
- It should be stocked with sufficient paper for the recording – tissues, clinical wipes, alcohol wipes, and a container for disposing of used items.
- Female patients should be asked to remove tights and should be offered a cover for their chest once the electrodes and ECG leads are placed and connected.
- Male patients with hairy chests may be required to have the electrode areas shaved, with permission; this will ensure good skin contact.
- The skin should be cleaned and dried, according to local procedure and protocol, prior to placing the electrodes.
- The patient should be supine. If this is not possible, for example if a patient is breathless or has back problems, then the bed back may be raised, and the nurse must note this on the ECG.

- Limb electrodes must be placed on the limbs – not the trunk.
- Ideally arm electrodes at the wrist and limb electrodes at the ankles
- In the case of a person who has an amputation or has a dressing in place, the electrodes should be placed further up the affected limb but on the same side.
- After each recording the electrodes and ECG leads should be cleaned with clinical wipes in accordance with local procedure and policy.

So far

The aim of assessment is to exclude a life-threatening cause, which needs immediate treatment, from other causes of chest pain. Diagnosis of chest pain can be difficult. However, the history often gives an indication of the underlying cause. As the nurse meets the patient pay attention to general appearance/status, including any confusion, anxiety, shortness of breath, pain, distress, whether pale or sweaty, and if there is any vomiting. If there is any serious cause for concern regarding the patient's general wellbeing, then the nurse must (if not in the hospital setting) arrange urgent hospital assessment and admission. If there is concern when in the hospital setting, then the nurse must escalate these concerns to a higher authority. At all times keep the patient (and if appropriate, the family) informed of what is happening.

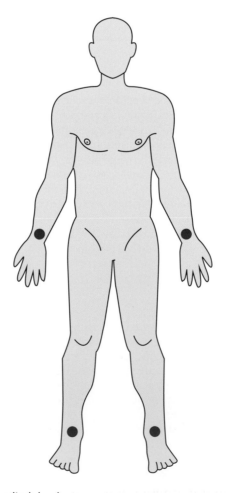

Figure 11.12   Placement of the limb leads.

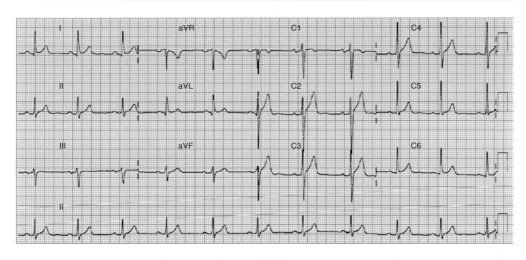

Figure 11.13 A 12-lead normal electrocardiogram (ECG). Source: Davey (2008).

Table 11.3 Possible causes of chest pain.

System	Potential cause
Cardiovascular	Myocardial infarction Unstable angina pectoris Pericarditis Dissecting aortic aneurysm Myocarditis
Pulmonary	Pleurisy Pulmonary embolism Pneumothorax Pneumonia
Haematological	Sickle cell anaemia
Musculoskeletal	Costochondritis Trauma
Gastrointestinal	Gastro-oesophageal reflux Peptic ulcer disease Gallstones Pancreatitis
Non-organic	Anxiety Depression

Source: Gaunt (2014), Tough (2004).

Assessing chest pain

Cardiac pain is intense and a rapid nursing response (intervention) is required. Chest pain is a common symptom and is one of the most common presenting complaints seen in primary and secondary care; it is the leading cause of emergency department visits after abdominal pain (Oriolo and Albarran 2010). When the nurse performs a structured nursing assessment it can be possible to identify those patients who are at high risk. It can be challenging to assess and distinguish between the various types of chest pain and presentation as a result of variation in the clinical presentation, the patient's history of the symptom, as well as the potential for atypical presentation in women, older people, and those with diabetes or chronic kidney disease. Some causes of chest pain are outlined in Table 11.3.

Acute coronary syndrome is a potentially more serious cause of chest pain that requires the nurse to act rapidly so as to identify this type of pain and to implement treatment in order to preserve myocardial function and prevent the development of arrhythmias, heart failure, or cardiogenic shock.

Table 11.4   The mnemonic OLDCARTS used as a framework when assessing chest pain.

OLDCARTS	Directed towards the patient
Onset	When did the pain begin?
Location	Where is the pain?
Duration	How long does the pain last?
Characteristics	Describe the pain (crushing, stabbing, dull ache, indigestion)
Associated factors	Other symptoms associated with the pain such as nausea and/or vomiting, weakness, fatigue, breathlessness, syncope (fainting), cold, and clammy?
Relieving factors/ radiation	Does the pain radiate, for example down the arm or up into the neck? Are there any relieving factors, for example does the pain stop when activity stops, and is it relieved by sitting forward or resting?
Treatment/temporal factors	Use of GTN, was the pain relieved by rest or a decrease in physical activity? When does the pain come on? Pain non-comparable to previous ischaemic chest pain?
Severity (intensity)	Use a numerical pain scale (1 no pain – 10 worst pain experienced) in order to gauge pain severity

The European Society of Cardiology (2007) note that 'acute coronary syndromes' is an umbrella term describing the clinical presentation of ischaemic heart disease and encompasses unstable angina pectoris, non-ST segment elevation myocardial infarction (NSTEMI), and ST segment elevation myocardial infarction (STEMI). Acute coronary syndrome is a life-threatening manifestation of atherosclerosis that is caused by rupture of a vulnerable atherosclerotic plaque with subsequent thrombus formation. This causes an abrupt complete or critical reduction in coronary blood flow, resulting in the clinical presentation of chest pain.

Cardiac chest pain is characteristically visceral, meaning it is a deep and diffuse kind of pain as opposed to localised and superficial pain. When asking the patient to locate the pain, they will typically point to a wide area of the chest, often being unable to point to a specific point on the chest. Cardiac chest pain varies in location depending on each individual. However, it is generally felt in the centre of the chest (or to the left of the sternum) (NICE 2010). It can extend down to the epigastrium or up to the neck and the jaw. In some cases, there is a pattern of referred pain that can extend down the left arm. The nurse should note that not everybody will experience chest pain in acute coronary syndromes. Those people with diabetes mellitus are specifically likely not to make a complaint of chest pain due to the neuropathy accompanying the condition.

The nurse should focus on the history of the pain, cardiovascular risk factor profile, a previous personal history of ischaemic heart disease, and prior relevant investigations when assessing chest pain (Oriolo and Albarran 2010). There are various types of chest pain assessment tools and scores available. Table 11.4 uses the mnemonic OLDCARTS as a framework that can be used when assessing chest pain.

In assessing chest pain the nurse needs to use a variety of skills, effective use of communication is essential, and this will include verbal and non-verbal communication. The person experiencing excruciating chest pain, who is fearful for their life may not want to, or not be able to, communicate in depth about their pain. A systematic approach is required using assessment tools to help make the assessment as objective as possible. The assessment has to be augmented by assessing vital signs,

Review

PQRST chest pain

Compare the assessment tool in this review box to the tool that has been presented in Table 11.4. What do you think are the similarities and differences (compare both)? Have you seen either of the tools used in clinical practice?

P	Precipitating or provoking factors
Q	Quality (intensity/pain score)
R	Radiation, region
S	Severity/symptoms/duration
T	Timing
C	Commenced when
H	History/evidence of risk factors
E	Extra/additional symptoms
S	Stays/radiation
T	Timing/how long has it lasted
P	Place/location
A	What alleviates/aggravates the pain
I	Intensity scoring
N	Nature and characteristics

Source: Seidel et al. (2011).

ECG, and the relevant bloods; this will aid in diagnosis, identify risk (and in so doing priorities), as well as suggesting treatment options.

Chest pain is a symptom associated with other clinical pathologies. As such, a thorough assessment of any chest pain is required to exclude a non-cardiac cause. Table 11.5 can help with interpreting what it is that the patient is saying about chest pain and what inferences the nurse can make regarding causation. Figure 11.14 provides information associated with typical areas of the body where cardiac pain may be experienced.

So far

Often it is difficult to be certain as to whether the chest pain the patient is complaining of is of a cardiac or non-cardiac cause. The nurse must take a full history from the patient to assess the need for immediate intervention or another form of referral.

There is an urgent need to diagnose the cause of any patient presenting with chest pain to ensure that serious and life-threatening conditions do not get missed.

Take note

If not in a hospital setting, urgent hospital referral is indicated if there is any indication of a severe underlying disorder or if the patient is acutely unwell. A 999 ambulance should be called and the incident must be treated as an emergency.

Table 11.5   Inferences that can be made regarding cardiac pain, type, and location.

What the patient says it is	Possible cause	Location of pain
Aching, squeezing, pressure, heaviness burning pain that usually subsides within 10 minutes	Angina pectoris	Substernal, may radiate to neck, jaw, back, arms
Tightness, pressure, burning, aching pain, maybe accompanied by shortness of breath, diaphoresis, weakness, fatigue, anxiety, nausea. 'Feels like there is a tight belt across my chest.' Onset is sudden, can last between 30 minutes and 2 hours. A feeling of impending death.	Acute myocardial infarction	Usually across the chest, may radiate to neck, jaw, back, arms
Sharp and continuous sudden onset	Pericarditis	Substernal may radiate to neck or left arm
Excruciating pain, tearing pain, sudden onset blood pressure difference in right and left arms	Dissecting aortic aneurysm	Retro sternal, upper abdomen, epigastric may radiate to back, neck, shoulders
Sudden stabbing like pain, which may be accompanied by cyanosis, dyspnoea, cough, and haemoptysis	Pulmonary embolism	Over the lung area
Sudden and severe pain can be accompanied by dyspnoea, tachycardia. Breath sounds decreased (particularly over one side)	Pneumothorax	Lateral chest
Burning feeling after eating, maybe accompanied by haematemesis, melena, sudden onset may subside after 20 minutes	Peptic ulcer	Epigastric
Dull stabbing pain, maybe accompanied by hyperventilation, breathlessness, onset is sudden can last between a minute and for several days	Acute anxiety	Anywhere in the chest and neck

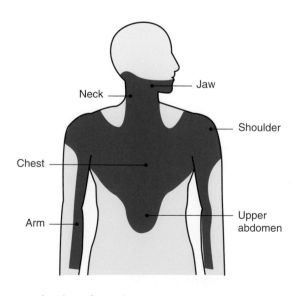

Figure 11.14   Areas associated with cardiac pain.

Maurice Samuda (Father)

This evening whilst Maurice was having supper, he felt unwell, he was sweaty, and he collapsed. He then regained consciousness. He had been working in his shed earlier and had pain then, but he thought that it was related to his back problems. Shahine, his wife, called for an ambulance.

He was seen by paramedics at his home, who took a 12-lead ECG and administered GTN. He was then transported to the emergency department.

Maurice was still complaining of chest pain when he arrived at the emergency department, telling the advanced nurse practitioner that the pain was spreading to the shoulders, neck, and arms. He said it felt like he was being choked or that somebody was 'sitting on my chest'. His pain, assessed using a visual analogue scale, is 9. The pain started about four hours ago a 'niggling, burning pain' he felt just after he had a bite of lunch and he thought it was indigestion and ignored it. He has had similar 'indigestion pain' before. Now he is sweating profusely, he is short of breath and nauseous. Maurice is anxious and has told the nurse that he is scared.

How would you assess Maurice using OLDCARTS?

Onset

Location

Duration

Characteristics

Associated factors

Relieving factors/radiation

Treatment/temporal factors

Severity (intensity)

Shahine, his wife states that he complained of not feeling too good when he got up that morning, he had vomited a couple of times in the toilet. She tells the nurse, I thought it was another one of his hangovers as he was out late last night and he has been in a foul mood lately. Things at home have not been as good as they might be.

His wife informs that he has been unwell recently. He has had a bad back and a few months ago the GP had put him on pills for his blood pressure and he has been putting on so much weight. She informs you that Maurice has a family history of diabetes and blood pressure and that things at home have been a mess, he is under a lot of pressure as he fears he will lose his job as a result of his poor performance, and they are behind in their mortgage payments. Shahine breaks down and says she feels she can't go on.

The 12-lead ECG reveals Maurice has had a STEMI. He is receiving analgesia, anti-emetic, and supplementary oxygen. The interventional cardiologist is now with him.

Plan the care required for Maurice in the next 48 hours as Maurice is admitted to the coronary care unit.

Conclusion

To ensure patient safety, it is essential that the nurse has an understanding of the anatomy and physiology of the collective cardiovascular system as well as the various skills required to undertake a competent patient-centred assessment of needs. Ongoing assessment of needs is essential as a nursing diagnosis is made, goals are set, and care is implemented and effectively evaluated.

It is essential that the skills described in this chapter related to assessment are perfected so as to ensure patient safety. It can take time and much practice to be deemed proficient in the skills required to assess the patient's cardiovascular status.

Experiencing chest pain can cause much anxiety for the patient and family. The way the nurse manages and works with the patient and family can often alleviate concerns and anxiety, so working in a calm and systemic way is advocated.

References

British Heart Foundation (2012). *Coronary Heart Disease Statistics: A Compendium of Health Statistics*. London: BHF.

Davey, P. (2008). *ECG at a Glance*. Oxford: John Wiley & Sons.

Gaunt, H. (2014). Is chest pain always an emergency? *Nursing Times* 110 (44): 12–14.

Jones, B., Higginson, R., and Santos, A. (2010). Critical care: Assessing blood pressure, circulation and intravascular volume. *British Journal of Cardiac Nursing* 19 (3): 153–159.

Marieb, E.N. and Hoehn, K. (2016). *Human Anatomy and Physiology*, 10e. San Francisco: Pearson Benjamin Cummings.

McCance, K.L. and Heuther, S.E. (2018). *Pathophysiology: The Biologic Basis for Disease in Adults and Children*, 8e. St Louis: Mosby.

National Institute of Health and Care Excellence (2010). Chest pain of recent onset: Assessment and diagnosis. www.nice.org.uk/guidance/cg95 (accessed July 2018).

O'Neill, D. (2003). Using a stethoscope in clinical practice in the acute sector. *Nursing Times* 18 (7): 391–394.

Oriolo, V. and Albarran, J.W. (2010). Assessment of acute chest pain. *British Journal of Cardiac Nursing* 5 (12): 587–593.

Rhoads, J. and Wiggins Petersen, S. (2018). *Advanced Health Assessment and Diagnostic Reasoning*, 3e. Burlington: Nelson Bartlett.

Seidel, H.M., Stewart, R.W., Ball, J.W. et al. (2011). *Mosby's Guide to Physical Examination*, 7e. St Louis: Mosby.

Task force for Diagnosis and Treatment of Non ST-Segment Elevation Acute Coronary Syndromes of European Society of Cardiology, Bassand, J.P., Hamm, C.W. et al. (2007). Guidelines for the diagnosis and treatment of non ST-segment elevation acute coronary syndromes. *European Heart Journal* 28 (12): 1598–1660.

Tortora, G.J. and Derrickson, B.H. (2014). *Principles of Anatomy and Physiology*, 14e. Hoboken: Wiley.

Tough, J. (2004). Assessment and management of chest pain. *Nursing Standard* 18 (26): 45–53.

Waugh, A. and Grant, A. (2018). *Ross and Wilson's Anatomy and Physiology in Health and Illness*, 13e. Edinburgh: Elsevier.

Chapter 12

Assessing the gastrointestinal system

Aim

This chapter introduces the reader to the assessment of the gastrointestinal system and the care required for people who experience problems associated with this system.

Learning outcomes

By the end of the chapter the reader will be able to:

1. Provide a brief overview of the gastrointestinal system and its functions
2. Discuss a number of conditions affecting the gastrointestinal system
3. Outline ways in which the nurse assesses the gastrointestinal system
4. Describe care planning related to the gastrointestinal system

Introduction

The functions of the gastrointestinal system and its accessory organs are essential for life. The gastrointestinal system is also known as the gastrointestinal tract, the digestive system, or the alimentary canal. The process of digestion provides nutrients to every cell in the body. If there is a disruption in any of these mechanisms, then the whole body will experience the ramifications. As with other systems, a detailed patient history is required and during the physical examination techniques such as inspection, palpation, percussion, and auscultation will be required. Any deviation that has been highlighted in the assessment could indicate potential gastrointestinal problems.

The gastrointestinal system can be affected primarily by specific disorders and also as a result of pathology elsewhere in the body (secondary). Primary and secondary disturbance can result in a medical/surgical emergency. The nurse has a key role to play in assessing and monitoring the patient with gastrointestinal signs and symptoms in order to identify the potential for the patient's condition to deteriorate as a result of the altered pathophysiological processes or as a result of a life-threatening complication such as infection or haemorrhage (hypovolaemia).

This chapter will provide an overview of the gastrointestinal system, the skills required by the nurse in order to undertake a comprehensive assessment of the system that will enable a diagnosis to be made, and care to be planned, implemented and evaluated. A number of conditions affecting the gastrointestinal system will be discussed.

Fundamentals of Assessment and Care Planning for Nurses, First Edition. Ian Peate.
© 2020 John Wiley & Sons Ltd. Published 2020 by John Wiley & Sons Ltd.

The gastrointestinal system

McErlean (2017) notes that this vast system is approximately 10 m long and traverses the length of the body originating in the mouth through the thoracic, abdominal and pelvic cavities and terminates at the anus (see Figure 12.1). The one major function of the gastrointestinal system is to convert the food eaten into a form that can be used by the cells of the body to carry out their specific functions. The nurse must remember that not all food is eaten (ingested), some patients will receive their nutrition parenterally or enterally.

Review

Provide examples of nutrition that is provided parenterally or enterally.

There are five categories that the activity of the digestive system can be organised into (see Table 12.1). See also Figure 12.2, showing the digestive processes.

Structures and organs make up the gastrointestinal system. The structures of the main gastrointestinal system include:

- Mouth
- Pharynx
- Oesophagus
- Stomach
- Small intestine
- Large intestine

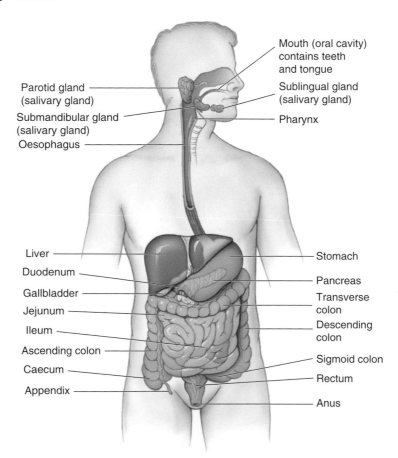

Figure 12.1   The gastrointestinal system.

Table 12.1   The five processes of the gastrointestinal system and their categories.

Activity	Description
Ingestion	The taking of food into the gastrointestinal system.
Propulsion	Transporting the food along the length of the gastrointestinal system. This includes the voluntary process of swallowing and the involuntary process of peristalsis.
Digestion	Breaking down food. This can be achieved mechanically as the person chews (mastication) the food, moving it through the digestive system (a physical process), or chemically by the work of enzymes as they are mixed with the food as it moves through the digestive system. The mechanical process continues in the stomach, where food is further broken apart and more of its surface area is exposed to digestive juices.
Absorption	The products of digestion leave the digestive system, entering the blood or lymph capillaries for distribution to where they are required. Absorption takes place primarily in the small intestine.
Elimination	The waste products of digestion (undigested matter) are excreted from the body as faeces, via the anus.

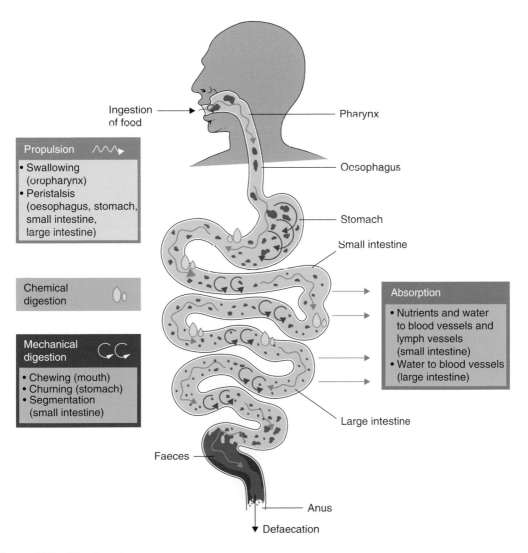

Figure 12.2   The digestive processes.

There are also a number of accessory organs that contribute to the function of the gastrointestinal system and these are:

- Salivary glands
- Liver
- Gall bladder
- Pancreas

Organs of the gastrointestinal system
The Mouth

The mouth (or oral cavity) is where food enters, and it is here where the process of digestion begins. The oral cavity comprises several structures (see Figure 12.3). Food enters the oral cavity in a process called ingestion, the food mixes with saliva. The lips and cheeks are made of muscle and connective tissue; this allows the lips and cheeks to move food that is mixed with saliva around the mouth, as mechanical digestion begins. The teeth contribute to mechanical digestion by the grinding and tearing of food. The process of chewing and mixing food with saliva is known as mastication. The oral cavity is lined with mucous-secreting, stratified squamous epithelial cells, offering some protection against abrasion, the effects of heat, and continuous wear and tear. The lips and cheeks form part of the ability to speak and facial expression.

Tongue

The large, voluntary muscular structure that occupies most of the oral cavity is the tongue. It is attached posteriorly to the hyoid bone and inferiorly by the frenulum (see Figure 12.3). The superior surface of the tongue is covered in stratified squamous epithelium for protection against wear and tear. This surface also contains a number of small projections called papillae. The papillae (or taste buds) contain the nerve endings that are responsible for the sense of taste (Tortora and Derrickson 2014). As well as taste, the tongue is also involved in swallowing (deglutition), holding and moving food around the oral cavity, and speech.

The palate

The palate forms the roof of the mouth consisting of two parts: the hard palate and the soft palate. The hard palate is located anteriorly and is bony. The soft palate lies posteriorly consisting of skeletal muscle and connective tissue (see Figure 12.3). The palate is involved in swallowing. The palatine tonsils lie laterally and are formed of lymphoid tissue. The uvula, a fold of tissue, hangs down from the centre of the soft palate.

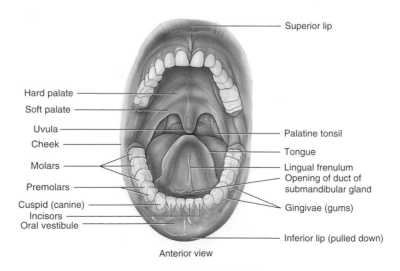

Anterior view

Figure 12.3   The mouth.

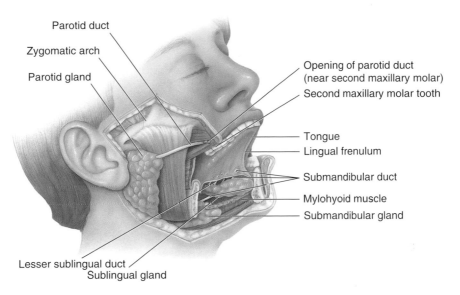

Figure 12.4 The salivary glands.

Teeth

There are 32 permanent teeth. Sixteen are located in the maxilla arch (upper) and 16 are located in the mandible (lower). Canines and incisors are cutting and tearing teeth. Premolars and molars are used for the grinding and chewing of food.

On all teeth, the visible part of the tooth is called the crown. The crown sits above the gum or gingiva. The centre of the tooth is called the pulp cavity. Blood and lymph vessels as well as nerves enter and leave the tooth here. Surrounding this is a calcified matrix, not unlike bone, called the dentine. Surrounding the dentine is a protective material called enamel. The teeth are anchored in a socket with cementum (a bone-like material). The function of the teeth is to chew (masticate) food.

Salivary glands

The three pairs of salivary glands are depicted in Figure 12.4. The parotid glands are the largest, located anterior to the ears. The submandibular glands are located below the jaw on each side of the face. The sublingual glands are the smallest, located in the floor of the mouth.

Saliva is continuously secreted in order to keep the oral cavity moist, parasympathetic fibres that innervate the salivary glands leading to an increased production of saliva in response to the sight, smell or taste of food. Sympathetic fibre activity causes a decreased secretion of saliva. Approximately 1–1.5 l of saliva is secreted daily (in health). Saliva consists of:

- Water
- Salivary amylase
- Mucus
- Mineral salts
- Lysozyme
- Immunoglobulins
- Blood clotting factors

The saliva performs a number of important functions:

- Salivary amylase, a digestive enzyme, is responsible for beginning the breakdown of carbohydrate molecules from complex polysaccharides to the disaccharide maltase.

(a)   (b)

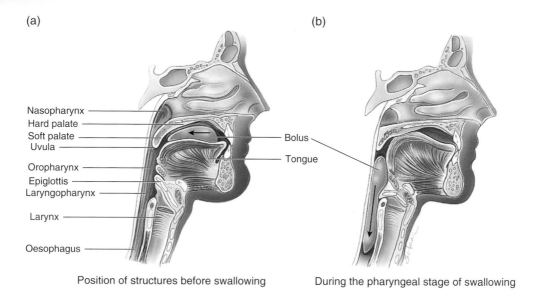

Nasopharynx
Hard palate
Soft palate ——————————————————— Bolus
Uvula
——————————————— Tongue
Oropharynx
Epiglottis
Laryngopharynx

Larynx

Oesophagus

Position of structures before swallowing   During the pharyngeal stage of swallowing

Figure 12.5   Swallowing.

- The fluid nature of saliva helps moisten and lubricate food.
- The continuous secretion of saliva is cleansing, helping to maintain moisture in the oral cavity.
- The oral cavity is an entry route for pathogens from the external environment. Lysozyme, a constituent of saliva, has an antibacterial action.
- Taste is only possible when food substances are moist.

Pharynx

The pharynx consists of three parts:

1. Oropharynx
2. Nasopharynx
3. Laryngopharynx

The nasopharynx is considered a structure of the respiratory system. The oropharynx and the laryngopharynx are passages for food and respiratory gases (see Figure 12.5). The epiglottis is closest to the entrance to the larynx during swallowing and this essential action prevents food from entering the larynx and obstructing respiratory passages.

Swallowing (deglutition)

Once ingested, food has been adequately chewed and formed into a bolus and is ready to be swallowed. Swallowing (deglutition) occurs in three phases.

1. The voluntary phase: The voluntary muscles serving the oral cavity manipulate the food bolus into the oropharynx. The tongue is pressed against the palate, preventing the food from moving forward again.
2. The pharyngeal phase: During this phase, a reflex action is initiated in response to the sensation of the food bolus in the oropharynx. This reflex is coordinated by the swallowing centre in the medulla oblongata and the motor response is contraction of the muscles of the pharynx. The soft palate elevates, closing the nasopharynx and preventing the food bolus from using this route. The larynx moves up and moves forward, allowing the epiglottis to cover the entrance to the larynx so the food bolus cannot move into the respiratory passages.
3. The oesophageal phase: The food bolus moves from the pharynx into the oesophagus. Waves of oesophageal muscle contractions move the food bolus down the length of the oesophagus into the stomach, known as peristalsis (see Figure 12.6).

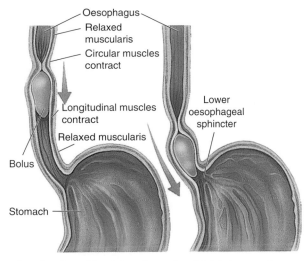

Oesophagus
Relaxed
muscularis
Circular muscles
contract
Longitudinal muscles
contract
Relaxed muscularis
Bolus
Stomach
Lower
oesophageal
sphincter

Anterior view of frontal sections of peristalsis in oesophagus

Figure 12.6   Peristalsis in the oesophagus.

The oesophagus

The food bolus leaves the oropharynx entering the oesophagus. The oesophagus extends from the laryngopharynx to the stomach and is a thick-walled structure, measuring approximately 25 cm in length, lying in the thoracic cavity, posterior to the trachea. Its function is to transport the food bolus from the mouth to the stomach. Thick mucus is secreted by the mucosa of the oesophagus. This aids the passage of the food bolus and protects the oesophagus from abrasion.

The upper oesophageal sphincter regulates the movement of substances into the oesophagus. The lower oesophageal sphincter (known as the cardiac sphincter) regulates the movement of substances from the oesophagus to the stomach. The muscle layer of the oesophagus differs from the rest of the digestive tract, as the superior portion consists of skeletal (voluntary) muscle and the inferior portion consists of smooth (involuntary) muscle. Breathing and swallowing cannot occur at the same time.

The organisation of the gastrointestinal tract

The four layers of tissue or tunicas that exist throughout the length of the digestive tract from oesophagus to anus are shown in Figure 12.7.

The mucosa is the innermost layer. The products of digestion are in contact with this layer as they pass through the digestive tract. The next layer is the lamina propria, which consists of loose connective tissue that has a role in supporting the blood vessels and lymphatic tissue of the mucosa. The outermost layer is the muscularis mucosa, consisting of a thin smooth muscle layer that helps form the gastric pits or the microvilli of the digestive system.

The stomach has three layers of smooth muscle and the upper oesophagus has skeletal muscle. Blood and lymph vessels and the myenteric plexus (a network of sympathetic and parasympathetic nerves) are located between the two layers of smooth muscle. The wavelike contraction and relaxation of this muscle layer (peristalsis) are responsible for moving food along the digestive tract. The outer layer of the digestive tract is the serosa (adventitia), the largest area of serosa is found in the abdominal and pelvic cavities, known as the peritoneum. The peritoneum is a closed sac. The visceral peritoneum covers the organs of the abdominal and pelvic cavity, the parietal peritoneum lines the abdominal wall. A small amount of serous fluid lies between the two layers. The peritoneum has a good blood supply and contains many lymph nodes and lymphatic vessels. It acts as a barrier, protecting the structures it encloses, and can take action to isolate areas of infection to prevent damage to neighbouring structures.

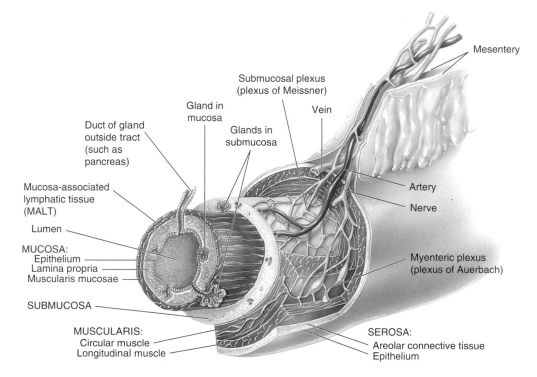

Figure 12.7   Structure of the digestive tract.

The stomach

The stomach is located in the abdominal cavity, lying between the oesophagus superiorly and the duodenum of the small intestine inferiorly. It is divided into regions (see Figure 12.8).

The entrance to the stomach from the oesophagus is via the lower oesophageal sphincter or cardiac sphincter, leading to the cardiac region or cardia in the stomach.

The fundus is the dome-shaped region in the superior aspect of the stomach. The body region occupies the space between the lesser and greater curvature of the stomach, the pyloric region narrows into the pyloric canal. The pyloric sphincter controls the exit of chyme (the food bolus as it leaves the stomach).

The vagus nerve innervates the stomach with parasympathetic fibres that stimulate gastric motility and the secretion of gastric juice. Sympathetic fibres from the celiac plexus reduce gastric activity.

The stomach has the same four layers of tissue as the digestive tract, but with some differences. The muscularis contains three layers of smooth muscle instead of two. It has longitudinal, circular, and oblique muscle fibres. The extra muscle layer enables the churning, mixing, and mechanical digestion of food, as well as supporting the onward journey of the food by peristalsis. The mucosa within the stomach is also different from the rest of the digestive tract. When the stomach is empty, the mucosal epithelia falls into long folds known as rugae. The rugae fill out when the stomach is full. A very full stomach can contain approximately 4 L, whilst an empty stomach contains only about 50 mL (Marieb and Keller 2017). The shape and size of the stomach varies from person to person and depending on the quantity of food stored within it. The mucosa also contains many gastric glands secreting a number of different substances.

Regulation of gastric juice secretion

This is divided into three phases:

1. The cephalic phase: Secretion of gastric juice by sight, taste, or smell of food stimulates gastric juice secretion

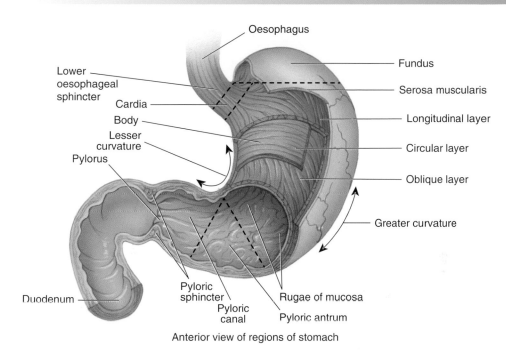

Anterior view of regions of stomach

Figure 12.8 The stomach.

2. The gastric phase: As food enters the stomach, the hormone gastrin is secreted into the bloodstream, stimulating the secretion of gastric juice. The secretion of hydrochloric acid reduces the pH of the stomach contents, when the pH drops below 2 the secretion of gastrin is inhibited.
3. The intestinal phase: As the acidic contents of the stomach enter the duodenum, the hormones secretin and cholecystokinin (CKK) are secreted. These hormones also act to reduce the secretion of gastric juice and gastric motility.

See Figure 12.9 for a diagrammatic representation of the phases of gastric juice secretion.

The small intestine

The primary function of the small intestine is to absorb water and nutrients. The small intestine is approximately 6 m long. When chyme is in the small intestine it is further broken down by mechanical and chemical digestion and absorption of the products of digestion takes place. The small intestine is divided into three parts (see Figure 12.10):

1. The duodenum is approximately 25 cm long and is the entrance to the small intestine.
2. The jejunum, the middle part of the small intestine, is about 2.5 m long.
3. The ileum is around 3.5 m long. It meets the large intestine at the ileocaecal valve. This valve prevents the backflow of the products of digestion from the large intestine back into the small intestine.

Partially digested food enters the small intestine, spending three to six hours moving through it. Smooth muscle activity in the small intestine continues the process of mechanical digestion. Chemical digestion completes the breakdown of the carbohydrates, fats, and proteins. Pancreatic juice, bile from the gall bladder, and intestinal juice contribute to this.

Around 1–2 L of intestinal juice is produced daily in the small intestine. Within the small intestine, any carbohydrates not broken down by the action of salivary amylase will be broken down by pancreatic amylase. Bile emulsifies fat and fatty acids, making it easier for lipase (also from

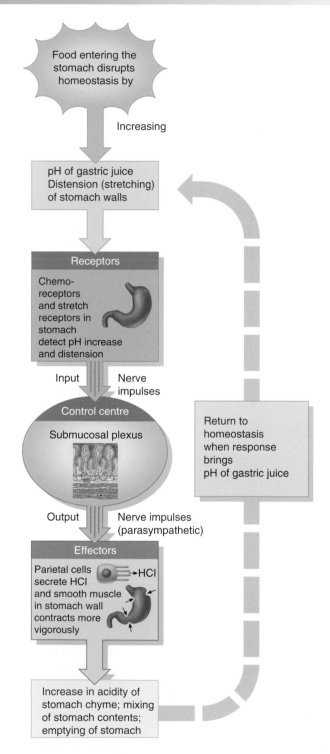

Figure 12.9   Phases of gastric juice secretion.

the pancreatic juice) to break the fats into fatty acids and glycerol. In the stomach proteins are denatured by hydrochloric acid and in the small intestine they are further acted upon by the enzymes trypsin, chymotrypsin, and carboxypeptidase. The end product of protein digestion is tripeptidases, dipeptidases, and amino acids. The functions of the small intestine are summarised in Table 12.2.

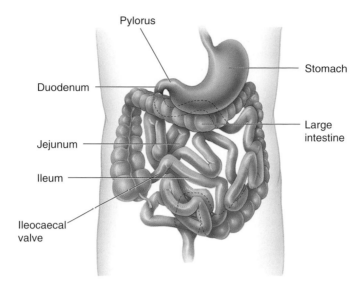

Figure 12.10 The stomach and small intestine.

Table 12.2 Functions of the small intestine.

- Production of mucus to protect the duodenum from the acidic effects of the chyme.
- Secretion of intestinal juice and pancreatic juice from the pancreas increases pH of chyme to facilitate the action of the enzymes.
- Bile enters the small intestine, emulsifying fat so it can be further broken down by the action of lipase.
- Many enzymes are secreted to complete the chemical digestion of carbohydrates, proteins, and fats.
- Mechanical digestion is by peristalsis and segmentation, slowing down to allow adequate mixing and maximum absorption.
- The small intestine is structurally designed with a large surface area for maximum absorption of the products of digestion.
- The majority of nutrients, electrolytes, and water are absorbed in the small intestine.

The pancreas

The pancreas is composed of exocrine and endocrine tissue and measures around 15–20 cm. It consists of a head, body, and tail (see Figure 12.11). The cells of the pancreas are responsible for making the endocrine and exocrine products.

The pancreas releases insulin and glycogen into the blood stream and produces pancreatic enzymes which are released into the duodenum, aiding chemical digestion.

The liver and bile production

The liver is the largest gland, weighing between 1 and 2 kg. It lies under the diaphragm, protected by the ribs, and occupies most of the right hypochondriac region, extending through part of the epigastric region into the left hypochondriac region. The right lobe is the largest of the four liver lobes. On the posterior surface of the liver there is an entry and exit to the organ called the portal fissure. Blood, lymph vessels, nerves, and bile ducts enter and leave the liver through the portal fissure.

The liver produces and secretes up to 1 L of yellow/green alkaline bile per day. Bile is composed of:

- Bile salts such as bilirubin from the breakdown of haemoglobin
- Cholesterol
- Fat-soluble hormones
- Fat
- Mineral salts
- Mucus

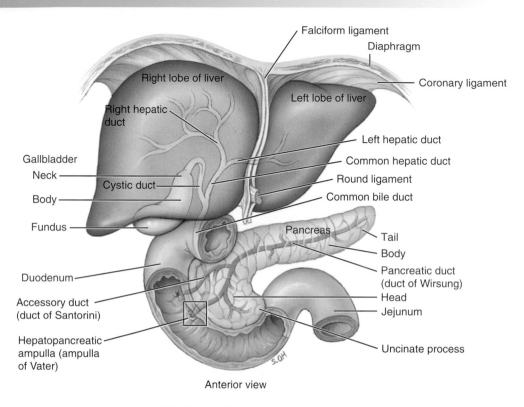

Figure 12.11   The pancreas, gall bladder and liver.

Box 12.1 Functions of the Liver

- Detoxification of drugs – the liver deals with medication, alcohol, ingested toxins as well as the toxins produced by the action of microbes
- Converting ammonia to urea for excretion
- Secretion of bile
- Recycling of erythrocytes
- Deactivation of many hormones, including the sex hormones, thyroxine, insulin, glucagon, cortisol, and aldosterone
- Production of clotting proteins
- Storage of vitamins, minerals, and glycogen
- Synthesis of vitamin A
- Synthesis of iron, vitamin D, K, and B$_{12}$
- Heat production

The function of bile is to emulsify fats, which provides the fat-digesting enzymes (trypsin, chymotrypsin, and carboxypeptidase) with a larger surface area to work on. Bile is stored and concentrated in the gall bladder.

As well as producing bile and the metabolism of carbohydrate, fat, and protein, the liver has a number of additional functions. Functions of the liver are displayed in Box 12.1.

The gall bladder

This is a small, green, pear-shaped, muscular sac, posterior to the liver, functioning as a reservoir for bile. It also concentrates bile by absorbing water. When the smooth muscle walls of the gall bladder contract, bile is expelled into the cystic duct and down into the common bile duct before entering the duodenum via the hepatopancreatic ampulla. CKK (a hormone) stimulates the secretion of pancreatic juice and the relaxation of the hepatopancreatic sphincter. When the sphincter is relaxed, both bile and pancreatic juice can enter the duodenum.

The large intestine

This is also called the colon, receives the contents of the small intestine. The key responsibilities of the large intestine are to:

- Absorb water and electrolytes
- Store food residue
- Eliminate waste products in the form of faeces

Entry to the large intestine is controlled by the ileocaecal sphincter. The sphincter opens in response to the increased activity of the stomach and the action of the hormone gastrin. Once food residue reaches the large intestine it is unable to backflow into the ileum (see Figure 12.12). The large intestine is approximately 1.5 m in length and 7 cm in diameter and is continuous with the small intestine from the ileocaecal valve, terminating at the anus. It usually takes food residue 24–48 hours to pass through the large intestine; 500 mL of food residue enters the large intestine daily and approximately 150 mL leaves as faeces.

Food residue enters the caecum passing up the ascending colon along the transverse colon, down the descending colon and out of the body via the rectum and anus. The caecum is a descending, sac-like opening into the large intestine. The vermiform appendix is a narrow, tube-like structure that leaves the caecum but is closed at its distal end. It is made up of lymphoid tissue and plays a role in immunity. The large intestine mucosa contains a number of goblet cells secreting mucus to ease the passage of faeces and protect the walls of the large intestine.

The food residue from the ileum is fluid when it enters the caecum and contains few nutrients. The small intestine has a responsibility for the absorption of some water. However, the primary function of the large intestine is to absorb water and turn the food residue into semi-solid faeces. The large intestine also absorbs some vitamins, minerals, electrolytes, and drugs.

Faeces are brown, semi-solid materials containing fibre, stercobilin (from the breakdown of bilirubin), water, fatty acids, shed epithelial cells, and microbes. Stercobilin gives faeces its brown colour. An excess of water in faeces results in diarrhoea. This occurs when food residue passes too quickly through the large intestine, failing to absorb water. Conversely, constipation occurs if food residue spends too long in the large intestine. Bacteria present in the colon are responsible for the production of flatus.

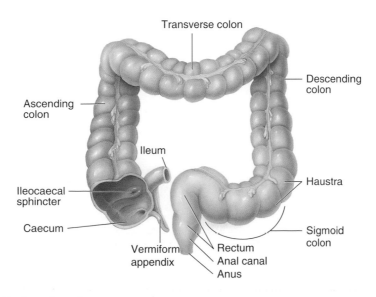

Figure 12.12 The large intestine.

So far

The maintenance of homeostasis is achieved through the ingestion of a balanced diet, containing a variety of elements from each of the food groups, and a fully functioning gastrointestinal system. The functions of the gastrointestinal system and its accessory organs are essential for life.

The gastrointestinal system processes ingested nutrients and breaks them down chemically and mechanically. Accessory structures have a key role to play in providing the digestive tract with bile and pancreatic juice to facilitate the digestion of protein, carbohydrate, and fat. The small intestine provides the large surface area available for the absorption of nutrients, the liver processes the products of digestion. The large intestine plays an excretory role, removing from the body the waste products from digestion and absorbing any remaining water back into the body.

Assessing needs

Understanding the anatomy and physiology of the gastrointestinal system will help the nurse become proficient in assessing this system, it will help the nurse understand some of the issues the person is presenting with and ensure that assessment is patient-centred.

When undertaking a focused gastrointestinal assessment with the patient, subjective and objective data are required. Components of the assessment may include:

- Chief complaint
- Present health status
- Past health history
- Current lifestyle
- Psychosocial status
- Family history
- Physical assessment

When communicating with the patient during history taking and physical examination the nurse must be respectful and ensure procedures are performed in a culturally sensitive manner. Privacy is essential and the nurse needs to be aware of posture, body language, and tone of voice whilst interviewing the patient (Jarvis 2015).

The history

It is important to begin by obtaining a thorough history of abdominal or gastrointestinal complaints. The nurse elicits information about any complaints of gastrointestinal disease or disorders. It is usual for gastrointestinal disease to manifest as the presence of one or more of the following:

- Abdominal or chest pain
- Eructation (belching)
- Gastroesophageal reflux
- Change in appetite
- Weight gain or loss
- Dysphagia
- Intolerance to some foods
- Nausea and vomiting
- Change in bowel habits

To investigate further the nurse should ask about:

- Quality
- Onset
- Location
- Duration
- Frequency
- Severity

Manifestations of gastrointestinal disease can be found in Table 12.3.

Also determine what it is that relieves or worsens the symptoms. Understanding what precipitates or relieves the patient's symptoms will help when undertaking the physical assessment, the planning of care, setting of goals, implementation of the care plan, and evaluation of interventions.

Past health history

Seeking a past health history helps the nurse determine if the patient's problems are new or a recurrence. Ask the patient about any past history of gastrointestinal disorders, for example ulcers, gall bladder disease, gastroesophageal reflux, hepatitis, diverticulitis, inflammatory bowel disease, rectal or gastrointestinal bleeding, appendicitis, hernias. Ask if treatment was received and if so, was it successful? History should also note any past abdominal surgery, trauma, any abdominal problems after the surgery, and tests performed such as X-rays and endoscopies and their results (Jarvis 2015).

Medication history

This is an important aspect of the history. There are many medications that can produce gastrointestinal symptoms. Almost every type of drug has the potential to cause gastrointestinal side effects. Many of the side effects will include nausea, vomiting, diarrhoea, and/or constipation. Ask the patient if they are taking opioids, antibiotics, or laxatives.

Aspirin and non-steroidal anti-inflammatory drugs (NSAIDs), for example, can cause abdominal pain and can also increase the likelihood of gastrointestinal bleeding. Dietary supplements and the use of over-the-counter medications should also be included in the medication history. Also ask about the patient's immunisation status.

At this point in the history taking ask about any known allergies to medications or foods; these allergies can often result in gastrointestinal symptoms

Review

Consult the British National Formulary or another pharmaceutical reference book and look at the side effects that are associated with three NSAIDS. How can the nurse help to reduce those side effects?

Social history and lifestyle risk factors

In taking a complete history, it is important to address lifestyle risk factors and social behaviours that could contribute to unhealthy lifestyles and as such may increase the risk of gastrointestinal disorders.

Ask the patient about the frequency and duration of alcohol consumption, their caffeine intake, and cigarette smoking. Alcohol can cause liver cirrhosis and oesophageal varices. Cigarette smoking and regular ingestion of caffeine can lead to gastroesophageal reflux and gastric ulcers. Also ask about recreational drug use, for example marijuana, opiates, or amphetamines. The use of these drugs can increase or suppress appetite and impact on gastrointestinal function (Shaw 2012).

Family history

There are some gastrointestinal disorders that may be heredity and because of this the nurse must seek a family history. Those disorders with a familial link include:

- Ulcerative colitis
- Colorectal cancer

Table 12.3 Some manifestations of gastrointestinal disease.

Manifestation	Line of investigation
Appetite	Ask if the patient has had any changes in appetite or food intake. If so, seek more information about the change. Appetite and eating can be influenced by a number of factors that could indicate gastrointestinal disease or may be attributed to socioeconomic considerations such as food availability, family norms, peers, and cultural practices. A loss of taste sensation can contribute to loss of appetite and this can result in poor nutrition, particularly in older people. Attempts at voluntary control can be a factor, such as dieting or eating disorders.
Weight gain/loss	If weight loss or gain is substantial or has happened rapidly, this requires further investigation. Dieting to a body weight leaner than recommended health standards is often highly promoted by fashion trends and media. Young people are especially at risk for diet-related alterations in normal gastrointestinal function. Weight loss may also be associated with illness, whilst weight gain could be attributed to fluid retention or a tumour (mass) (Jarvis 2015).
Dysphagia	Those with dysphagia have difficulty swallowing and can also experience pain whilst swallowing. Some people may be completely unable to swallow or may have trouble swallowing liquids, foods or saliva. Eating then becomes a challenge, making it difficult to take in enough calories and fluids to nourish the body. Ask the patient if they have any difficulty swallowing and when the difficulty first occurred. It is important to note what the patient has difficulty swallowing, is it more solids or liquids? Ask the patient about the area where it feels the food gets 'stuck' (Altman 2010). Those patients who have diseases of the nervous system, such as cerebral palsy or Parkinson's disease, frequently have problems swallowing. Stroke or head injury can also affect the coordination of the swallowing muscles or limit sensation in the mouth and throat. An infection or irritation can cause stenosis of the oesophagus. Cancer of the head, neck, or oesophagus can also cause swallowing problems. The treatment required for these types of cancers can cause dysphagia. Injuries or trauma of the head, neck, and chest may also result in swallowing problems (National Institute of Health 2014).
Food intolerance	Ask if the patient has any intolerance to certain foods, if so, determine which foods and the type of reaction. Do not confuse food intolerance and food allergies. An intolerance to certain foods is usually predicated on the presence of a gastrointestinal imbalance, for example having too little of a particular enzyme that can hamper effective breakdown and use of the food by the body. Food intolerance can be related to disorders such as coeliac disease, diabetes mellitus, and inflammatory bowel disease. Symptoms of intolerance to a specific food could include stomach discomfort, flatus, bloating, eructation, abdominal pain, and diarrhoea. Food intolerance can also increase with older adults (Ahmed and Haboubi 2010).
Nausea and vomiting	These can be side effects of medications and a manifestation of many diseases. Ask the patient about the frequency of these symptoms. Nausea and vomiting may also indicate food poisoning. Questions about types of food eaten in the past 24 hours should be asked to rule out potential poisoning. Also enquire about any recent travel abroad and where to, parasitic infection, hepatitis, and diarrhoea can result from ingesting contaminated food or water. If vomiting is present, seek information about the amount, frequency, colour, and odour of the vomitus. Ask if there is any blood in the vomit or if the vomit appears to be like coffee grounds. Haematemesis, or blood in the vomitus, is a common symptom of gastric or duodenal ulcers and could also indicate oesophageal varices. Coffee ground vomit signifies an 'old' gastrointestinal bleed. The old, partially digested blood resembles coffee grounds (Jarvis 2015).
Change in bowel habit	A common manifestation of gastrointestinal disease is a change in bowel habits, particular emphasis should be placed on these. The frequency, colour, and consistency of bowel movements should be assessed. Assess also the use of laxatives. Passing a black, tarry stool may indicate melaena, suggestive of an upper gastrointestinal bleed. However, they may simply be from the ingestion of iron supplements. Bright red blood in the stools could indicate haemorrhoids or localised lower gastrointestinal bleed. If the nurse has any concern about blood in the stool, then this must be reported immediately as the patient may be bleeding. The person's haemodynamic status must be assessed quickly.

- Peptic ulcers
- Gastric cancers
- Alcoholism
- Crohn's disease

Ask if anyone in the family has a gastrointestinal disorder.

Cultural considerations

In Europe (2012), the highest world age-standardised incidence rates for stomach cancer are in Belarus for men and Albania for women.

Source: Cancer Research UK (2014).

Ashkenazi Jews (originally from Central and Eastern Europe) are a particular population that is at high risk for Crohn's disease. Crohn's disease is two to four times more prevalent amongst people of Ashkenazi ancestry, compared to those of non-Jewish European ancestry.

Source: Kenny et al. (2012).

Psychosocial health

Stress is known to cause gastroesophageal reflux. Determine stress levels, type of employment (or not), exercise habits, and dental/oral hygiene. How does the person cope with increased stress levels, do they have and use coping mechanisms? Seek information about family life and support systems at home.

Nutritional assessment

A nutritional assessment is also required. The nutritional assessment is important for a number of reasons. A detailed nutritional assessment can help to identify those who are at risk for malnutrition and it can also provide a baseline for subsequent nutritional assessments that may take place.

Jarvis (2015) suggests that some patients will require a thorough nutritional assessment, including those:

- Who have recent unintentional weight loss
- Who are receiving chemotherapy or radiation
- With recent weight gain
- Who have food allergies or intolerance
- With decreased appetite
- Receiving multiple medications
- Experiencing alterations in the sense of taste
- With a dieting history
- Who may have difficulty chewing or swallowing
- Who are vomiting
- With mobility problems
- Who have diarrhoea
- Who are unable to feed themselves
- Who have recently undergone surgery or have a major illness or injury
- Who have substance abuse history
- With chronic conditions
- Who may be socially isolated or a potential for social isolation
- On a low income

The Malnutrition Universal Screening Tool (MUST) (BAPEN 2018) can be used to help with assessment and identification of those patients at risk of nutritional problems. The dietician may be the person who undertakes a detailed and thorough assessment, local policy and procedure must be adhered to.

Review

Revise how to calculate a BMI. What are the differences between these three categories?

1. Underweight
2. Overweight
3. Obese

The physical examination

Along with the health history, the physical examination can help the nurse arrive at a diagnosis and plan patient care accordingly. The physical examination should be undertaken in a systematic manner and will include examination of the mouth, abdomen, and rectum.

Prior to undertaking the examination, the nurse must ensure the room or wherever the examination is to take place is in a quiet private area that is warm, as the person being examined will have some aspect of the anatomy exposed during the procedure. A good light source is required and a pen torch will be needed. Explain to the person what is to happen and that there may be some aspects of the examination that may be uncomfortable.

6Cs

Throughout the procedure continually explain to the patient what is to happen, what is happening, and what is to happen next. Always seek permission from the patient and be guided by them as the examination proceeds.

When carrying out the assessment, the nurse uses a number of skills including inspection, auscultation, percussion, and palpation. Jarvis (2015) suggests that these techniques should be undertaken in an organised manner, from least disturbing or invasive to most invasive to the patient. Inspection is the first part of the sequence as this is non-invasive. This is followed by auscultation; the nurse should auscultate the abdomen prior to percussion or palpation as this will prevent production of false bowel sounds, which may lead to an inaccurate assessment.

For an accurate assessment of the abdomen the patient should be relaxed and comfortable, with the knees supported and arms at the sides, and the bladder should be empty.

The mouth

Wearing gloves, inspection and palpation are employed to examine the mouth. Inspect the mouth and jaw, noting colour, asymmetry, and any swelling. Inspect the inner and outer lips, observe for angular stomatitis. Using a pen torch, examine the oral mucosa (is it dry? (xerostomia)), mouth ulcers, oral candidiasis, teeth, and gums. Take note of any bleeding, ulcerations, caries, missing or loose teeth, and determine if there are any colour changes or rashes in the oral cavity. Is the patient edentulous? Do they wear dentures? If so, partial or full? Do the dentures fit? Palpate the gums inner lips and cheeks noting tenderness, lumps, and lesions. When assessing the tongue observe for glossitis (swelling), coating, tremor, and unusual halitosis (bad breath odours). In examining the pharynx, a tongue depressor is required. Gently press the tongue depressor down on the middle of the tongue (the patient may retch). When the patient says 'ahh' this reveals the pharynx, and this should be observed for any colour changes, uvular deviation, tonsillar irregularities, lesions, plaques, and exudate.

The abdomen

In order to promote clear communication, for instance about the location of a patient's abdominal pain or a suspicious mass, the abdomen is often divided up into four quadrants. For landmarks, see Table 12.4 and Figure 12.13.

Table 12.4 The abdominopelvic four quadrants.

Quadrant	Content
Right upper quadrant (RUQ) (Right hypochondriac)	Right lobe liver Gall bladder Pylorus Duodenum Head of pancreas Hepatic flexure colon Aspects of the ascending and transverse colon
Left upper quadrant (LUQ) (Left hypochondriac)	Left lobe liver Stomach Body of pancreas Splenic flexure of colon Aspects of transverse and descending colon
Right lower quadrant (RLQ) (Right iliac region)	Caecum and appendix Aspects of the ascending colon
Left lower quadrant (LLQ) (Left iliac region)	Sigmoid colon Aspects of the descending colon

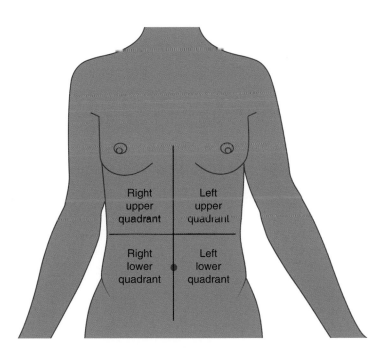

Figure 12.13 The four quadrants.

Prior to assessing the abdomen using inspection, auscultation, percussion, and palpation ensure that the patient's bladder is empty, wash your hands, and provide cover for the genitalia and chest. You are required to visualise the entire abdomen. Place a small pillow under the patient's knees so as to help relax the abdominal muscles. Request the patient keeps his/her arms at the sides. Explain clearly what you are going to do and during uncomfortable procedures ask the patient to take deep breaths. If the patient is experiencing pain ask them to point to the area where the pain is, assess these areas last as this can help prevent the patient from tensing the abdominal muscles. The hands and the stethoscope should be warmed prior to placing on the abdomen.

Using a four abdominal quadrants approach (this approach is most commonly used), imagine subdividing the abdomen with one horizontal and one vertical line that intersects at just above the umbilicus. This provides the four abdominal quadrants.

Inspect the abdomen with the four abdominal quadrants in mind and imagine the organs in each quadrant. Look at the abdomen and note colour and symmetry. Are there any bumps, bulges, lesions, scars, rashes, skin excoriation, or masses (there may be a malignancy or organomegaly)? Does the patient have a stoma? If there are any bulges this may indicate a hernia, a distended bladder. Observe for the presence of spider naevi, enlarged veins.

The abdomen in people of average weight should appear flat to rounded (in slim patients it can appear concave), and its shape and contour should be noted. A protruding abdomen may indicate ascites, abdominal distension, or pregnancy.

Ask the patient to raise the head and shoulders, if the umbilicus protrudes this could indicate an umbilical hernia. The skin covering the abdomen should be smooth and uniform in colour. Note that any signs of striae could be caused by pregnancy, weight gain or ascites. Observe and note any scars (surgical or otherwise) on the abdomen. Abdominal pulsations and movement cannot normally be seen (a central pulsatile mass may imply an abdominal aortic aneurysm). If the nurse observes visible, rippling waves of peristalsis, this should be reported immediately as it might indicate bowel obstruction.

Review

Complete the names of the nine regions in the abdominal chart:

1............................
2............................
3............................
4............................
5............................
6............................
7............................
8............................
9............................

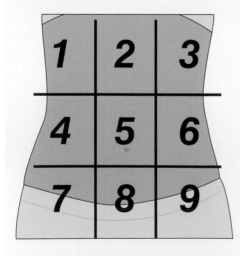

Auscultation

The patient should be positioned comfortably in the supine position (Plevris and Parkes 2018). The diaphragm of the stethoscope should be placed lightly on the right lower quadrant, just below and to the right of the umbilicus. The nurse auscultates each quadrant in a clockwise fashion and in so doing notes the character and quality of bowel sounds. Breum et al. (2015) have questioned the

Table 12.5 Bowel sounds.

Bowel sound	How it is produced	Potential cause
Normal bowel sounds, gurgling. Normal bowel sounds can sometimes be heard without the use of a stethoscope.	Occurs as the intestine is transporting fluid and digested food through the lumen of the intestine.	A normal functioning intestine
Hypoactive bowel sounds (silent abdomen). Low in frequency and volume. Tinkling-like sound.	As the intestine is transporting fluid and digested food through the lumen of the intestine, this is at a decreased rate.	Paralytic ileus Peritonitis Vascular obstruction Late intestinal obstruction can occur after the administration of certain drugs, for example opioids.
Hyperactive bowel sounds.	The intestine is transporting fluid, digested food, and possibly air through the lumen of the intestine at an increased rate.	Gastroenteritis/diarrhoea Inflammatory bowel disease Early intestinal obstruction Anxiety

Source: Jarvis (2015).

accuracy of assessing for bowel sounds specifically when attempting to determine if bowel sounds have returned, for example post-operatively. If bowel sounds are not heard, in order to determine if they are truly absent, listen for a total of five minutes (Jarvis 2015).

Bowel sounds echo the underlying movements of the intestines. It is normal to hear high-pitched clicking and gurgling sounds approximately every 5–15 seconds as air mixes with fluid during peristalsis. The noises vary in frequency, pitch, and intensity and are loudest before a meal.

It is suggested that the nurse listen to bowel sounds for a full minute before deciding if they are normal, hypoactive, or hyperactive. See Table 12.5 relating to the different bowel sounds produced and what they might indicate.

The abdomen should also be auscultated for vascular sounds using the bell of the stethoscope (see Figure 12.14 for the sites where abdominal vascular sounds can be heard). This skill needs to be perfected and it can take time to develop proficiency. Using firm pressure, listen over the aorta and renal, iliac, and femoral arteries for bruits, venous hums, and friction rubs. Bruits are 'swishing' sounds that are heard over major arteries during systole or, less commonly, systole and diastole. The areas should be examined carefully for bruits.

Percussion

Percussion is used to provoke tenderness or sounds that give clues to underlying problems. When the nurse percusses directly over suspected areas of tenderness, also monitor the patient's face for any signs of discomfort. Percussion requires skill and practice; it is an intricate aspect of the physical examination. Initially, you may find that this skill is a bit awkward to perform, so watch other skilled practitioners as they undertake percussion. It takes a while to develop an ear for what is resonant and what is not.

Review

Have you watched a colleague undertake percussion? If so, what skills and knowledge were required in order to carry out this activity effectively?

How might you develop your percussion skills?

When percussing, ask the patient to lie on a level examination table that is at a comfortable height for both of you. The patient should be dressed in a gown and underwear. Take a spare bed sheet (or cover) and drape it over the lower body so that it just covers the upper edge of their underwear (or so that it crosses the top of the pubic region if completely undressed). This allows you to fully expose

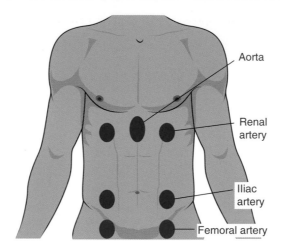

Aorta

Renal
artery

Iliac
artery

Femoral artery

Figure 12.14   Auscultating abdominal sounds.

the abdomen whilst at the same time ensuring patient dignity. The gown can be withdrawn so that the area extending from just below the breasts to the pelvic brim is entirely uncovered. Take note that the superior margin of the abdomen extends beneath the rib cage. Percussion is performed over the abdominal regions.

Percussion is based on the difference in pitch between the sounds caused by tapping on the body wall. The auditory response to tapping depends on the ease with which the body wall vibrates. It is influenced by underlying organs, strength of the stroke, as well as the state of the body wall. There are three main medical percussion sounds

1. Resonance (heard over lungs)
2. Tympany (heard over the air-filled bowel loops)
3. Dullness (heard over fluid or solid organs)

Take note

Think anatomically.
   When looking, listening, feeling, and percussing, imagine what organs are in the area that you are examining. When thinking in anatomical terms, this will remind you of what resides in a particular quadrant and as such what might be identifiable during normal and pathological states.

The contrast between dullness versus tympany or resonance allows for determination of the size and margins of organs and masses. It also allows for the identification of fluid accumulation and those areas of consolidation.

Prior to undertaking percussion, wash and warm the hands and explain to the patient what you intend to do. Place the left hand firmly against the abdominal wall so that only the middle finger is resting on the skin. Strike the distal interphalangeal joint of the left middle finger two or three times with the tip of the right middle finger. Special note should be made if percussion produces pain. This can occur if there is underlying inflammation, for example peritonitis. The liver and spleen are the two solid organs which are percussable in the normal patient. In most cases, the liver will be entirely covered by the ribs. Sometimes, an edge may protrude a centimetre or two below the costal margin. The spleen is smaller and is entirely protected by the ribs, when the spleen is enlarged (splenomegaly) percussion in the left upper quadrant (left hypochondriac region) will produce a dull tone.

Palpation

Another commonly used physical examination technique is palpation, which requires the nurse to touch the patient with different parts of the hand, employing variable degrees of pressure. Great care is required when palpating the abdomen. During light palpation, the nurse is required to press the skin about to 1.5–2 cm with the pads of the fingers. When using deep palpation, the finger pads are used to compress the skin about 3–5 cm.

Prior to palpating the nurse washes and warms the hands and begins by palpating lightly at first then deeply, noting any signs of muscle guarding, rigidity, masses, or tenderness.

Undertake palpation of tender areas last. Only if indicated, palpate the liver margins, the spleen, or the kidneys and percuss the abdomen for general tympany, liver span, splenic dullness, costovertebral angle tenderness, presence of fluid wave, or shifting dullness with ascites (Jarvis 2015).

When palpating this allows the nurse to assess for texture, tenderness, temperature, moisture, pulsations, masses, and the internal organs. Normally, you should not provoke tenderness when using light or deep palpation of the abdomen. If the inguinal lymph nodes are palpated, these should be small and freely moveable.

Local areas of tenderness can be identified on palpation, with rebound tenderness or guarding. If present, this may reflect an underlying pathological condition. There are many reasons why a person has a palpable mass, which may indicate a tumour or hernia. If the mass is palpable in the right iliac region this could signify Crohn's disease or an appendix abscess. A pulsatile mass may identify an abdominal aortic aneurysm.

Abdominal pain

Bates and Plevris (2013) suggest that abdominal pain is one of the most common presentations in those people who attend emergency departments. Al-Maqbali (2013) notes that there are a number of reasons why a person may have abdominal pain, for example abdominal trauma (road traffic collision, stabbing), gastric ulcers, bowel obstruction, peritonitis, inflammatory disease, or cholecystitis. Types of abdominal pain are discussed in Table 12.6.

Take note

Older people tend to show less-specific signs and symptoms and to present later in the course of their illness.

Source: Lyon and Clarke (2006).

Table 12.6   Types of abdominal pain and possible causes.

Type of Pain	Potential cause
Gnawing or burning pain	Gastritis, gastric ulcer, gastroesophageal reflux disease
Cramping, colicky	Biliary colic, irritable bowel disease, diarrhoea, constipation, flatulence, food allergy, menstruation, urinary tract infection
Chronic cramping	Appendicitis, Crohn's disease, diverticulitis
Sharp or stabbing	Pancreatitis, cholecystitis

If the patient is experiencing abdominal pain, request that they point, if possible, to the exact location of the pain, and ask how and when it began. Abdominal pain can be classified as:

- Visceral
- Parietal
- Referred

Visceral pain

This is often described as dull, crampy, squeezing, or aching. It may be continuous or sporadic. The patient may find it difficult to localise, it may be located over an abdominal organ (Jarvis 2015).

Take note

Visceral pain that is associated with conditions such as gallstones, acute pancreatitis, acute appendicitis and diverticulitis are the most common reasons for visits to outpatient and inpatient gastrointestinal clinics.

Source: International Association for the Study of Pain (2018).

Parietal pain

Parietal pain typically arises from inflammation over the peritoneum. Peritoneal inflammation frequently implies an underlying emergency, and this should be assessed swiftly (Jarvis 2015). Parietal pain is often intense, constant and on one side. It can be exacerbated by extension of the lower extremity on the affected side, by coughing, or causing rebound tenderness.

Referred pain

This kind of pain is usually visceral pain, felt in another area of the body when a common nerve pathway is shared. It happens with specific gastrointestinal disorders, for example appendicitis, gall bladder disease, and pancreatitis.

Take note

The brain sometimes gets confused and can lead you to think that one part of the body hurts, when actually another part of the body, far removed from the pain, is the real source of the problem. This important phenomenon is known as referred pain. Shoulder pain, for example, may be a sign of something subtly going on in the liver, gall bladder, stomach, or spleen. Conditions as varied as liver abscesses, gallstones, gastric ulcers, and ruptured spleen can all trigger shoulder pain.

Using PQRST for pain assessment

The use of the PQRST mnemonic can be helpful in assessing abdominal pain and other gastrointestinal symptoms. It provides an approach in which communication to other healthcare providers will be efficient and informative. The tool is valuable in accurately describing, assessing, and documenting a patient's pain. The method also helps in the selection of appropriate pain medication and evaluating the patient's response to treatment (see Table 12.7).

Locations of pain

Table 12.8 provides an overview of abdominal pain, location, and the possible causes.

When assessing abdominal pain, the patient history is very important in determining if the pain is chronic or acute and if it is related to inflammation, mechanical obstruction, or infection. Altman

Table 12.7   Using the PQRST tool to assess, describe, and document pain.

Aspect	Using the tool
Provocation/palliation	What were you doing when the pain began? What do you think caused it? What makes it better or worse? **What seems to trigger it:** Stress Position Certain activities **What relieves it?** Medications Massage Heat/cold Changing position Being active Resting **What aggravates it?** Movement Bending Lying down Walking Standing
Quality/quantity	What does it feel like? Use words to describe the pain, for example sharp, dull, stabbing, burning, crushing, throbbing, nauseating, shooting, twisting, or stretching.
Region/radiation	Where is the pain located? Does the pain radiate? Where? Does it feel as if it is travelling/moving around? Did it start elsewhere and is now localised to one spot?
Severity scale	How severe is the pain, on a scale of 0–10, with zero being no pain and 10 being the worst pain ever? Does it restrict your ability to perform the activities of living? How bad is it at its worst? Does it force you to sit down, lie down, slow down? How long does an episode go on for?
Timing	When/at what time did the pain begin? How long did it last? How often does it occur: Hourly Daily Weekly Monthly Is it sudden or gradual? What were you doing when you first felt it? When do you usually experience it: Daytime Night Early morning Are you ever woken by it? Does it lead to anything else? Are there other signs and symptoms that accompany it? Does it ever occur before, during, or after meals? Does it occur seasonally, for example is it worse in the winter than the summer?

213

(2010) notes that physical examination techniques can be employed to assist with the assessment in acute abdominal pain, such as the iliopsoas muscle test, obturator test, and Blumberg test.

As well as the history and the physical examination there are a number of blood tests (values) that can also help in undertaking an assessment of the patient's gastrointestinal system. The blood test results should be looked at closely and considered collectively in the context of the history and the examination.

Table 12.8 Abdominal pain, location, and potential causes.

Right		Left
Right hypochondriac region Gall stones Pancreatitis Gastric ulcer Hepatic and biliary tract disorders	*Epigastric region* Gastric ulcer Gastroesophageal reflux Gall stones Pancreatitis Epigastric hernia Hepatic and biliary tract disorder	*Left hypochondriac region* Gastric ulcer Gastritis Duodenal ulcer Biliary colic Pancreatitis Splenic disorders
Right lumbar region Renal stones Urine infection Constipation Lumbar hernia Hepatic and biliary tract disorders	*Umbilical region* Pancreatitis Gastric ulcer Inflammatory bowel disease Umbilical hernia	*Left lumbar region* Renal stones Diverticular disease Constipation Inflammatory bowel disease
Right iliac region Appendicitis Inguinal hernia Constipation Gynaecological disorders	*Hypogastrium* Urine infection Appendicitis Diverticular disease Inflammatory bowel disease Gynaecological disorders Prostatitis	*Left iliac region* Diverticular disease Inguinal hernia Gynaecological disorders

Source: Adapted Tintinalli et al. (2011) and Talley and Connor (2013).

So far

There are many causes of abdominal pain, ranging from non-acute presentations such as a urinary tract infection to acute life-threatening presentations such as an abdominal aortic aneurysm. The intricacies of some abdominal disorders mean that those with abdominal pain may have various physiological and psychological needs. Nurses have a key role in assessing the holistic needs of patients who experience abdominal pain. The type of abdominal pain may give clues to the nurse as to the cause of the pain.

The nurse should try to obtain as complete a history as possible, this is usually the foundation of an accurate diagnosis. The history should include a complete description of the patient's pain and associated symptoms. The physical examination and the assessment of blood tests can help make a diagnosis.

Oswald (Ossie) Samuda (Son)

Ossie's mother brought Ossie to the Emergency Department (ED) as she was concerned about him. His mother told staff in the ED that Ossie 'has not been right' for a few days. Ossie's chief complaint was abdominal pain. Analgesia was prescribed and administered.

Ossie was off school for two days. Ossie had experienced several episodes of nausea and vomiting and had pain in his right iliac region radiating to the umbilical area, he looked unwell. Ossie had previously enjoyed good health with no relevant past medical history. Ossie had not eaten for 48 hours, he was constipated, his skin was dry, he was dehydrated and had a pyrexia of 38.2 °C. His other vital signs were taken, reported, and recorded. Ossie's clinical history was gained, a physical examination was undertaken and various other diagnostic tests (including an abdominal ultrasound) were carried out. Blood was obtained for various investigations (Ossie had an elevated white blood count (leucocytosis)).

Working with Ossie and his mother, when asked where the pain was Ossie pointed to the right iliac region and he also moved his finger towards the umbilical region. Ossie was reluctant to move. As well as including details of the location and radiation, type, onset, duration, and severity of the pain during history taking, it was also ascertained if there were any other symptoms. From an emotional perspective, Ossie was clearly upset and not saying very much, he held his mother's hand throughout the assessment. The severity of pain and its duration, from onset to presentation and other findings, were reported and recorded and local policy and procedure concerning documentation was adhered to.

Auscultation of the abdomen was undertaken, which revealed borborygmi that could be heard loudly. Percussion was undertaken. Palpation was performed gently and with warm hands, beginning with light palpation. Rebound tenderness was noted during examination of Ossie. A digital rectal examination was not performed due to the possibility of exacerbating his pain and discomfort.

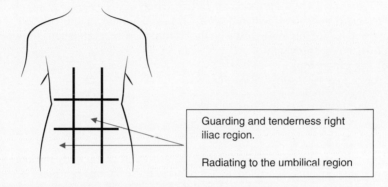

Guarding and tenderness right iliac region.

Radiating to the umbilical region

The Alvarado (1986) scoring system was used as a part of Ossie's assessment, the tool can help to confirm a diagnosis of appendicitis. This scoring system considers signs, symptoms, and laboratory findings in suspected cases of acute appendicitis.

Ossie presented with pain in the right iliac region migrating to the umbilical region, he was nauseous and had vomited, palpation revealed tenderness in the right iliac region with rebound pain, Ossie was pyrexial with anorexia and had a high white blood count.

Andersson and Andersson (2008) and Jang et al. (2008) have determined that the Alvarado scoring system has high sensitivity and accuracy when making a diagnosis of appendicitis. The Alvarado scoring system uses the acronym MANTRELS to aid diagnosis (see Table 12.9).

Using the Alvarado scoring system, calculate a score for Ossie.

In a systematic review of the Alvarado score and prediction Ohle et al. (2011) suggest that a score of:

1–4 Discharge
5–6 Observe and admit
7–10 Surgery

Table 12.9   The Alvarado scoring system using he acronym MANTRELS.

		Score
Symptoms	**M**igration to right iliac region	1
	Anorexia	1
	Nausea and vomiting	1
Signs	**T**enderness of right iliac region	2
	Rebound pain	1
	Elevated temperature	1
Laboratory	**L**eucocytosis	2
	or **S**hift of leucocyte count to the left (this indicated an increase in the percentage of neutrophils)	1
	Total	

A diagnosis of appendicitis was made, and this was explained to Ossie and he was admitted for surgery. A laparoscopic appendectomy was performed under general anaesthetic and Ossie made an uneventful recovery.

The DisDAT assessment tool

The DisDAT is a disability distress assessment tool and is intended to help identify distress cues in those who as a result of cognitive impairment or physical illness have severely limited communication. The tool has been designed to describe a person's usual content cues, thereby enabling distress cues to be identified in a clearer way. The tool is not a scoring tool. It documents a record against which subtle changes can be compared. This information can be transferred with the person to any environment. This is just the first step in the process. When distress has been identified, the usual clinical decisions are made by professionals, but this tool assists with the client/patient/nurse relationship, which in turn will help you improve the care provision.

The DisDAT assessment tool:
http://prc.coh.org/PainNOA/Dis%20DAT_Tool.pdf.

Conclusion

The gastrointestinal system supplies nutrients to every cell of the body through the processes of digestion, transport, and absorption. If disruption to these various processes occurs, then there is potential for deterioration in the person's health and wellbeing.

When the nurse asks explicit questions regarding the patient's gastrointestinal history, undertaking focused abdominal examination techniques will help in being able to assess for changes in gastrointestinal function. Any alterations noted in the nurse's findings could indicate actual or potential problems. When the nurse has an understanding of the gastrointestinal system and is skilled in undertaking a focused gastrointestinal assessment this provides for speedy interventions that could have a positive impact on the patient's health and wellbeing.

Assessing abdominal pain can be complex. This chapter has provided some insight into how pain might be assessed in the care setting using a range of tools and a focus on a person with a learning disability.

References

Ahmed, T. and Haboubi, N. (2010). Assessment and management of nutrition in older people and its importance to health. *Clinical Interventions in Ageing* 5: 207–216.

Al-Maqbali, M.A. (2013). Appendicitis: a case study. *Nursing Standard* 27 (42): 35–41.

Altman, G.B. (2010). *Fundamental and Advanced Nursing Skills*, 3e. New York: Delmar.

Alvarado, A. (1986). A practical score for the early diagnosis of acute appendicitis. *Annals of Emergency Medicine* 15 (5): 557–564.

Andersson, M. and Andersson, R.E. (2008). The appendicitis inflammatory response score: a tool for the diagnosis of acute appendicitis that outperforms the Alvarado score. *World Journal of Surgery* 32 (8): 1843–1849.

BAPEN (2018). Introducing MUST. www.bapen.org.uk/screening-and-must/must/introducing-must (accessed July 2018).

Bates, C.M. and Plevris, J.N. (2013). Clinical evaluation of abdominal pain in adults. *Medicine* 41 (2): 81–86.

Breum, B.M., Rud, B., Kirkegaard, T., and Nordentoft, T. (2015). Accuracy of abdominal auscultation for bowel obstruction. *World Journal of Gastroenterology* 21 (34): 10018–10024.

Cancer Research UK (2014) Stomach cancer incidence statistics. www.cancerresearchuk.org/health-professional/cancer-statistics/statistics-by-cancer-type/stomach-cancer/incidence#heading-Eleven (accessed July 2018).

International Association for the Study of Pain (2018) Visceral pain. www.iasp-pain.org/GlobalYear/VisceralPain (accessed July 2018).

Jang, S.O., Kim, B.S., and Moon, D.J. (2008). Application of Alvarado score in patients with suspected appendicitis. *The Korean Journal of Gastroenterology* 52 (1): 27–31.

Jarvis, C. (2015). *Physical Examination and Health Assessment*, 7e. St Louis: Elsevier.

Kenny, E.E., Pe'er, I., Karban, A. et al. (2012). A genome-wide scan of Ashkenazi Jewish Crohn's disease suggests novel susceptibility loci. *PLoS* https://doi.org/10.1371/journal.pgen.1002559. (accessed July 2018).

Lyon, C. and Clarke, D.C. (2006). Diagnosis of acute abdominal pain in older patients. *American Family Physician* 174 (9): 1537–1544.

Marieb, E. and Keller, S. (2017). *Essentials of Human Anatomy and Physiology*, 12e. Boston: Pearson.

McErlean, L. (2017). The digestive system. In: *Fundamentals of Anatomy and Physiology for Nursing and Healthcare Students*, 2e (ed. I. Peate and M. Nair), 257–297. Oxford: Wiley.

National Institute of Health (NIH) (2014) Dysphagia. www.nidcd.nih.gov/sites/default/files/Documents/health/voice/NIDCD-Dysphagia.pdf (accessed July 2018).

Ohle, R., O'Reilly, F., Obrien, K. et al. (2011) The Alvarado Score for predicting acute appendicitis: A systematic review. *BMC Medicine* www.ncbi.nlm.nih.gov/pmc/articles/PMC3299622

Plevris, J. and Parkes, R. (2018). The gastrointestinal system. In: *Macleod's Clinical Examination*, 14e (ed. J.A. Innes, A.R. Dover and K. Fairhurst), 93–117. Edinburgh: Elsevier.

Shaw, M. (2012). *Assessment Made Incredibly Easy*, 5e. Philadelphia: Lippincott.

Talley, N.J. and Connor, S. (2013). *Clinical Examination: A Systematic Guide to Physical Diagnosis*, 7e. Sydney: Elsevier.

Tintinalli, J.E., Stapczynski, J.S., Ma, J.S. et al. (2011). *Tintinalli's Emergency Medicine: A Comprehensive Study Guide*, 8e. New York: McGraw-Hill.

Tortora, G.J. and Derrickson, B.H. (2014). *Principles of Anatomy and Physiology*, 14e. New Jersey: Wiley.

Chapter 13

Assessing the renal system

Aim

This chapter introduces the reader to the assessment of the renal system and the care required for people who may experience problems related to this system.

Learning outcomes

By the end of the chapter the reader will be able to:

1. Provide a brief overview of the renal system and its functions
2. Discuss a number of conditions that can affect the renal system
3. Outline the various ways in which the nurse undertakes an assessment of the renal system
4. Describe care planning that is related to the renal system

Introduction

The renal system has a number of components and plays a key role in maintaining homeostasis. It is the responsibility of the kidneys to filter the blood, remove waste products, and produce urine. The formation of urine is achieved through the processes of filtration, selective reabsorption, and excretion. The kidneys also have an endocrine function, secreting hormones such as renin and erythropoietin. The urinary bladder stores the urine and releases this during the act of micturition.

Having an understanding of the various roles and functions of the renal system including those component parts can help the nurse undertake a holistic assessment as they strive to provide safe and effective care to those they offer care to.

The renal system

The renal system is also known as the urinary system consists of the:

- Kidneys
- Ureters
- Urinary bladder
- Urethra

The organs of the renal system ensure that a stable internal environment is maintained for the survival of cells and tissues in the body (see Figure 13.1).

Fundamentals of Assessment and Care Planning for Nurses, First Edition. Ian Peate.
© 2020 John Wiley & Sons Ltd. Published 2020 by John Wiley & Sons Ltd.

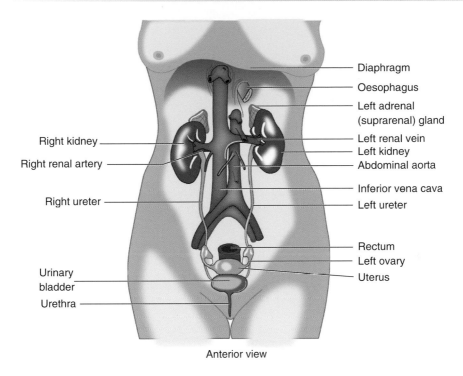

Anterior view

Figure 13.1   The renal system.

Table 13.1   Functions of the kidneys.

- Filtration
- Regulation of blood volume
- Regulation of osmolarity
- Secretion of renin and erythropoietin
- Maintenance of acid–base balance
- Synthesis of vitamin D
- Detoxification of free radicals and drugs
- Gluconeogenesis

Source: Adapted Waugh and Grant (2018) and Adam et al. (2017).

The kidneys

There are two kidneys, one on each side of the spinal column. The functions of the kidney are to maintain fluid, electrolyte, and acid–base balance of the blood. Functions of the kidney have been summarised in Table 13.1.

The kidneys are approximately 11 cm long, 5–6 cm wide, and 3–4 cm thick (Marieb and Hoehn 2016) and are bean-shaped organs. The outer border is convex. The inner border is known as the hilum and it is from here that the renal arteries, renal veins, nerves, and ureters enter and leave the kidneys. The right kidney is in contact with the liver's right lobe and as such the right kidney is approximately 2–4 cm lower than the left kidney. There are three different regions inside a kidney (see Figure 13.2):

- Renal cortex
- Renal medulla
- Renal pelvis

The outermost part of the kidney is the renal cortex. It is reddish brown with a granular appearance as a result of the capillaries and the structures of the nephron. The medulla is lighter in colour and has an abundance of blood vessels and tubules of the nephron (Figure 13.3). The medulla consists of

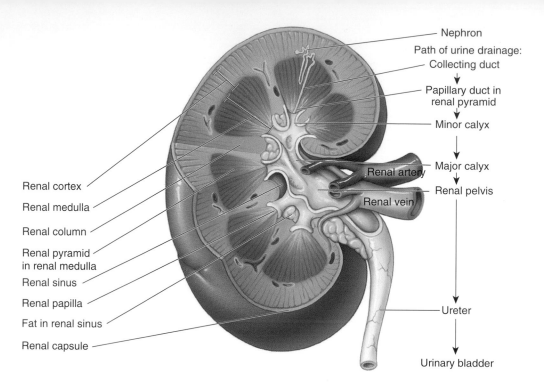

Figure 13.2 External layers of the kidney.

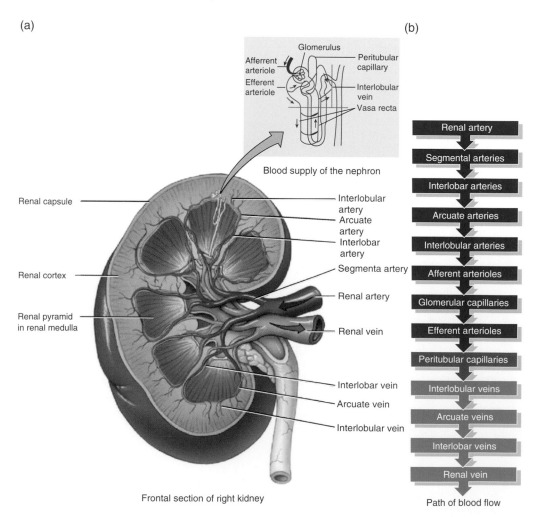

Frontal section of right kidney

Figure 13.3 Internal structures showing blood vessels.

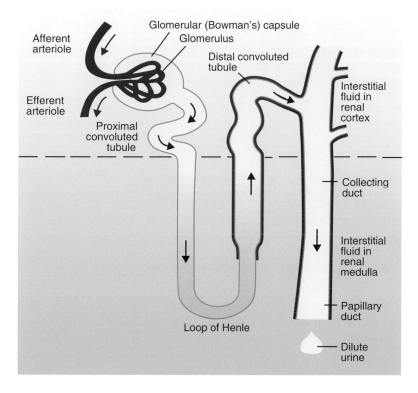

Figure 13.4   Nephron.

approximately 8–12 renal pyramids (Figure 13.2). The renal pelvis is formed from the expanded upper portion of the ureter and is funnel-shaped. It collects urine from the calyces (Figure 13.2) and transports it to the urinary bladder.

Nephrons

The nephrons are small structures found in the kidney, there are over one million nephrons per kidney and urine is formed within these structures. The nephrons are responsible for:

- Filtering blood
- Performing selective reabsorption
- Excreting unwanted waste products from the filtered blood

The nephron is divided into numerous sections, each performing a different function (Figure 13.4).

Bowman's capsule

This is the first portion of the nephron (Figure 13.5). The network of capillaries called the glomerulus are found in this section (Marieb and Hoehn 2016). Filtration of the blood occurs in this portion of the nephron.

Proximal convoluted tubule

From the Bowman's capsule, the filtrate drains into the proximal convoluted tubule. Those cells that line this portion of the tubule actively reabsorb water, nutrients, and ions into the peritubular fluid (the interstitial fluid surrounding the renal tubule).

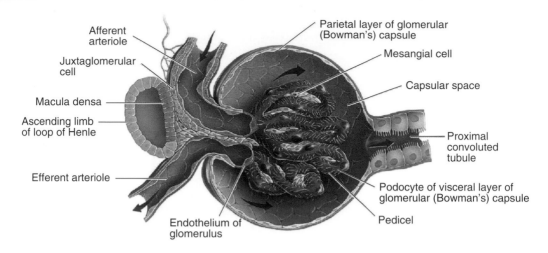

Afferent arteriole
Juxtaglomerular cell
Macula densa
Ascending limb of loop of Henle
Efferent arteriole
Endothelium of glomerulus
Parietal layer of glomerular (Bowman's) capsule
Mesangial cell
Capsular space
Proximal convoluted tubule
Podocyte of visceral layer of glomerular (Bowman's) capsule
Pedicel

Figure 13.5 Bowman's capsule.

Loop of henle

The proximal convoluted tubule then bends and becomes the loop of Henle. The loop of Henle is divided into the descending and ascending loop. The ascending loop of Henle is much thicker than the descending portion.

Distal convoluted tubule

The thick ascending portion of the loop of Henle leads into the distal convoluted tubule. The distal convoluted tubule is an important for:

- Active secretion of ions and acids
- Selective reabsorption of sodium and calcium ions
- Selective reabsorption of water

Collecting ducts

The distal convoluted tubule then drains into the collecting ducts. There are several collecting ducts that converge and drain into a larger system known as the papillary ducts, these empty into the minor calyx (plural – calyces). From here the filtrate, now called urine, drains into the renal pelvis.

Blood supply

Around 1200 mL of blood flows through the kidney per minute. The kidneys receive their blood supply directly from the aorta via the renal artery which divides into the anterior and posterior renal arteries. Two large veins emerge from the hilus and empty into the inferior vena cava.

Urine formation

There are three processes involved in the formation of urine:

- Filtration
- Selective reabsorption
- Secretion

Filtration

This takes place in the glomerulus, lying in the Bowman's capsule. The blood for filtration is supplied by the renal artery. In the kidney, the renal artery divides into smaller arterioles, the arteriole entering

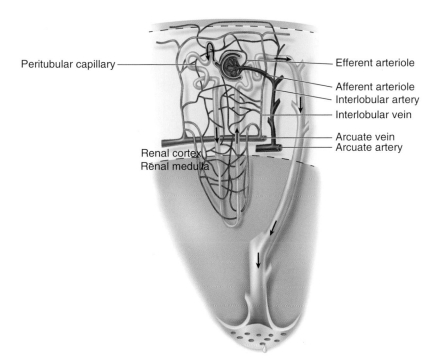

Figure 13.6   The nephron with capillaries.

the Bowman's capsule is the afferent arteriole, which further subdivides into a cluster of capillaries called the glomerulus. Fluid from the filtered blood is protein free and contains electrolytes, for example sodium chloride, potassium chloride, and waste products of cellular metabolism, e.g. urea, uric acid, and creatinine (McCance et al. 2018). The filtered blood then returns to the circulation via the efferent arteriole and finally the renal vein.

Selective reabsorption

Processes associated with selective reabsorption ensure that any substances in the filtrate that are essential for body function are reabsorbed into the plasma. Sodium, calcium, potassium, and chloride, for example, are reabsorbed to maintain the fluid and electrolyte balance and the pH of blood. However, if these substances are in excess of body requirements, they are excreted in the urine.

Secretion

Any substances not removed through filtration are secreted into the renal tubules from the peritubular capillaries (Figure 13.6) of the nephron. These include drugs and hydrogen ions.

Urine

Urine is a sterile and clear fluid that contains nitrogenous waste and salts, it is transparent with an amber or light yellow colour. It is slightly acidic and the pH may range from 4.5 to 8. The pH is affected by an individual's dietary intake. Diet that is high in animal protein tends to make the urine more acidic, whilst a vegetarian diet may make the urine more alkaline. Urine is 96% water and approximately 4% solutes. The solutes include organic and inorganic waste products.

Ureters

The ureters extend from the kidney to the bladder and are approximately 25–30 cm in length and 5 mm in diameter (Mader 2004), they terminate at the bladder and enter obliquely through the muscle wall of the bladder. They pass over the pelvic brim at the bifurcation of the common iliac arteries (Figure 13.7).

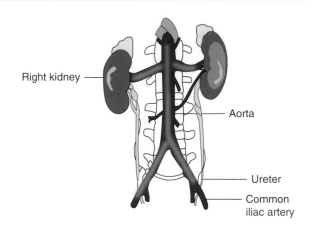

Right kidney

Aorta

Ureter

Common
iliac artery

Figure 13.7   Common iliac vessels and ureter.

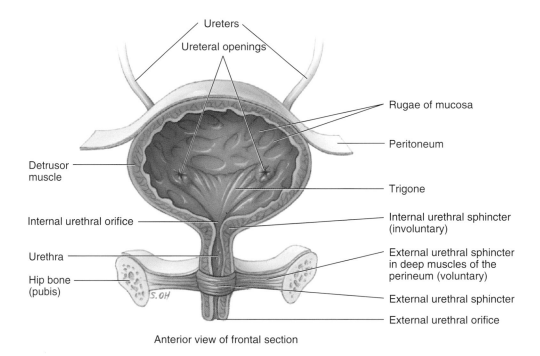

Ureters

Ureteral openings

Rugae of mucosa

Peritoneum

Detrusor
muscle

Trigone

Internal urethral orifice

Internal urethral sphincter
(involuntary)

Urethra

External urethral sphincter
in deep muscles of the
perineum (voluntary)

Hip bone
(pubis)

External urethral sphincter

External urethral orifice

Anterior view of frontal section

Figure 13.8   Layers of the urinary bladder.

The ureters have three layers:

- Inner layer – transitional epithelial mucosa
- Middle layer – smooth muscle layer
- Outer layer – fibrous connective tissue

The peristaltic contraction of the ureters propels the urine from the kidney to the bladder.

Urinary bladder

The urinary bladder is located in the pelvic cavity posterior to the symphysis pubis. In men, the bladder lies anterior to the rectum and in women it lies anterior to the vagina and inferior to the uterus. It is a smooth muscular sac which stores urine. As urine accumulates, the bladder expands without a

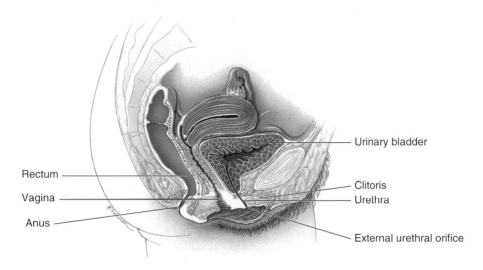

Figure 13.9   Location of the female urethra.

significant rise in the internal pressure of the bladder. The bladder normally distends and holds approximately 350 mL of urine. The urinary bladder has three layers (Figure 13.8):

- Transitional epithelial mucosa
- A thick muscular layer
- A fibrous outer layer

Urethra

The urethra is a muscular tube draining urine from the bladder, conveying it out of the body. It varies in length in males and females. Sphincters keep the urethra closed when urine is not being passed. The internal urethral sphincter is under involuntary control and lies at the bladder–urethra junction. The external urethral sphincter is under voluntary control. The male urethra passes through three different regions:

- Prostatic region – passes through the prostate gland
- Membranous portion – passes through the pelvic diaphragm
- Penile region – extends the length of the penis.

The female urethra is bound to the anterior vaginal wall. The external opening of the urethra is anterior to the vagina and posterior to the clitoris (Figure 13.9).

So far

The renal system (sometimes called the urinary system) is made up of a number of organs (kidneys, ureters, bladder, and urethra). The renal system contributes to homeostasis through management of blood volume and waste excretion, balance of body pH, regulation of blood pressure, and erythropoiesis (this controls red blood cell production in the bone marrow).

When functioning effectively this system removes waste products from the body, for example urea, as well as excess ions and water from the blood. The kidneys contain many nephrons, which remove any waste before reabsorbing substances that the body needs. Waste is stored in the bladder before being removed as urine via the urethra.

Working with the other systems of the body, the renal system helps to maintain homeostasis. The kidneys are the key organs of homeostasis as they maintain the acid–base balance and the water salt balance of the blood. Kidneys also regulate the acid–base balance and conserve fluids.

Cultural considerations

Different ethnic groups have different risk levels of kidney failure that requires renal replacement therapy (RRT), with patients from a Black, Asian or Minority Ethnic (BAME) background at most risk. Those from a BAME background make up approximately 15% of the whole population in England. However, about 22% of those who started RRT in England in 2012 were from a BAME background. This indicates a higher risk of starting RRT in these ethnic groups compared to White patients.

Source: National Kidney Federation (2014).

Assessing needs

The renal system is essential to the function of the entire body. When the nurse undertakes an accurate assessment, it will help ensure that any impact on the renal system is recognised quickly and steps are taken to prevent damage to the kidneys or other components of this system. Treating renal failure early will make a difference to the health and wellbeing of the individual and their family. The nurse needs to be aware of those people who are at risk so as to purposefully target those in need.

As with the assessment of all systems, there are two types of data that the nurse can collect. Subjective data includes reports from the patient (primary data) and data from other sources (secondary data). Objective data will include data derived from the physical examination and any diagnostic tests. When the data is considered together this provides an understanding of how the renal system is functioning (or not). It should be noted that the absence of signs or symptoms does not always mean that the system is functioning normally.

Obtaining a patient history

The patient with a renal condition may present asymptomatically or they may present with non-specific conditions such as fatigue or breathlessness (Dhaun and Kluth 2018). In some cases of advanced renal disease there may be few or vague symptoms.

The data gathered when gaining a health history is subjective data. This is what the person tells the nurse, how the patient describes or explains perceptions, feelings, or experiences. A health history will accompany the physical assessment (here the data becomes more objective). As with most health histories, the nurse gathers data that includes biographical data, current health problems, past health history, family history of health challenges, current medication and treatments, allergies, personal social history, cultural beliefs, and practices related to health (health promotion with attention to exercise undertaken, diet, and so forth).

The nurse systematically gathers data and organises it, focusing on reviewing the renal system and in particular noting any impact that ill health may have on the activities of living. A focused history-taking activity (assessment) helps identify patient expectations and concerns and provides the patient's perspective and meaning of the data. The identification of strengths and limitations guide the planning of nursing care. See Table 13.2 urinary elimination patterns.

Table 13.2   Renal system assessment and urinary elimination patterns.

- Route: via urethra, use of assistive devices (catheter, ureterostomy) dialysis: peritoneal catheter, haemodialysis: arteriovenous fistula
- Character of urine: amount, colour, dilute, concentrated, timing, odour, pH, frothy, sediment, haematuria, albuminuria, ketonuria
- Voiding pattern: frequency, urgency, hesitancy, burning, pain, dribbling, nocturia, oliguria, change in stream, enuresis, back pain, polyuria
- Urinary control: continence, retention, incontinence, stress incontinence, bladder distention
- Fluid balance: positive/negative (intake/output) fluid balance, weight gain, presence of oedema

Review

Ask a colleague to assess you/rate you as you undertake a patient history specifically relating to the renal system (you could also do this exercise through simulation).

Action	Performed yes/no	Observations/ comments
Makes an introduction		
Checks patient details		
Uses open questioning technique to determine presenting complaint		
Asks about pain (systematically assesses this)		
When did the symptoms start		
Severity of symptoms		
Extent/duration of symptoms		
Course of systems		
Aggravating /relieving factors/actions		
Previous episode of symptoms		
ICE (elicits patients Ideas, Concerns, and Expectations)		
Dysuria		
Frequency of micturition		
Nocturia		
Hesitancy and terminal dribbling		
Poor urinary stream		
Urinary incontinence		
Pyrexia/rigours		
Nausea/vomiting		
Previous urological disease		
Other medical history		
Surgical history		
Use of prescribed medications		
Use of over-the-counter medications (including herbal remedies)		
Known allergies		
Family history of urological disease		
Smoking/alcohol/recreational drug history		
Social history (home situation, ability to function independently)		
Occupation (or previous occupation)		
Reviews other body systems		
Summarises		
Actively listens		
Summarises		
Signposts (what's next)		
Thanks patient and closes consultation		

Source: Adapted Talley and O'Connor (2013) and Dhaun and Kluth (2018).

A focused health history for those with renal problems will alert the nurse to any actual or potential renal or urinary problems the patient may have. Jarvis (2015) suggests that these are some of the renal or urinary system-focused questions to ask patients:

- Are you urinating more frequently than usual, do you experience urgency, nocturia?
- When you urinate do you have pain, where is the pain?
- When urinating, do you experience a burning-like sensation?
- Do you have any difficulty in starting or maintaining the stream of urine?
- Is there any blood in your urine?
- Do you have any difficulty controlling your urine?

If the patient is experiencing difficult or painful urination (dysuria) then further information/detail is required. In order to illicit this information the nurse might ask:

- Is there any pain as you urinate or after you have urinated?
- How much fluid do you normally have in a day (fluid intake)?

There may be a number of possible causes when a patient presents with dysuria and these can include:

- Urinary tract infection (UTI)
- Urinary tract obstruction
- Urethral obstruction
- Bladder calculi
- Prostatitis
- Sexually acquired infection

If haematuria is a symptom, determine:

- Does the blood appear at the beginning, end or throughout urination?
- Have you noticed any new bruises or experienced bleeding from the gums?
- What medications are you taking?
- Have there been any changes in exercise pattern?
- Have you had any recent abdominal trauma?
- Any recent sore throat or infection?
- Are you having a period?

The may be several possible causes of blood in the urine:

- Renal cell carcinoma
- Trauma to the kidney
- Thrombocytopenia
- Bladder infection
- Renal calculi
- Glomerulonephritis
- Anticoagulant use
- Smoking
- Strenuous exercise
- Menstruation

Take note

The language the nurse uses to ask patients about intimate activities such as urination must be appropriate and meaningful, and communicated in language and formats that are easily accessible. Using language that is open and transparent can help to promote understanding, and provide the patient with a rationale for current and future action.

Table 13.3 Some imaging and biopsy investigations.

Plain abdominal X-ray

Ultrasound scan

Doppler ultrasound of renal vessels

Intravenous urography

CT urogram

Angiography/CT or MRI angiography

Isotope scan

Renal biopsy

Source: Plevris and Parkes (2018).

Patients with alteration in their renal function may be asymptomatic or symptomatic. Asking focused questions during assessment from a patient with a history of renal dysfunction can establish the degree of renal dysfunction experienced and current treatment modalities. Ask the patient about the following:

- What treatments have you received for your illness (medications, X-rays, chemotherapy, dyes used in therapeutic diagnostics)?
- What are your current prescribed medications?
- What over-the-counter medications do you use (including herbal preparations)?
- What food do you eat?
- Do you have any sleep disturbances?
- Do you experience general malaise, fatigue, or headaches?
- Have you noticed that you are bruising easily?
- Is there a delay noted in any wound healing?
- How often are you passing urine and when (polyuria, nocturia, and urine output)?
- Do you have high blood pressure or experience palpitations or chest pain?
- Do you have any heartburn, nausea, vomiting, constipation, or diarrhoea (gastrointestinal symptoms)?

The objective data that is collected will include data from the physical examination and any additional tests such as imaging (see Table 13.3) or blood tests. When all sources of data are brought together (subjective and objective) this can provide the nurse and others with a picture of how the renal system is functioning. To reiterate, it should be noted that the absence of signs or symptoms will not always signify a normally functioning system. In some cases of advanced renal disease, they may be few, vague, or disparate symptoms.

So far

As with other systems the nurse needs to adopt a systematic approach to undertaking an assessment of the renal system. The most common complaints about the urinary system include output changes, for example amount of urine passed (polyuria, oliguria), voiding patterns such as frequency, incontinence, hesitancy, urgency, and nocturia.

The urine

The nurse should pay attention to the patient's urine. The amount of urine output and its colour can indicate renal concerns. Dutton and Finch (2018) note that normally approximately 1–2 L of urine is produced in a 24-hour period. A minimum of 0.5–1 mL/kg/h is needed to indicate good renal perfusion and function (however, normal urine output depends on a number of factors). Too little urine output can indicate dehydration or renal insufficiency, with too much urine being produced indicating diabetes mellitus, diabetes insipidus, or renal failure. Normal urine should be clear and a straw yellow colour (Thomas 2015). Cloudy or malodorous urine haematuria require further testing as they could indicate infection or other problems.

Review

Define these terms:

Anuria

Oliguria

Polyuria

Dysuria

Haematuria

Proteinuria

Strangury

Urinary lithiasis

Pyuria

Urinalysis

There are many reasons why urine is screened either routinely or selectively. Dipstick urinalysis is often undertaken by the nurse. Urinalysis is the testing of urine as an assessment of wellbeing. When abnormalities are identified, depending on the circumstances, the nurse may need to refer abnormalities to another member of the multidisciplinary team. There may also be a requirement to undertake the monitoring of vital signs and/or blood tests to assist in the generation of a diagnosis.

Analysis of urine provides valuable information about the kidney function and other biological processes within the body. Organic compounds found in the urine include urea, uric acid, creatinine, and hippuric acid. Inorganic substances found are sodium, chloride, phosphate, potassium, and ammonia. Urine composition varies according to the person's fluid intake and diet; therefore, the time the specimen is obtained may influence the results.

When performing urinalysis, the dipstick should be dipped in the urine briefly. After waiting the appropriate amount of time for each component, the dipstick is cross-referenced against the manufacturer's chart (usually on the container) for each individual colour change, which will then give a result (Lindsay 2018). Understanding of specific manufacturer's instructions should be ensured prior to performing the test. As visual dipsticks are associated with a high level of false positive results (Waugh and Clark 2004), a more common way of analysing is by using automated readers. Care of dipsticks will optimise their effectiveness, for example, noting on the bottle containing the dipsticks the date the bottle was opened, replacing the cap, and storing within temperatures that the manufacturer advises.

All testing must be carried out on fresh urine in a clean container. The constituents of urine change as it ages, and contamination from containers may impact the results. Bacteria can also multiply at room temperature and this can compromise results. All specimens that are to be sent to the laboratory must be sent immediately or placed in a medical specimen fridge, and local policy and procedure must be adhered to. When completing documentation on urine the nurse should include:

- Time
- Date
- Appearance
- Odour
- Colour
- Results of any testing carried out

See Table 13.4.

Take note

All urine samples that are to be tested must be fresh.

Table 13.4   Urinalysis.

Component	Description
Colour	Urochrome gives urine its colour. Factors that may alter colour include specific gravity, foods, bilirubin and drugs (e.g. pyridium-orange stains that are permanent).
Character	If urine is cloudy or hazy as opposed to its normal clear character, this could be due to white blood cells, bacteria, faecal contamination, prostatic fluid, or vaginal secretions.
Specific gravity	This is the weight of urine. A low specific gravity signifies diluted urine whereas urine with a high specific gravity indicates concentrated urine.
pH	Values increase with urinary tract infections (UTIs) and if the urine specimen is old, changes that are seen are associated with acid–base imbalances
Glucose	The renal threshold for blood sugar is 160–180 mg/dL. Pregnancy, endocrine, and renal disorders can lower the renal threshold for glucose.
Ketones	Ketones are a product of fat metabolism. Ketonuria can be caused by diabetic ketoacidosis (DKA), starvation, fasting, vomiting, strenuous exercise, and dehydration.
Protein	The presence of protein in the urine (proteinuria) may be induced by benign conditions such as stress, pregnancy, pyrexia, strenuous exercise, and vaginal secretion. However, hypertension, diabetes mellitus, post renal infection, or multiple myeloma may also be responsible for proteinuria
Bilirubin	When there is bilirubin present in the urine this is typically as a result of hepatobiliary obstruction
Urobilinogen	The occurrence of urobilinogen in the urine is normal. When urobilinogen is decreased, or absent it can indicate hepatobiliary duct obstruction. Increased amounts of urobilinogen could point to hepatic damage or haemolytic disease
Blood	Haematuria may make the urine cloudy, if tested positive using a dipstick then further microscopic analysis is needed The microscopic presence of red blood cells: UTI, urinary calculi, cystitis, pyelonephritis, glomerular nephritis, renal cancer, bladder cancer, strenuous exercise, menses The presence of myoglobulin: myocardial infarction, trauma, burns Haemoglobin: hypertension, sickle cell anaemia, reaction to blood transfusion, disseminated intravascular coagulation
Nitrate	If the urine is positive to nitrates, bacteria are present in the urine. Bacteria is broken down into nitrate and urinary nitrates
Leucocyte esterase	Denotes the presence of white blood cells, suggestive of UTI, renal disease, urinary tract disease

Source: Adapted Fischbach (2015), Royal College of Nursing (2015), and Pagana and Pagana (2017).

231

Urine analysis (urinalysis) can often provide clues to renal disease. Normally, only traces of protein are found in urine and when higher amounts are found, this can indicate damage to the glomeruli. When a patient is passing unusually large quantities of urine this could signify diseases such as diabetes mellitus or hypothalamic tumours that cause diabetes insipidus. Yates (2016) notes that there are a number of ways in which the urine can be analysed. The type of analysis chosen will depend on the reason why analysis is required (see Table 13.5).

6Cs

The patient must give their consent for their urine to be tested. They must also be told what their urine is being tested for.

Take note

Urine testing can indicate the amount of sugar in the urine, providing an indirect indication of how much is the blood. However, testing blood for sugar levels provides much more up-to-date and accurate results and is the preferred testing option.

Table 13.5   Types of urine analysis.

Type of urine analysis	Reason
24-hour collection	The patient is asked to void into the toilet, emptying the bladder, then after this point all urine is collected for the next 24 hours. As the body chemistry alters continually, this test is used to measure substances, such as steroids, white cells, electrolytes or to determine urine osmolarity
First-morning specimen	The first urine specimen of the morning (or eight hours after being in a lying position). This test is the best sample for pregnancy testing
Fasting specimen	The second voided urine specimen after a period of fasting
Mid-stream specimen of urine (MSSU) or mid-stream urine (MSU)	This test is used to obtain urine for bacterial culture. First and last part of urine stream is voided into the toilet, this avoids contaminating the specimen with organisms present on the skin
Random specimen	Used for chemical or microscopic examination, a randomly collected specimen is suitable for most screening purposes
Catheter specimen of urine (CSU)	A CSU is obtained and collected for bacteriological examination if a patient's symptoms suggest the presence of a urinary tract infection (UTI). Evidence-based local policy and procedure must be used for the sampling technique.

Source: Adapted Tortora and Derrickson (2014), Dougherty and Lister (2015), and Yates (2016).

The colour of urine is determined primarily by the breakdown products of red blood cell destruction. The liver converts the 'haem' of haemoglobin into water-soluble forms that can be excreted into the bile and indirectly into the urine. This yellow pigment is called urochrome. The colour of urine can also be affected by some foods, for example beetroot, berries, and fava beans. Kidney stone(s) or a cancer of the urinary system can produce enough bleeding to make the urine pink or even bright red. Diseases of the liver or obstructions of bile drainage from the liver produce a dark 'tea' or 'cola' tone to the urine. Dehydration results in darker, concentrated urine that can also produce a slight odour of ammonia. A distinctive odour can also be found in the urine after a person consumes food such as asparagus.

So far

The urine can reveal a number of clues about the health and wellbeing of a patient. When the nurse undertakes an analysis of a person's urine it can be a useful way of identifying or ruling out some conditions and infections. The use of a reagent stick is the most popular way to carry out urinalysis. Urinalysis is an important screening and diagnostic tool. However, the nurse must know how to perform the test and to interpret results correctly if the analysis is be of any use.

Focused patient examination

The patient's blood pressure should have been checked and recorded. The examination of the patient begins as the nurse approaches the foot of the bed, looking for the presence of a catheter bag (if present, note urine volume and colour). Determine if there are any alternative vascular access routes present, and assess whether there are any arteriovenous fistulae present (this may determine that the patient has/is receiving renal dialysis).

Prior to the examination the nurse must wash his/her hands, explain the process, and gain consent. Ensure privacy; the patient should lie flat and the abdomen should be exposed, but dignity maintained.

Perform an abdominal assessment by inspecting the abdomen for any signs of distention or swelling, which might indicate kidney enlargement or bladder distention. Take note of any abdominal scars and ask the patient about them. The nurse should then auscultate the abdomen for any bruit. A bruit is a buzzing-like sound occurring when there is an abnormal blood flow within a vessel. An abdominal bruit might indicate renal artery stenosis or narrowing.

The abdominal assessment also includes palpation of the abdomen and flank for tenderness or enlargement of the kidneys (see also Chapter 12). When palpating the kidney, the nurse places one hand anterior and one posterior. Ask the patient to take a deep breath out and press up into renal angle with posterior hand and press down with the anterior hand. As the patient breathes in, the kidney may be felt between the hands. The nurse can palpate for the abdomen for signs of bladder distention. Assess the abdomen for trauma and palpate for the presence of abdominal masses.

Table 13.6 provides an overview of the signs and symptoms of chronic renal failure. The signs and symptoms outlined in Table 13.6 arise from a failing kidney, they are all associated with the various roles of the kidney.

Table 13.6 Signs and symptoms associated with chronic renal failure.

System	Manifestations
Neurological	Seizures Asterixis Restlessness leg syndrome Burning of the soles of feet Changes in behaviour Weakness and fatigue Confusion Inability to concentrate Disorientation Tremors
Dermatological	Grey-bronze skin colour Dry, flaky skin Pruritus Ecchymosis Purpura Thin, brittle nails Coarse, thinning hair
Cardiovascular	Hypertension Pitting oedema (feet, hands, sacrum) Periorbital oedema Pericardial rub Distended neck veins Pericarditis Pericardial effusion Pericardial tamponade Hyperkalaemia Hyperlipidaemia
Musculoskeletal	Muscle cramps Loss of muscle strength Renal osteodystrophy Bone pain Bone fractures Foot drop
Reproduction	Amenorrhoea Testicular atrophy Infertility Decreased libido
Haematological	Anaemia Thrombocytopenia
Gastrointestinal	Ammonia odour to breath ('uremic fetor') Metallic taste in mouth Mouth ulcerations and bleeding Anorexia, nausea, and vomiting Hiccups Constipation or diarrhoea Gastrointestinal tract bleeding

233

(Continued)

Table 13.6   (Continued)

System	Manifestations
Respiratory	Crackles Thick, tenacious sputum Depressed cough reflex Pleuritic pain Shortness of breath Tachypnoea Kussmaul respirations Uremic pneumonitis

Source: Adapted Hinkle and Cheever (2017).

Bob Coleman (Grandad)

Mr Coleman was admitted to the acute medical admissions ward after a referral from the practice nurse.

UTIs are common in the community and in hospitals. Infections in men and recurrent, drug-resistant, or complicated UTIs will always require further evaluation. Confirming the cause is key to ensuring the best treatment. Mr Coleman's chief complaint: 'It hurts when I pee and I am going to the toilet more and more.'

Mr Coleman gives a history of four days of pain with urination. He describes his urine as cloudy in appearance and with foul odour. He is complaining of going to the toilet to urinate frequently and is urinating only small amounts each time he passes urine. Mr Coleman has no fever, rigours, vomiting, or night sweats. He tells the nurse in the acute medical admissions unit that he needs to urinate more during the night.

You have been asked to undertake an assessment of Mr Coleman's needs.

Describe the assessment process here:

Check Table 13.2. Did you consider the issues that Mr Coleman describes with Table 13.2?

What observations would you make on Mr Coleman's urine?

What other tests and investigations would be required to ensure that a definitive diagnosis is made?

Having assessed Mr Coleman's needs, now write a plan of care. In the plan of care a discharge plan should also be included. Describe what health education and health promotion activities would be included in the care plan.

So far

The nurse undertakes a focused assessment of needs related to the renal system. Ascertain the patient's reason for seeking help with their health care. This is usually the presenting complaint. The patient is asked about their past history of renal system disease and this includes a history of hypertension and diabetes mellitus. The kidneys are associated with drug metabolism, so ask the patient about their drug history as drugs may affect renal function. Some renal conditions are inherited, and this is why it is important to gather a family history. Other risk factors may be associated with lifestyle, such as smoking and excessive alcohol consumption, which are related to hypertension. Undertake a dietary history and establish patient diet and intake of water and other fluids such as milk. Ask the patient about their occupation; some occupations can predispose a person to renal disease.

A systematic physical examination is required.

Dysuria and urinary tract infection

UTI is an infection of any part of the urinary tract, usually caused by bacteria, but seldom by other micro-organisms, for example fungi, viruses, or parasites. UTIs are classified in several ways. Lower UTI is infection of the bladder. Urethritis and prostatitis are also considered lower UTIs. Cystitis is often referred for lower UTI (particularly in the case of women). It means 'inflammation of the bladder' and there may be rare non-infectious causes, for example radiation- and chemical-induced cystitis. Upper UTI includes pyelitis and pyelonephritis.

Uncomplicated UTI is an infection of the urinary tract usually by a micro-organism in a patient with a normal urinary tract and normal kidney function. A complicated UTI is when one or more risk factors are present that will predispose the patient to persistent infection, recurrent infection, or treatment failure.

Recurrent UTI is a repeated UTI. This may be due to relapse or reinfection and may be defined as two or more episodes of confirmed UTI in three months. Relapse is a recurrent UTI with *the same strain* of micro-organism. Relapse is the likely cause if infection recurs within a short period after treatment (within two weeks, for example). Reinfection is a recurrent UTI with *a different strain or species* of micro-organism. Reinfection is the likely cause if UTI recurs more than two weeks after treatment. Asymptomatic bacteriuria is defined as the presence of significant bacteria in the urine without symptoms or signs of infection (COMPASS 2012; European Association of Urology 2015).

When a patient complains of dysuria, this will usually suggest a UTI. However, the nurse needs to ask questions regarding the pain the patient is experiencing. This can help to provide a differential diagnosis. See Table 13.7 for suggested questions to be asked when a patient presents with dysuria.

235

Table 13.7   Questions to ask in relation to dysuria with rationale.

Concern	Question	Rationale/Discussion
Onset	Did the dysuria occur suddenly or was it a slow progression of pain?	If gradual onset, this may be related to a more chronic problem
Duration	How long has the patient experienced the pain	Some patients describe dysuria as a burning sensation
Frequency of incidence, regularity	Is this the first time the patient has experienced dysuria? If not, how many times in the past? Does the patient experience pain each time they urinate? When does the pain occur: just before urination, at the beginning, during the whole period of urination, or at the end?	If pain occurs just before urinations this might indicate bladder irritation. Pain experienced at the beginning of urination could point to bladder outlet obstruction. If pain occurs at the end of urination this can suggest bladder spasm. When pain occurs throughout the whole activity of urination, pyelonephritis may be suspected.
Severity	Does the dysuria impact negatively on the patient's lifestyle, is it interfering with their ability to perform the activities of living? A visual analogue scale should be used to assess pain.	Severe pain could imply kidney stone or kidney trauma.
Related symptoms	Does the patient experience pain in other parts of the body? Does the pain radiate to other parts of the body: ● Back ● Supra-pubic area ● Testicles/scrotal sac ● Abdomen Is there any haematuria, urgency, urethral discharge, rigor, pyrexia, nausea, vomiting, shortness of breath, changes to colour and odour of the urine?	Lower back pain could infer cystitis or pyelonephritis. Changes in the colour of urine could point to issues within the urinary system and these changes might provide the nurse with pointers to other problems in the body, such as hepatic, cardiac, or endocrine problems. If the patient is passing large amounts of clear and diluted urine this could indicate diabetes insipidus. Dysuria and malodourous urine could be an indication of kidney infection.

(Continued)

Table 13.7   (Continued)

Concern	Question	Rationale/Discussion
Alleviating factors	Has the patient tried to ease the pain? Is the patient taking any prescribed medication, over-the-counter medications (including herbal remedies)? Has the treatment been successful?	These questions ensure that the patient is being assessed from a holistic patient-centred perspective.

Source: Adapted Rhoads and Wiggins Petersen (2018), Jarvis (2015), and Jarvis et al. (2014).

So far

There are several ways to classify a UTI. Understating the various classifications can help the nurse plan, implement, and evaluate care in a patient-centred way.

When dysuria is the presenting complaint this is usually suggestive of a UTI. The nurse needs to ask the patient questions regarding the pain being experienced. When appropriate questions are asked, this can help with a differential diagnosis.

Conclusion

Treating renal disease early will make a difference. One aspect of the focused assessment will be to recognise who is at risk of renal disease and provide information to the other health care providers that will ensure appropriate testing is carried out, a definitive diagnosis is made, and the most appropriate treatment offered to the patient. In conjunction with gathering information about a patient's history (and this includes a history of hypertension and diabetes), nurses should also understand that heredity can also play a part in the potential of developing renal and urinary disease.

The urine that the patient produces should always be considered carefully by the nurse as it can point to a number of abnormal renal conditions. The signs and symptoms of renal disease vary and may be disparate. The nurse must take this into account when undertaking a holistic patient-centred assessment.

References

Adam, S., Osbourne, S., and Welch, J. (2017). *Critical Care Nursing: Science and Practice*, 3e. Oxford: Oxford University Press.

COMPASS (2012) Therapeutic notes on the management of bacterial urinary tract infections in primary care. Northern Ireland Health and Social Care Board. www.medicinesni.com/assets/COMPASS/uti_2012.pdf (accessed August 2018).

Dhaun, N. and Kluth, D. (2018). The renal system. In: *Macleod's Clinical Examination*, 14e (ed. J.A. Innes, A.R. Dover and K. Fairhurst), 237–250. Edinburgh: Elsevier.

Dougherty, L. and Lister, S. (eds.) (2015). *The Royal Marsden Hospital Manual of Clinical Nursing Procedures*, 9e. Oxford: Wiley.

Dutton, H. and Finch, J. (2018). *Acute and Critical Care at a Glance*. Oxford: Wiley.

European Association of Urology (2015) Guidelines on urological infections. https://uroweb.org/wp-content/uploads/19-Urological-infections_LR2.pdf (accessed August 2018).

Fischbach, F. and Dunning, M.B. (2015). *Manual of Laboratory and Diagnostic Tests*, 8e. Philadelphia: Wolters Kluwer.

Hinkle, J.L. and Cheever, K.H. (2017). *Brunner and Suddarth's Textbook of Medical-Surgical Nursing*, 14e. Philadelphia: Lippincott Williams and Wilkins.

Jarvis, C. (2015). *Physical Examination and Health Assessment*, 7e. St Louis: Elsevier.

Jarvis, T.R., Chan, L., and Gottlieb, T. (2014). Assessment and management of lower urinary tract infection in adults. *Australian Prescriber* 37: 7–9. https://doi.org/10.18773/austprescr.2014.002.

Lindsay, P. (2018). Urinalysis. In: *Midwifery Skills at a Glance* (ed. P. Lindsay, C. Bagness and I. Peate), 102–103. Oxford: Wiley.

Mader, S.S. (2004). *Understanding Human Anatomy and Physiology*, 5e. Maidenhead: McGraw-Hill.

Marieb, E.N. and Hoehn, K. (2016). *Human Anatomy and Physiology*, 10e. San Francisco: Pearson Benjamin Cummings.

McCance, K.L., Huether, S.E., Brashers, V.L., and Rote, N.S. (2018). *Pathophysiology: The Biologic Basis for Disease in Adults and Children*, 8e. St Louis: Mosby.

National Kidney Federation (2014) Facts and figures for kidney patients. www.kidney.org.uk/assets/Uploads/documents/Facts-Figures-web.pdf (accessed July 2018).

Pagana, K.D. and Pagana, T. (2017). *Mosby's Manual of Diagnostic and Laboratory Tests*, 6e. St Louis: Mosby.

Plevris, J. and Parkes, R. (2018). The gastrointestinal system. In: *Macleod's Clinical Examination*, 14e (ed. J.A. Innes, A.R. Dover and K. Fairhurst), 93–117. Edinburgh: Elsevier.

Rhoads, J. and Wiggins Petersen, S. (2018). *Advanced Health Assessment and Diagnostic Reasoning*, 3e. Burlington: Nelson Bartlett.

Royal College of Nursing. (2015) Urine testing. http://rcnhca.org.uk/clinical-skills/observation/urine-testing (accessed August 2018).

Talley, N.J. and O'Connor, S. (2013). *Clinical Examination: A Systematic Guide to Physical Diagnosis*, 7e. Sydney: Elsevier.

Thomas, R.K. (2015). *Practical Medical Procedures at a Glance*. Oxford: Wiley.

Tortora, G.J. and Derrickson, B.H. (2014). *Principles of Anatomy and Physiology*, 14e. New Jersey: Wiley.

Waugh, J.J. and Clark, T.J. (2004). Accuracy of urinalysis dipstick techniques in predicting significant proteinuria in pregnancy. *Obstetrics and Gynecology* 103: 769–777.

Waugh, A. and Grant, A. (2018). *Ross and Wilsons Anatomy and Physiology in Health and Illness*, 13e. Edinburgh: Elsevier.

Yates, A. (2016). Urinalysis: How to interpret results. *Nursing Times Online* (92): 1–3. www.nursingtimes.net/clinical-archive/continence/urinalysis-how-to-interpret-results/7005353.article (accessed March 2019.

Chapter 14

Assessing the respiratory system

Aim

This chapter introduces the reader to the assessment of the respiratory system and the care required for people who may experience problems related to this system.

Learning outcomes

By the end of the chapter the reader will be able to:

1. Provide a brief overview of the respiratory system and its functions
2. Consider a number of conditions that can affect the respiratory system
3. Describe the various ways in which the nurse undertakes an assessment of the respiratory system
4. Outline care planning related to the respiratory system

Introduction

Alterations in respiratory function may have a negative impact on other body systems. Abnormalities of the respiratory system are often manifestations of other systemic disease processes (Heuer and Scanlan 2017). This means that the nurse needs to be aware that assessment of the respiratory system cannot be restricted to assessment of the chest only; the nurse needs to undertake an inclusive assessment of the patient's entire health status.

Respiratory assessment requires the nurse to understand the anatomy and physiology of the respiratory system, clinical knowledge, skills, confidence, and competence. Structural changes in anatomy can impact on chest expansion, reduced respiratory muscle strength that can inhibit efficient airway clearance by coughing and increased physiological demand, such as in pneumonia or heart failure, that can lead to an inadequate compensatory response to hypoxia.

The respiratory system

The respiratory system (sometimes called the respiratory tract) is usually discussed in terms of upper and lower parts. The upper respiratory tract is related to the nasopharynx and larynx (the portion above the vocal cords) and the lower relates to the larynx (the portion below the vocal cords), trachea, bronchi, and lungs.

The respiratory system is located in the thorax and is responsible for gaseous exchange between the circulatory system and the atmosphere. Air is taken in via the upper airways through the lower airways and into the small bronchioles and alveoli within the lung tissue (Figure 14.1).

Fundamentals of Assessment and Care Planning for Nurses, First Edition. Ian Peate.
© 2020 John Wiley & Sons Ltd. Published 2020 by John Wiley & Sons Ltd.

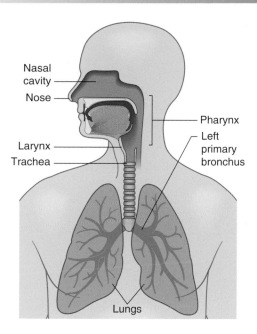

Figure 14.1   Respiratory organs.

The upper respiratory system

The organs of the upper respiratory tract include the mouth, nose, nasal cavity and pharynx. The functions of this aspect of the respiratory system are to warm, filter, and moisten the inhaled air. The nasal septum divides the nasal cavity into two equal sections. This structure is formed out of the ethmoid bones and the vomer of the skull. The vestibule is the space where air enters the nasal cavity just inside the nostrils.

The nasal cavities are subdivided into three air passageways which are formed by three shelf-like projections known as the superior, middle, and inferior conchae or turbinates. The incoming air bounces off the conchal surface and swirls. Small particles in the air are then trapped in the mucosa of the nasal cavity (Figure 14.2).

The pharynx is a chamber that is shared by the digestive and respiratory systems and connects the nasal and oral cavity with the larynx and is divided into three regions called the nasopharynx, the oropharynx, and the laryngopharynx. The nasopharynx is located behind the nasal cavity and contains two openings that lead to the auditory (eustachian) tubes. The oropharynx and the laryngopharynx are passageways for food and drink as well as air, they are lined with non-keratinised stratified squamous epithelium.

The lower respiratory system

The lower respiratory system includes the larynx (the portion below the vocal cords), the trachea, the right and left primary bronchi and all the parts of both lungs (Figure 14.3). The lungs are two cone-shaped organs, almost filling the thorax. They are protected by a framework of bones, the thoracic cage, consisting of the ribs, sternum (breast bone), and vertebrae (spine). The air passages are lined with mucous membrane composed mainly of ciliated epithelium. The cilia are constantly cleaning the tract and transporting foreign matter upwards for swallowing or expectoration.

The larynx

The larynx is made up of nine pieces of cartilage tissue, three single pieces and three pairs. The single pieces of cartilage are the thyroid, epiglottis, and cricoid cartilage. The thyroid cartilage is

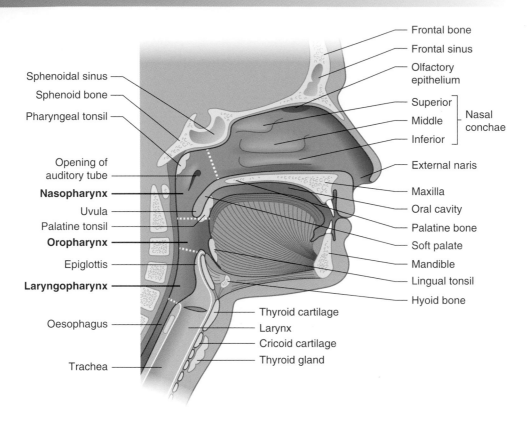

Figure 14.2   Detailed structures of the upper respiratory tract.

more commonly referred to as the Adam's apple and, along with the cricoid cartilage, provides protection of the vocal cords. The epiglottis is a leaf-shaped piece of elastic cartilage that is attached to the top of the larynx, functioning to protect the airway from food and water. When swallowing, the epiglottis blocks entry to the larynx and food and liquids are then diverted towards the oesophagus, which is situated nearby.

Trachea

The trachea (referred to also as the windpipe) extends from the laryngopharynx at the level of the cricoid cartilage at the top to the carina (also called the tracheal bifurcation). The trachea is made up of 15–20 C-shaped cartilage rings that reinforce and protect the trachea and prevent it from collapsing or over-expanding as pressure changes within the respiratory system. The carina is a ridge-shaped structure at the level of T6 or T7. The carina possesses sensory nerve endings that will usually cause the person to cough if food or water is accidently inhaled.

Bronchi and bronchioles

The trachea (sometimes called the windpipe) divides into two main bronchi (also main stem bronchi), the left and the right, at the level of the sternal angle and of the fifth thoracic vertebra or up to two vertebrae higher or lower, depending on breathing, at the anatomical point known as the carina.

The right main bronchus is more vertical, wider, shorter, and subdivides into three lobar bronchi, the left main bronchus, which divides into two. The segmental bronchi divide into many primary bronchioles that divide into terminal bronchioles, each of which then gives rise to several respiratory bronchioles, which then go on to divide into and terminate in tiny air sacs that are known as the alveoli (Figure 14.4).

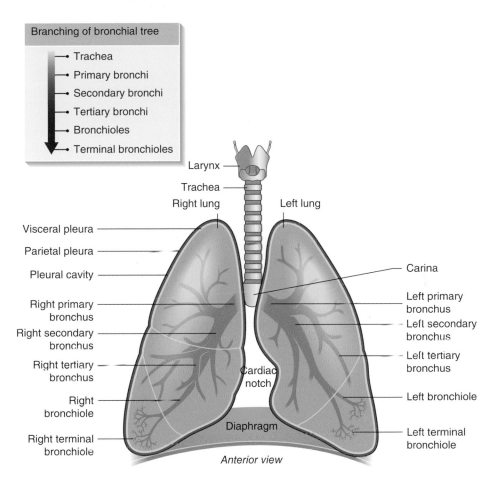

Branching of bronchial tree

- Trachea
- Primary bronchi
- Secondary bronchi
- Tertiary bronchi
- Bronchioles
- Terminal bronchioles

Larynx

Trachea

Right lung

Left lung

Visceral pleura

Parietal pleura

Pleural cavity

Right primary bronchus

Right secondary bronchus

Right tertiary bronchus

Right bronchiole

Right terminal bronchiole

Carina

Left primary bronchus

Left secondary bronchus

Left tertiary bronchus

Left bronchiole

Left terminal bronchiole

Cardiac notch

Diaphragm

Anterior view

Figure 14.3 The lower respiratory system.

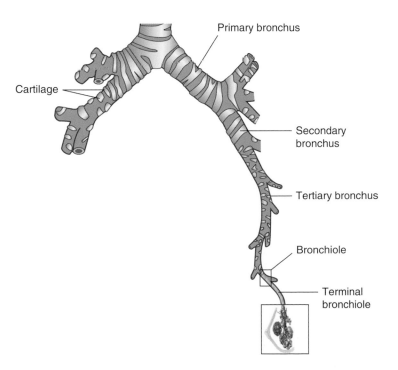

Primary bronchus

Cartilage

Secondary bronchus

Tertiary bronchus

Bronchiole

Terminal bronchiole

Figure 14.4 The bronchial tree.

Lungs

There are two lungs that are divided into distinct regions known as lobes. There are three lobes in the right lung and in left lung there are two. Each lung is surrounded by two thin protective membranes called the parietal and visceral pleura. The parietal pleura line the wall of the thorax and the visceral pleura line the lungs themselves. The space between the two pleura, is called the pleural space, this is minute and contains a thin film of lubricating fluid. This reduces friction between the two pleura, allowing both layers to slide over one another during breathing. The pleural fluid also helps the visceral and parietal pleura to adhere to each other.

The lungs receive blood from different arteries. The conduction region of the lungs receives oxygenated blood from capillaries that arise from the bronchial arteries, which originate from the aorta. Some of the bronchial arteries are connected to the pulmonary arteries. However, the majority of blood returns to the heart via the pulmonary or bronchial veins.

Pulmonary ventilation

Breathing (pulmonary ventilation) involves the physical movement of air in and out of the lungs. The principal function of pulmonary ventilation is to maintain adequate alveolar ventilation. This prevents the build-up of carbon dioxide in the alveoli and a constant supply of oxygen to the tissues.

Air flows between the atmosphere and the alveoli of the lungs as a result of pressure difference that is created by the contraction and relaxation of the respiratory muscles. The rate of air flow and the effort needed for breathing is influenced by the alveoli surface tension and the integrity of the lungs.

Inspiration

Just prior to breathing (inhalation) the pressure in the lungs equals the atmospheric pressure (760 mmHg or 101.33 kilopascals [kPa]). Therefore, for air to flow into the lungs, the pressure inside the alveoli has to be lower than the atmosphere. This is achieved by increasing lung volume.

When inspiration occurs, the thorax will expand and intrapulmonary pressure will fall below atmospheric pressure. Because intrapulmonary pressure is now less than atmospheric pressure, air will naturally enter the lungs until the pressure difference no longer exists. This phenomenon is explained by Boyle's law (Figure 14.5) and Dalton's law. Gases exert pressure and Boyle's law states that the amount of pressure exerted is inversely proportional to the size of its container.

Dalton's law states that in a mixture of gases each gas will exert its own individual pressure that is proportional to its size. Atmospheric air, for example, contains a mixture of gases and each individual gas will exert its own pressure dependent upon its quantity. Nitrogen, for example, will exert the greatest pressure as it is the most abundant gas. Together all the gases in the atmosphere exert a pressure –atmospheric pressure is 101.33 kPa at sea level. On inhalation the thorax expands, intrapulmonary pressure falls below 101.33 kPa, and air enters the lungs.

A range of respiratory muscles are needed to achieve thoracic expansion during inspiration. The major muscles of inspiration are the diaphragm and external intercostal muscles. The diaphragm, a dome-shaped skeletal muscle is found beneath the lungs at the base of the thorax. There are 11 external intercostal muscles, sitting in the intercostal spaces (the spaces between the ribs). During inspiration the diaphragm contracts downwards, pulling the lungs with it (Figure 14.6). At the same time the external intercostal muscles pull the rib cage outwards and upwards. The thorax is now bigger than before and as a result intrapulmonary pressure is reduced below atmospheric pressure. The most important muscle of inspiration is the diaphragm, 75% of the air that enters the lungs is as a result of diaphragmatic contraction.

Exhalation

Breathing out (exhalation) is also as a result of pressure gradient but it is converse to inhalation, that is, the pressure in the lungs is greater in the lungs than the atmosphere. At rest the normal exhalation is a passive process, no skeletal muscles are involved in the process. The process results from elastic recoil of the chest walls and the lungs.

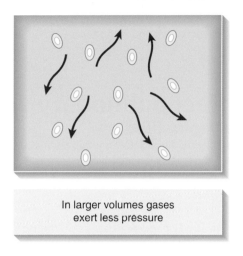

In larger volumes gases
exert less pressure

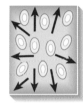

In smaller volumes gases
exert more pressure

Figure 14.5   Boyle's law.

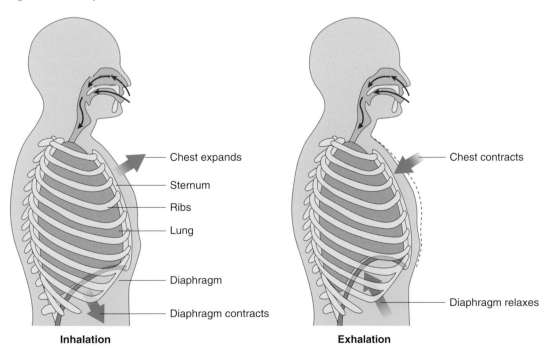

Chest expands

Sternum

Ribs

Lung

Diaphragm

Diaphragm contracts

Inhalation

Chest contracts

Diaphragm relaxes

Exhalation

Figure 14.6   Inspiration and expiration.

During exercise, the muscles of exhalation, which are the abdominals and intercostal muscles contract, the inferior ribs move downwards and compresses the abdominal viscera and the diaphragm moves upwards.

Factors that affect pulmonary ventilation

Surface tension of alveolar fluid

Surface tension is provided by the fluid surfactant, this is a mixture of phospholipids and lipoproteins. During inhalation, the surface tension must be overcome to expand the lungs, it also aids in the lungs elastic recoil.

Airway resistance

The flow of air through the airway passage depends on the resistance and pressure difference. The walls of the airways offer some resistance to the flow of air into and out of the lungs. During inspiration, the bronchioles dilate because their walls are pulled in all directions. The diameter of the airway passage is also dependent on the smooth muscles. Stimulation from the sympathetic nerve fibres cause the smooth muscles to relax resulting in bronchodilation and decreased resistance.

Lung compliance

Compliance refers to the effort that is required for lung and chest expansion. The higher the compliance the less effort is needed in chest and lung expansion and low compliance means that more effort is needed. In the lungs, there are two factors playing a part in compliance; the surface tension and elasticity.

Normal lungs have a high compliance and expand easily because the elastic fibres stretch readily and the surfactant in the lungs reduces surface tension. In pulmonary diseases, for example emphysema, there is decreased compliance as a result of the loss of elastic fibres of the alveolar walls.

Lung volumes

At rest, a healthy adult normally has a respiration rate of 12 to 18 breaths per minute and with each respiration 500 mL of air is moved in or out of the lungs. The volume of air in one breath is called tidal volume. By taking a deep breath, the tidal volume can be increased above 500 mL (inspiratory reserve volume). In adult males, this could be up to 3100 mL and in females is approximately 1900 mL.

How breathing is controlled

Pneumotaxic area

The pneumotaxic area (Figure 14.7) is another important area of the respiratory centre. This area is in the pons and is important for regulating the amount of air taken in with each breath. Yet, the inspiratory musculature is controlled by the dorsal respiratory group. The pneumotaxic area alters the bursting pattern of the dorsal respiratory group. When there is a need to breath faster, the pneumotaxic area tells the dorsal respiratory group to speed it up. and when longer breaths are needed, the pneumotaxic area tells the dorsal respiratory group to prolong its bursts. All the information from the body that needs to feed into the control of breathing converges in the pneumotaxic area, in order for it to properly adjust breathing.

Apneustic area

The apneustic area is another part of the brain situated in the lower pons that coordinates transition between inhalation and exhalation, (Figure 14.7). This area sends signals to the inspiratory area, activating and prolonging inhalation, resulting in long, deep inhalation. When the pneumotaxic area is active, it overrides the signals from the apneustic area.

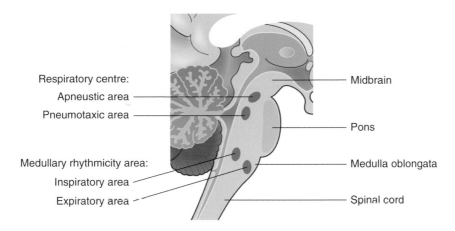

Respiratory centre:
  Apneustic area ——————
  Pneumotaxic area ——————

Medullary rhythmicity area:
  Inspiratory area ——————
  Expiratory area ——

—— Midbrain

—— Pons

—— Medulla oblongata

—— Spinal cord

Figure 14.7 The respiratory centre.

Medullary rhythmicity area

This area controls respiratory rhythm. There are inspiratory and expiratory areas within the medullary rhythmicity area (Figure 14.7). During quiet breathing, the inhalation is around two seconds, expiration is three seconds. Impulses from the inspiratory area maintain this rhythm. When the inspiratory area is active, the expiratory area is inactive.

However, during forceful breathing the expiratory area is stimulated by nerves from inspiratory area. Stimulation by the expiratory area causes the intercostal and abdominal to contract, which causes a decrease in the thoracic cavity and forceful exhalation.

Central chemoreceptors

These areas are found in the brainstem and contain neurons within them, central chemoreceptors, detecting changes in the carbon dioxide levels. When the carbon dioxide levels rise, this means that the respiration rate has to increase, getting rid of the carbon dioxide and taking in more oxygen. Carbon dioxide does not tend to remain CO_2 gas in water. Instead, it changes into a bicarbonate ion, producing hydrogen ions as a by-product of this conversion.

In blood, when carbon dioxide is converted into bicarbonate ions, the hydrogen ions are not a problem because they immediately associate with haemoglobin (the globin acts to buffer the hydrogen ions). However, in the brain, in the chemosensitive areas, there is no haemoglobin. The cerebrospinal fluid (CSF) of the brain does not have proteins to buffer the hydrogen ions, and when levels of CO_2 in the brain begin to increase, much of it is converted into bicarbonate ions and hydrogen ions. The central chemoreceptors are sensitive to hydrogen ion levels, so they indirectly recognise the increase in carbon dioxide levels.

However, a change in plasma pH alone will not stimulate central chemoreceptors as H^+ are not be able to diffuse across the blood–brain barrier into the CSF. Only CO_2 levels affect this as it can diffuse across, reacting with H_2O to form carbonic acid and thus decreases pH. Central chemoreception remains, in this way, distinct from peripheral chemoreceptors.

Peripheral chemoreceptors

Where the common carotid artery branches into the internal and external carotid arteries, there is a small swelling (Figure 14.8), the carotid sinus, containing regions called carotid bodies. The aorta contains regions called aortic bodies. These regions contain peripheral chemoreceptors, which detect oxygen levels directly.

Inflation reflex

This reflex is a type of negative feedback. As the lungs expand, there are sensory neurons detecting lung stretching; stretch receptors, but they are not like the stretch receptors in muscle. These neurons are sensory neurons that detect stretch. The more these neurons are active, the more they send signals

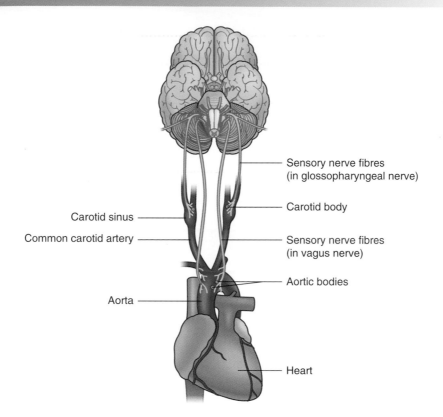

Figure 14.8   Peripheral chemoreceptors.

Table 14.1   Other influences on respiration.

Influence	Impact
Limbic system	Increases rate and depth of ventilation in times of stress through inspiratory area stimulation.
Temperature	Increase or decrease in body temperature can result in increase or decrease of the respiration rate, for example fever and hypothermia respectively.
Pain	Sudden severe pain can cause a brief period of apnoea, whilst a prolonged somatic pain increases respiration rate
Irritation of airways	Cessation of breathing can result from physical or chemical irritation of the pharynx. This is followed by coughing and sneezing.

into the pneumotaxic area to tell it to end this round of inspiration, this prevents the lungs from ever overinflating. Other influences on respiration can be found in Table 14.1.

Gas exchange

The principal function of pulmonary ventilation is to maintain adequate alveolar ventilation and for this to occur effective gas exchange is required. Gas exchange in the lungs and in the alveoli occurs between the alveolar air and the blood in the pulmonary capillaries. This exchange is a result of increased concentration of oxygen and a decrease of CO_2. This process of exchange is done through diffusion (see Figure 14.9).

External respiration

External respiration (pulmonary gas exchange) is the diffusion of oxygen from the alveolar sac to the lung capillaries and the diffusion of carbon dioxide from the lung capillaries to the alveolar sac to be exhaled. External respiration converts the oxygenated blood in the lungs to oxygenated blood before the blood returns to the left side of the heart.

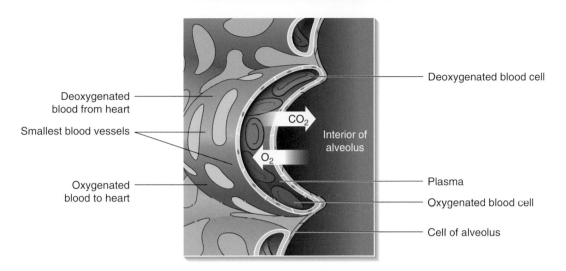

Deoxygenated blood from heart

Smallest blood vessels

Oxygenated blood to heart

Deoxygenated blood cell

CO_2

Interior of alveolus

O_2

Plasma

Oxygenated blood cell

Cell of alveolus

Figure 14.9 Gas exchange in the lungs.

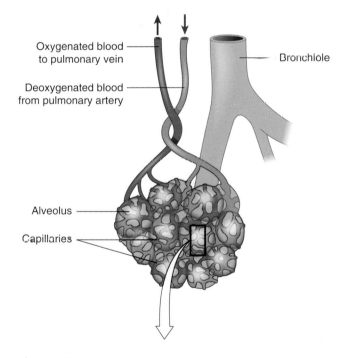

Oxygenated blood to pulmonary vein

Deoxygenated blood from pulmonary artery

Bronchiole

Alveolus

Capillaries

Figure 14.10 External respiration.

External respiration only occurs beyond the respiratory bronchioles. External respiration is the diffusion of oxygen from the alveoli into pulmonary circulation (blood flow through the lungs) and the diffusion of carbon dioxide in the opposite direction (Figure 14.10). Diffusion occurs because gas molecules always move from areas of high concentration to low concentration.

Internal respiration

Internal respiration describes the exchange of oxygen and carbon dioxide between blood and tissue cells (Figure 14.11), governed by the same principles as external respiration. Cells utilise oxygen when manufacturing the cells' prime energy source, adenosine tri-phosphate (ATP). In addition to ATP the cells also produce water and carbon dioxide. Because cells are continually using oxygen, its concentration within tissues is always lower than within blood. Similarly, the

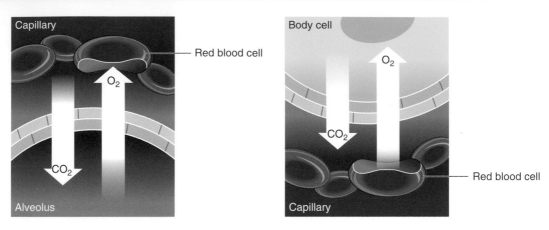

Figure 14.11   Internal respiration.

repeated use of oxygen ensures that the level of carbon dioxide within tissue is always higher than within blood. As blood flows through the capillaries oxygen and carbon dioxide follow their pressure gradients, continually diffusing between blood and tissue. The concentration of oxygen in blood flowing away from the tissues, back towards the heart is described as being de-oxygenated.

Transportation of gases

Oxygen and carbon dioxide are transported from the lungs to body tissues in blood. Both gases travel in blood plasma and haemoglobin, found within erythrocytes. Each erythrocyte contains approximately 280 million haemoglobin molecules and each haemoglobin molecule has the potential to carry four oxygen molecules. The delivery of oxygen, therefore, is also reliant upon the presence of an adequate supply of erythrocytes and haemoglobin.

So far

The respiratory system consists of a series of organs that are responsible for taking in oxygen and expelling carbon dioxide. The main organs of the respiratory system are lungs, carrying out the exchange of gases as we breathe.

Oxygen is exchanged for carbon dioxide through external respiration. This takes place through microscopic sacs called alveoli. Oxygen binds to haemoglobin molecules in red blood cells and is transported through the bloodstream. Carbon dioxide from deoxygenated blood diffuses from the capillaries into the alveoli, expelled through exhalation.

The bloodstream delivers oxygen to cells and removes waste carbon dioxide through internal respiration, red blood cells carry oxygen absorbed from the lungs around the body, through the vasculature. The red blood cells release the oxygen through the narrow capillaries diffusing through the capillary walls into body tissues. Carbon dioxide diffuses from the tissues into red blood cells and plasma. Carbon dioxide is carried back to the lungs for release.

Cultural considerations

In order to provide care that is culturally appropriate, the key issue is to know what cultural competency is. Cultural competence is a developmental process developed over time with the intention of enhancing understanding and knowledge of cultural differences that impact on the health care experience. Factors of cultural competence include cultural awareness, cultural knowledge, cultural skill, cultural encounters, and cultural desire (a willingness to engage in cultural competence).

The patient history

Undertaking a health examination and patient history provides the nurse with an opportunity to explore the patient's subjective symptoms and objective signs, to screen for diseases and identify risk for future health problems. According to Verghese and Horwitz (2009), skilled physical assessment may lead to fewer unnecessary diagnostic tests and increased patient satisfaction. There are many clinical signs that cannot be fully appreciated without a physical assessment being carried out, which is required to recognise slight changes and improve the patient experience (Zambas 2010).

The nurse is required to undertake a comprehensive respiratory assessment. One important aspect of this wide-ranging assessment will include the gathering of a medical history. The details gleaned from the medical history may help to explain physical assessment findings and can help with making the definitive diagnosis. Older adults may have a long respiratory history that can include smoking or exposure to second-hand smoke, environmental exposure to pollutants (inclusion asbestos), and illnesses that can include chronic obstructive pulmonary disease (COPD), congestive heart failure (CHF), or pneumonia.

During the gathering of the medical history the nurse should also determine if the patient has been vaccinated against influenza and pneumonia. It may also be appropriate for the nurse to offer education on the benefits of vaccination for the older person as well as discussing with the patient smoking cessation activities.

Review

What vaccination programmes are run in the area where you work? How are people made aware of the various vaccination programmes and what is the uptake?

Influenza is an acute viral infection of the respiratory tract. There are three types of influenza virus: A, B and C. Influenza A and influenza B are responsible for majority of clinical illnesses. Influenza is highly infectious and has a usual incubation period of one to three days (Public Health England and Department of Health 2013). The influenza immunisation programme aims to protect those who are most at risk of serious illness or death should they develop influenza and to reduce transmission of the infection, thus contributing to the protection of vulnerable patients who may have a suboptimal response to their own immunisations.

The pneumococcal vaccine offers protection against serious and potentially fatal pneumococcal infections. The vaccination is also known as the 'pneumo jab' or pneumonia vaccine. A pneumococcal infection can affect anyone. However, there are some people at higher risk of serious illness, these include:

- Babies
- Adults aged 65 or over
- Children and adults with certain long-term health conditions, such as a serious heart or kidney condition

The influenza vaccination is given annually. However, the pneumococcal vaccine should be given just once to those adults who are over the age of 65, and this will offer protection for life. Those people with a long-term health condition may need just a single one-off pneumococcal vaccination or a five-yearly vaccination, depending on the individual's underlying health problem.

The nurse is required to take a thorough family history, review current medications, enquire about the patient's energy levels, and determine their ability to perform the activities of living, and, if appropriate, their degree of dependence on others. Also take a smoking history. Is there any environmental exposure that can be a cause or exacerbate the condition? What is the patient's past medical and family history and current medications? Ask about shortness of breath, or wheezing. Also ask about symptoms such as coughing and if the patient is producing any sputum, the timing of a cough and the characteristics of sputum produced could indicate

Table 14.2   Some respiratory symptoms.

Symptom	Discussion
Cough	Is the cough productive or non-productive, hoarse, or barking?
Sputum	Is sputum clear, purulent, bloody (haemoptysis), rust-coloured, or pink and frothy?
Dyspnoea	Does the patient experience dyspnoea with or without activity, is there any wheezing (inspiratory of expiratory) or stridor?
Chest pain	If there is chest pain, does this occur on inspiration, expiration, or with coughing. Where is the pain? Ask the patient to point.

specific problems. A nocturnal cough may be a sign of pulmonary oedema associated with CHF, the sputum produced can be pink-tinged or frothy, rust-coloured, currant jam-like sputum might indicate pneumonia (see Table 14.2).

Review

When observing a sputum specimen think about and make notes on the following:

Characteristic	Potential meaning
Is the specimen: Frothy Watery Thick Tenacious	
Is there any haemoptysis?	
Does the specimen appear purulent (pus, yellow, green?)	
Foul-smelling	
The amount of sputum being produced	

Review

Revise local policy and procedure related to the collection of a sputum specimen and the transportation to the laboratory.

A guide to questioning using the mnemonic OLDCART in relation a cough (see Table 14.3).

The nurse should also ask about associated symptoms, for example cold symptoms, fever, night sweats, and fatigue. If the patient describes any of these symptoms enquire about the duration, when did the symptoms start, where, the location, how severe, the setting, the time of day, were there any alleviating factors as well as any aggravating factors, making the condition worse (Mansen and Gabiola 2015).

Take note

Because older adults are at increased risk for respiratory diseases as a result of loss of elasticity and decreased ventilation of the lower lobes of the lungs, specifically enquire about fatigue, weight change, dyspnoea on exertion, influenza and pneumonia vaccine status, and change in number of pillows that the patient uses at night.

Source: Hogstel and Curry (2005).

Table 14.3   A cough OLDCART.

O	Onset: When was the cough first noticed, did anything precipitate it? Has the patient been on new medications?
L	Location: Does the cough come from the throat or the chest?
D	Duration: Does the cough happen at a particular time of the day? Does it come and go or does it last all of the time? Does it wake the patient at night? Does it occur at rest or when undertaking exercise or activity?
C	Characteristic symptoms: Does the patient cough when inhaling or exhaling? Does the cough come in spasms, making breathing difficult? Is the patient coughing up mucous or phlegm and if so, what is the colour, odour, consistency, and amount? Is there any blood in the sputum? If the patient is actively coughing request a sample in a tissue so it can be examined
A	Associated manifestations: Are there any other symptoms such as shortness of breath, wheezing?
R	Relieving factors: Is there anything that makes it better?
T	Treatment: Has the patient seen another health care professional? Was any treatment prescribed?

Source: Adapted Hogan-Quigley et al. (2016).

So far

A detailed history should be gathered. The nurse should also be aware of the patient's current condition, i.e. they may be breathless. So as not to cause an exacerbation of their current health, ask only pertinent questions.

Respiratory problems may be caused by disorders of other systems therefore a full systems assessment may be needed.

How to use a stethoscope

Prior to undertaking a physical examination, a number of skills have to be honed and developed and one is the use of a stethoscope (see Figure 14.12). Stethoscopes are used for a number of reasons and nurses use them in all spheres of practice, for example to listen to a baby's first breath and sometimes to listen to a patient's last heartbeat.

Take note

When caring for people, the nurse must be able to gather and interpret physical assessment data that goes beyond the stethoscope, including knowledge of changes that can affect the person to determine the most appropriate interventions for care provision.

As well as the traditional binaural stethoscope, electronic stethoscopes are also available which provide amplification so that it is easier to hear heart and lung sounds. This can be a significant advantage since heart sounds and lung sounds are very faint.

The nurse uses the stethoscope to auscultate, this is the listening to sounds produced by the body, for example the lungs, abdomen, heart, and blood vessels. There are some sounds that can be heard by the ear alone, for example a rumbling stomach, a person with a wheezy chest or congested, snuffled breathing. Some sounds are soft and to be heard they have to be channelled through a stethoscope, so the nurse can assess the sounds. To get the most out of the stethoscope the nurse needs to learn how to use it, the ear can be trained to listen accurately. Stethoscopes do not magnify sound they will, however, block out some extraneous room noise.

It is important that the nurse uses a high-quality and well-fitting stethoscope so as to hear clearly and in so doing assess effectively. Choose ear tips that fit comfortably and painlessly (if they hurt

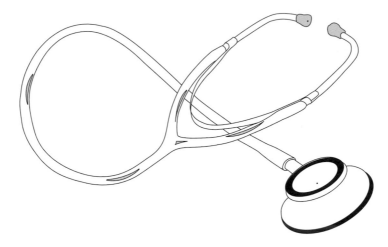

Figure 14.12   The stethoscope.

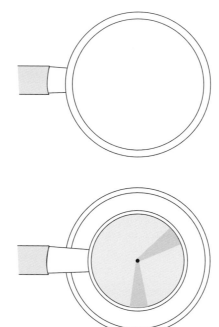

Figure 14.13   The bell and diaphragm.

then they are inserted too far). The slope of the ear pieces point forward, matching the natural shape of the ear canals. Point them towards your nose; this can eliminate any ambient noise. Use tubing that is thick-walled and as short as is practicably possible so as to augment the transmission of sound; longer tubing has the potential to distort sound.

At the disk end of the stethoscope is the bell and diaphragm (see Figure 14.13). The smaller component is the bell, this is cupped and transmits lower-pitched sounds (such as extra heart sounds or murmurs). Hold the bell lightly against the person's skin so that it forms a perfect seal. Be careful not to hold the bell too hard against the skin as this will obliterate low-pitched sounds. The diaphragm is flatter and larger transmitting higher-pitched sounds (for example, breath, bowel, normal heart sounds). Hold the diaphragm firmly against the person's skin. The bell and diaphragm can be changed by rotating the disk. To determine which end is open for transmission, lightly tap on the disk.

Auscultation (see Box 14.1) is a skill that many novice nurses are keen to learn. However, it can be difficult to master. The nurse must first learn the wide range of normal sounds, so that they can

Box 14.1 Auscultation

1. Explain the process to the patient and seek consent.
2. Wash hands.
3. Inspect the stethoscope for quality and damage. Also, make sure that tubing is free of leaks.
4. Prior to evaluating body sounds, the nurse must endeavour to remove any confusing artefacts. Find a relatively quiet area to ensure that the body sounds are not overpowered by background noise.
5. Use the stethoscope on bare skin to avoid picking up the sound of rustling fabric. The examination room should be kept warm. If the patient is shivering, then the involuntary muscle contractions can reduce the quality of other sounds.
6. Do not talk into the round part whilst the stethoscope is in the ears. It can also cause hearing impairment or loss, depending on the volume of the noise emitted.
7. The stethoscope end piece must be cleaned with an alcohol wipe. The bell should be warmed by rubbing it in the palm.
8. The friction on the endpiece from a man's chest hair causes a crackling sound that sounds like an abnormal breath sound called *crackles*. To reduce this problem, wet the hair prior to auscultating.
9. Never listen through a gown. Listening through clothing will create artifactual sounds and will muffle any diagnostically valuable sound from the heart or lungs. With consent and explanation reach under a gown to listen, but avoid any clothing rubbing on the stethoscope.
10. Finally, avoid your own 'artefact', such as breathing on the tubing, or the 'thump' from bumping the tubing together.
11. Thank the patient.
12. Wash hands.
13. Record and report findings.

Source: Adapted Haro and Olivera (2012).

discriminate the abnormal sounds and extra sounds. In some body locations, there may be more than one sound heard and this can cause confusion. Mastering the skill means the nurse will need to be selective in what they are listening to, so as to hear only one thing at a time. Periodic stethoscope disinfection helps to reduce bacterial contamination.

Review

Take time to observe an experienced health care professional as they use the stethoscope during a clinical consultation.

Take note

When listening selectively, the nurse should ask:

- What is it that I am *actually* hearing?
- What is it that I *should* be hearing at this location?

Take note

Prerequisites for auscultation:
   A good-quality stethoscope, the ability and patience to listen to the sounds, along with a detailed understanding of anatomy, physiology, and pathophysiology of the sound-producing organ.

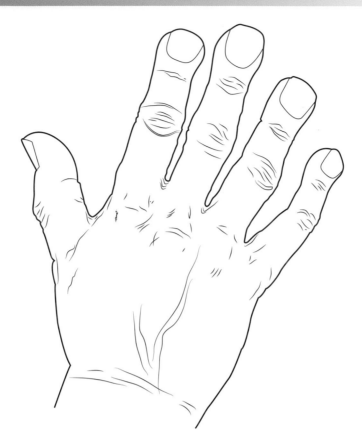

254

Figure 14.14   Clubbing.

Physical examination

The physical examination yields the objective data, and this together with the subjective data (the patient history) can help make a differential diagnosis with the ensuing development of a care plan. The physical examination begins with inspection/observation.

Take note

Prior to an examination, the nurse should introduce themselves, explain to the patient what is to occur and the reason why, wash hands and gain consent.

When meeting the patient observe the level of consciousness, facial expression, skin colour, moisture, and temperature. The patient's facial expression should be relaxed, showing no signs of distress or anxiety, are the lips pursed as the patient breathes, is there any nasal flaring. If there is any indication that breathing is a conscious effort hence this could be an indication that something is wrong. Observe the nail beds, lips, mouth, ears, and the conjunctiva for oxygen saturation, bluish tinge signifies cyanosis and hypoxia. Clubbing of the fingers may indicate chronic hypoxaemia (see Figure 14.14). Determine whether the patient is using any accessory muscles of respiration, observe the neck for contraction of the sternomastoid muscles. If so, this can mean difficulty with breathing (Mansen and Gabiola 2015).

Explain clearly to the patient what you intend to do as part of the physical examination and gain consent. With the patient properly prepared and exposing only what is necessary to examine the chest and back, the patient should be sitting upright, observe the respiratory rate and rhythm for a full minute. The patient's breathing is considered abnormal if the rate is irregular, too fast (tachypnoea), too slow (bradypnoea), or shallow (see Table 14.4).

Table 14.4   Characteristics of breathing.

Type	Characteristic	Related conditions
Tachypnoea	Regular respirations with a rate above 20 breaths per minute	Pneumonia, pulmonary oedema, pain, chronic obstructive pulmonary disease (COPD), heart failure
Bradypnoea	Regular respiratory rate that is less than 12 breaths per minute	Central nervous system depression, over-sedation, raised intracranial pressure
Hyperventilation	Over-breathing, rapid, shallow respiratory rate.	May be due to a physical or psychological cause, for example pain or anxiety. Can be caused by exercise, asthma, COPD, metabolic disorder
Hypoventilation	Shallow respirations	Brain stem disorder, over sedation. Rib fracture, pain. Minimal movement of the breath can sometimes be seen in asthma
Kussmaul	Regular rapid, deep, and laboured breathing	Diabetic ketoacidosis, metabolic acidosis, renal disease, poisoning
Cheyne Stokes	Apnoea, associated with a crescendo and decrescendo type of breathing. Deeper and faster breathing accompanied with shallow and slower breathing with apnoea up to 60 seconds	Often observed in the dying patient. Acid–base balance disturbance, neuromuscular disease
Apnoea	Cessation of breathing	Respiratory arrest

Source: Adapted Rawles et al. (2015).

Take note

The assessment of vital signs is essential for identifying acute changes in a patient's condition. Vital sign assessment allows for the identification of signs of improvement or if the patient is deteriorating. Assessment of these clinical parameters will play an important role in early detection of a patient who is deteriorating but only if the nurse understands the basis of the signs and they are measured, communicated, and acted upon.

Source: Armstrong et al. (2008).

Respiratory rate assessment is essential for detecting acute changes in a patient's condition. Elliott (2016) notes that despite this it has been shown that it is the most neglected vital sign in clinical practice.

Take note

Assessment of vital signs is essential for detecting acute changes in a patient's condition. Vital sign assessment allows for the identification of signs of improvement or if the patient is deteriorating, alternate, or emergency care to be initiated. Assessment of these clinical parameters plays a fundamental role in early detection of patient deterioration, but only if nurses understand the basis of the signs, and they are measured, communicated, and acted upon.

Hogan-Quigley et al. (2016) informs that the nurse should observe the shape of the thorax, this should be symmetrical with uniform chest movement. If there is retraction or bulging of the intercostal spaces this could indicate obstructed airways. There may be flail chest. Flail chest often occurs after trauma where a segment(s) of the rib cage brakes and the injured area may cave inward on inspiration and outward on expiration. Observe the anterior and posterior chest for evidence of scaring (surgery), bruising, and abnormality.

If the patient is unable to sit up, the nurse can perform the respiratory assessment by gently rolling the patient from one side, then to the other.

Auscultation of the chest

Being able to competently auscultate the chest requires much skill. When undertaking lung auscultation, it is important to be consistent in preparing and auscultating the patient, this enables a complete assessment that will be more accurate and increases the chances of identifying subtle breath sound change. The nurse should always compare equivalent positions on each side of the chest as this permits identification of asymmetry in the quality or loudness of the breath sounds. It is imperative that the nurse knows the lung anatomy so as to ensure that the stethoscope is being placed in the correct position for auscultation. As the intensity of sound may vary depending upon location, it is important to always auscultate the opposite sides of the thorax successively. The most common sites are shown in Figures 14.15 and 14.16.

There are usually four types of breath sound heard in a normal chest (see Table 14.5).

Adventitious breath sounds are abnormal sounds that can be heard over the patient's lungs and airways (Ford et al. 2005). These sounds include abnormal sounds, for example, fine and coarse crackles (crackles are also known as rales). Crackles are discontinuous and soft pitched, popping sounds and are more common during inspiration. The sounds come from fluid in the airways or from the opening of alveoli that have collapsed. Wheezes are caused by air movement through a narrowed or partially obstructed airway, for example in asthma. The sounds are continuous and persist through the respiratory cycle. Rhonchi, a continuous low-pitched, rumbling breath sound, can indicate the presence of secretions in the larger airways. Pleural rubs and stridor can also be heard through auscultation.

Percussion of the chest

The nurse uses percussion to assess underlying structures of the chest wall. The patient should be lying at 45° with the chest and back fully exposed (privacy and dignity must be maintained). The anterior chest should be examined first and then the posterior chest.

6Cs

The patient should always be given the opportunity to have a chaperone present during the examination. The nurse should also consider privacy, modesty, and dignity.

Percussion is an assessment technique which produces sounds by the nurse tapping on the patient's chest wall. Tapping on the chest wall produces sounds that are based on the amount of air in the lungs, percussion producing audible sounds and palpable vibrations, helping to determine whether the underlying tissues are filled with air, fluid, or solid material.

To percuss, wash the hands and place the first part of the middle finger of your non-dominant hand firmly on the patient's skin. Then strike the finger placed on the patient's skin with the end of the middle finger of the dominant hand. Working from the upper part of the chest downward, compare sounds heard on the right and left sides of the chest. As this is done, visualise the structures underneath as you progress. After the assessment ensure the patient is comfortable, wash hands, document, and report your findings. Figure 14.17 demonstrates the technique for percussion and Figure 14.18 the sites for percussion: the anterior and lateral chest wall. Figure 14.19 shows the sites for percussion of the posterior chest wall.

A normal lung will produce a resonant note. Rawles et al. (2015) suggest, however, that normal percussion does not confirm the absence of important pathology. In Table 14.6 percussion sounds (notes) are presented.

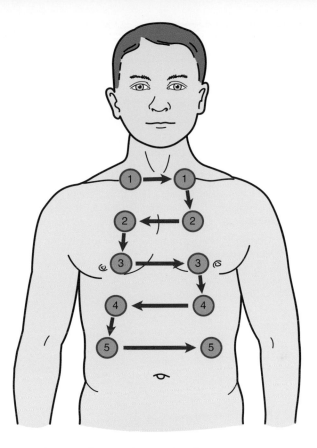

Figure 14.15 Common sites for auscultation, the anterior chest.

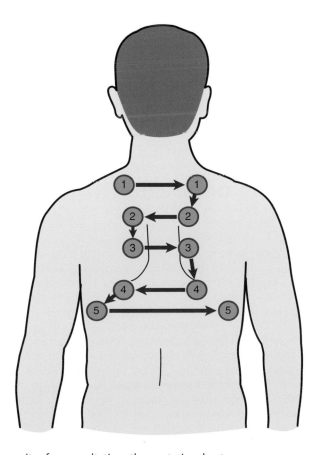

Figure 14.16 Common sites for auscultation, the posterior chest.

Table 14.5   Breath sounds.

Type of breath sound	Description
Vesicular	Quiet and low-pitched, there is a longer inspiratory than expiratory phase heard, these sounds are heard in most fields
Bronchovesicular	Medium sound in pitch, inspiratory and expiratory phases equal in length
Bronchial	This is higher-pitched and louder than the vesicular sounds. Expiration is longer than the inspiratory phase, anteriorly sounds are heard at the second and third intercostal space
Tracheal	A loud, high-pitched sound with equal inspiratory and expiratory phase, this is heard over the trachea

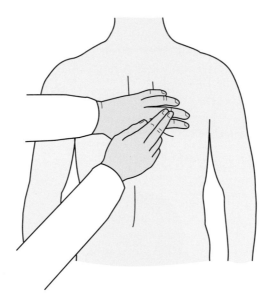

Figure 14.17   Technique for percussion.

Palpation of the neck and thorax

Palpating the neck and thorax can provide the nurse with important information about the respiratory system. If the patient is complaining of pain, ask them to point where this is and inspect in more detail.

To assess the respiratory system using palpation, gently place the palm of the hand lightly over the thorax. Palpate for tenderness, alignment, bulging, and retractions. Inspect in more detail. Check the position of the trachea, locate the two clavicle heads, Preston and Kelly (2017) suggests that any deviation may indicate a tumour or pneumothorax. Determine if the chest is expanding equally. Do this by placing the hands on the chest wall with thumbs meeting at the midline (see Figure 14.20).

Tactile fremitus refers to the ability to palpate vibrations that are produced by the voice in the large airways and transmitted to the chest wall. Ask the patient to say 'ninety nine' or 'one, one, one' (this is known as broncophony) and as this is done, at the apex above the clavicle, moving downward for the upper to the lower lobes, check for symmetry between the left and the right. Palpate for sound vibrations, which are reduced in, for example, pleural effusion or pleural thickening; this can muffle the transmission of the vibrations from the lung to the chest wall (see Figure 14.21). If there is consolidation of the lung this may enhance transmission of the vibration.

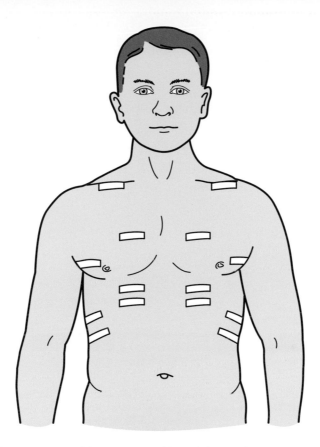

Figure 14.18   Sites for percussion of the anterior and lateral chest wall.

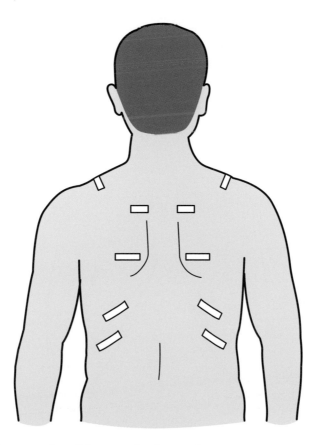

Figure 14.19   Sites for percussion of the posterior chest wall.

So far

The physical examination should take place after a detailed history has been obtained. Dignity and privacy are essential as the upper aspect of the patient will need to be exposed. The physical examination comprises:

- Inspection
- Auscultation
- Percussion
- Palpation

Table 14.6 Lung sounds.

Type	Clinical significance
Resonant sounds. Low-pitched, hollow sounds	Normal lung tissue
Dull or thud like sounds. Medium in intensity and pitch, moderate length	These are normally heard over dense areas, for example the heart or liver. Dullness substitutes resonance when fluid or solid tissue replaces air-containing lung tissues, this occurs with pneumonia, pleural effusions, pulmonary collapse, fibrosis, or tumours
Hyperresonant. These are louder and lower pitched than resonant sounds	An area of hyperresonance on one side of the chest may indicate a pneumothorax.
Stony, dull or flat. Short high-pitched very dull	Pleural effusion or haemothorax.

Source: Adapted Devereux and Douglas (2013), Innes and Tiernan (2018), Rawles et al. (2015).

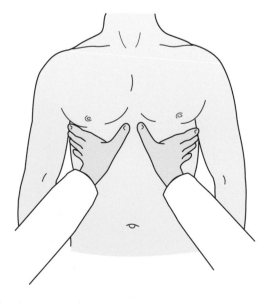

Figure 14.20 Checking for chest expansion.

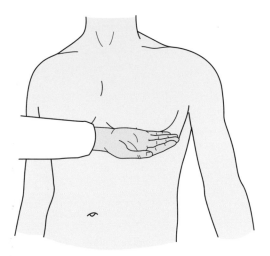

Figure 14.21   Tactile fremitus.

261

Ruby Coleman (grandmother)

Ruby described her chief complaint as, 'My cough is getting worse and it is now hurting.'

The nurse gathered information as a history was taken. Being aware that Mrs Coleman was short of breath, she also gathered information from Mrs Coleman's husband, Bob. The nurse also asks closed-ended questions that would require a nod, shaking of the head or a 'yes' or 'no'.

Mrs Coleman presents with a three-day history of left-sided pleuritic chest pain, dyspnoea, ortho-pnoea, with an intermittent pyrexia and chills. Mrs Coleman has a productive cough. She is coughing up yellow sputum and since yesterday this has become brown. Her pleuritic chest pain is radiating to the proximal left upper quadrant (LUQ) when she coughs. This morning she also experienced a runny nose (rhinorrhoea) as well as a sore throat.

Mrs Coleman has had asthma since childhood. Usually this has been under good control. She had run out of her Ventolin inhaler, she has not been using it for some time. Four years ago, Mrs Coleman had a left inguinal hernia repaired under spinal anaesthesia, and she was diagnosed with pneumonia during her recovery period.

Mrs Coleman's father had been diagnosed with hypertension. He died aged 67 from 'a heart condition'. Her mother died in childbirth. There is a family history for coronary artery disease, asthma, diabetes, and cancer. Mrs Coleman does not smoke. She reports alcohol use, two bottles of Guinness on a Friday and Saturday.

Since Mrs Coleman has pain, assess her pain using the PQRST approach (remember, though, she is dyspnoeic):

	Your assessment findings
Provocation/palliation	
Quality/quantity	
Region/radiation	
Severity scale	
Timing	

Now you have a medical history you will need to perform a physical examination. Describe your actions with regard to:

- Inspection
- Palpation
- Percussion
- Auscultation

Whilst you are inspecting Mrs Coleman's chest, look for these characteristics that may put a *CRAMP* in Mrs Coleman's respiratory system.

Chest wall asymmetry

Respiratory rate and pattern (abnormal)

Accessory muscle use

Masses or scars

Paradoxical movement

What investigations are required in this case that will help you make a definitive diagnosis?

Write a care plan for Mrs Coleman for the first 72 hours after she has been admitted to the medical assessment unit.

Conclusion

As the role of the nurse has continued to evolve, nurses are expected to take on additional duties that may have been traditionally associated with the medical profession. In taking on these additional duties this means that the nurse must be able to demonstrate proficiency when carrying out the additional skills that are required to assess a person holistically including the respiratory system.

Respiratory assessment is essential for detecting acute changes in a patient's condition. Inspection, palpation, percussion, and auscultation of the lungs should form part of the respiratory assessment as well as obtaining a detailed medical history. These activities will provide a baseline for patients with respiratory and lung disease. The nurse needs to hone and develop the various skills associated with assessment in order to offer care that is evidence-based.

References

Armstrong, B., Walthall, H., Clancy, M. et al. (2008). Recording of vital signs in a district general hospital emergency department. *Emergency Medical Journal* 25: 799–802.

Devereux, G. and Douglas, G. (2013). The respiratory system. In: *Macleod's Clinical Examination* (ed. G. Douglas, F. Nicol and C. Robertson), 137–163. Edinburgh: Elsevier.

Elliott, M. (2016). Why is respiratory rate the neglected vital sign? A narrative review. *International Achieves of Nursing Health Care* 2: 50.

Ford, M., Hennessey, I., and Japp, A. (2005). *Introduction to Clinical Examination*. Oxford: Elsevier.

Haro, B. and Olivera, L. (2012). *Nursing Profession and Basic Medical Care Techniques*. Delhi: Academic Press.

Heuer, A.J. and Scanlan, C.L. (2017). *Wilkins' Clinical Assessment in Respiratory Care*, 8e. St Louis: Mosby.

Hogan-Quigley, B., Palm, M.L., and Bickely, L.S. (2016). *Bate's Nursing Guide to Physical Examination and History Raking*, 2e. Philadelphia: Lippincott.

Hogstel, M. and Curry, L. (2005). *Health Assessment Through the Life Span*, 4e. Philadelphia: F.A. Davis.

Innes, J.A. and Tiernan, J. (2018). The respiratory system. In: *Macleod's Clinical Examination* (ed. J.A. Innes, A.R. Dover and K. Fairhurst), 75–92. Edinburgh: Elsevier.

Mansen, T. and Gabiola, J. (2015). *Patient-Focused Assessment*. Boston: Pearson.

Preston, W. and Kelly, C. (2017). *Respiratory Nursing at a Glance*. Oxford: Wiley.

Public Health England and Department of Health (2013) Immunisation against infectious disease. https://assets.publishing.service.gov.uk/government/uploads/system/uploads/attachment_data/file/660902/Green_book_cover_and_contents.pdf (accessed August 2018).

Rawles, Z., Griffiths, B., and Alexander, T. (2015). *Physical Examination Procedures*, 2e. London: CRC Press.

Verghese, A. and Horwitz, R.I. (2009). In praise of the physical examination. *British Medical Journal* 339: https://doi.org/10.1136/bmj.b5448.

Zambas, S.I. (2010). Purpose of the systematic physical assessment in everyday practice: critique of a 'sacred cow'. *Journal of Nursing Education* 49 (6): 305–310.

Chapter 15

Assessing the male reproductive system

Aim

This chapter introduces the reader to the assessment of the male reproductive system and the care required for men who may experience problems related to this system.

Learning outcomes

By the end of the chapter the reader will be able to:

1. Provide a brief overview of the male reproductive system and its functions
2. Discuss a number of conditions that might affect the male reproductive system
3. Outline the various ways in which the nurse may undertake an assessment of the male reproductive system
4. Describe care planning that is related to the male reproductive system

Introduction

The male reproductive system is considered in this chapter. Chapter 16 considers the female reproductive system. Whilst these two systems are very different there are some fundamental issues that concern both systems, for example the approach the nurse takes when obtaining a health history.

There are a number of diseases and medications that have the potential to have a negative impact on the male reproductive system and its function. Assessment of the male genitalia is undertaken with inspection and palpation. The nurse must document what the patient reports during the data-gathering phase (the history), what is seen (inspection), and what is felt (palpation).

The physiological and anatomical facets of the reproductive tract are predominately associated with procreation, the psychological and social aspects of reproduction are also important, the pleasure that is often provided by the reproductive organs should also be given due consideration. Ill health that is related to the reproductive tract can result in loss of life, acute and chronic illness, and also physical and emotional distress.

The male reproductive system

The male reproductive tract produces spermatozoa, depositing it inside the vagina, this contributes to reproduction. The spermatozoa are responsible for the fertilisation of the female egg. Whilst the female genitalia are found primarily inside of the body, this is not the same for the male (see Figure 15.1).

Fundamentals of Assessment and Care Planning for Nurses, First Edition. Ian Peate.
© 2020 John Wiley & Sons Ltd. Published 2020 by John Wiley & Sons Ltd.

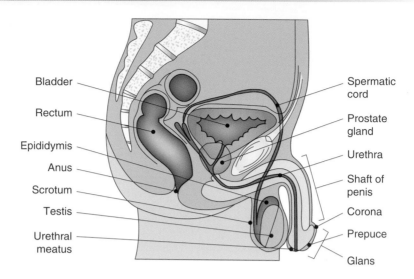

Figure 15.1 The male reproductive system.

264

Male reproductive organs work together with other body systems, such as the neuroendocrine system, that produce the hormones that are key in biological development and sexual behaviour, performance, and actions. These reproductive organs also include and are essential for the functioning of the urinary system.

The male genitalia

The penis and scrotum are the male external genitalia. The scrotal sac is a loose bag like sac of skin which is suspended by the spermatic cord located between the thighs. Within the scrotal sac are the testes approximately 4.5 cm long, 2.5 cm in breath, and 3 cm diameter. They feel smooth and move easily within the scrotal sac (Waugh and Grant 2018). The testes are located outside the abdominal cavity, in the scrotum. However, they develop in the abdominal cavity and usually descend into the scrotal sac during the last two months of foetal development. The testes traverse the inguinal canal and inguinal rings and into the scrotum, where they are suspended.

It is common for one of the testicles to hang lower than the other. As the cremasteric muscle contracts, the spermatic cord shortens and the testes move upwards towards the abdomen. This movement towards the abdomen provides the testes with more warmth. For sperm to develop effectively, the testes have to be at a lower temperature than the body; this is why the testes are located externally (outside the body) (see Figure 15.2).

There are two functions associated with the testes: to secrete the hormone testosterone and produce sperm. Testosterone is required for the development of the male secondary sex characteristics, such as deep voice, beard growth, body hair, as well as the function of the male reproductive system in the production of spermatozoa (Tortora and Derrikson 2014) (see Figure 15.3). Levels of testosterone are regulated by a negative-feedback mechanism with the hypothalamus. The testes are the essential organs of reproduction.

The testes situated under a membranous shell are glandular tissue composed of several lobules of differing size. Each lobule consists of around 660 to 1200 seminiferous tubules, which are small, convoluted structures responsible for sperm production. The spermatozoa develop in different stages in different parts of the tubules. Sperm is formed continuously in a young man and is produced at the rate of 120 million per day. The sperm moves from the seminiferous tubules to the rete testes, to the efferent ducts, and on towards to the epididymis, where spermatogenesis occurs and newly created mature sperm cells are formed. Spermatogenesis is complex and according to Heffner and Schust (2014) can be divided into three phases

1. Mitotic proliferation, producing large numbers of cells
2. Meiotic division, producing genetic diversity
3. Maturation, manufacturing sperm for transit and penetration of the oocyte

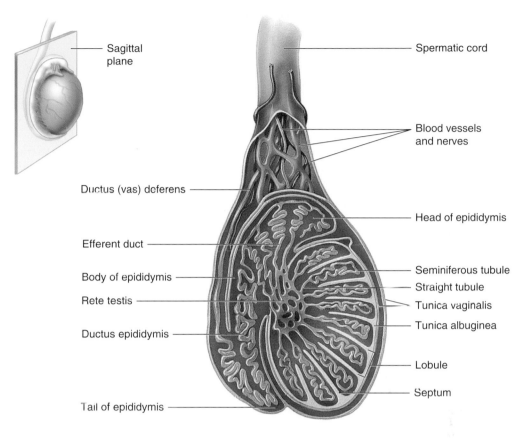

Sagittal plane

Spermatic cord

Blood vessels and nerves

Ductus (vas) deferens

Head of epididymis

Efferent duct

Body of epididymis

Rete testis

Seminiferous tubule

Straight tubule

Tunica vaginalis

Tunica albuginea

Ductus epididymis

Lobule

Septum

Tail of epididymis

Figure 15.2 The teste.

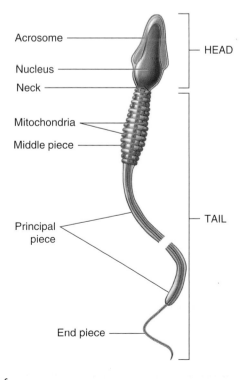

Acrosome

Nucleus

Neck

HEAD

Mitochondria

Middle piece

Principal piece

TAIL

End piece

Figure 15.3 Components of a sperm.

The sperm is then relocated on to the vas deferens and expelled through the urethra as a result of rhythmic peristaltic contractions.

Review

What does the surgical procedure vasectomy involve?

The Leydig cells are situated between the seminiferous tubules, it is here where testosterone and other androgens are formed. The stages of spermatogenesis are detailed in Figure 15.4. Figure 15.5 provides details concerning physical changes in the male related to testosterone.

The penis is the external male reproductive organ and located within the penis is the urethra. The penis provides a route for the elimination of ejaculate and urine via the urethra orifice situated at the end of the penis, the enlarged aspect is known as the glans penis. The glans penis is akin to the female clitoris. The penis is made up of three columns of erectile tissue (see Figure 15.6):

- Two corpora cavernosa
- One corpus spongiosum

The end of the corpus spongiosum is the bulbous glans penis, covered with a thin layer of skin allowing for erection and in the uncircumcised male the skin at the glans folds over on itself to form the prepuce (or foreskin). The area where the foreskin is attached, underneath the penis, is the frenulum. The foreskin is homologous with the female clitoral hood. The urethra, the terminal end of the urinary tract, is at the tip of the glans and is known as the urethral meatus. Erection requires complex vascular activity. This includes dilation of the arteries supplying blood to the penis and sympathetic nervous system activity.

The prostate gland lies at the base of the urinary bladder, surrounded by the upper part of the urethra (Marieb and Hoehn 2016). The function of the prostate gland is not well understood. The gland is said to be chestnut-shaped, made up of 20–30 compound tubuloalveolar glands which are embedded in a mass of smooth muscle and dense connective tissue. A thin milky fluid is secreted, adding bulk to semen on ejaculation. During orgasm sperm are conveyed from the urethra via the ejaculatory ducts situated in the prostate gland. Smooth muscle in the prostate gland contracts during ejaculation, expelling semen.

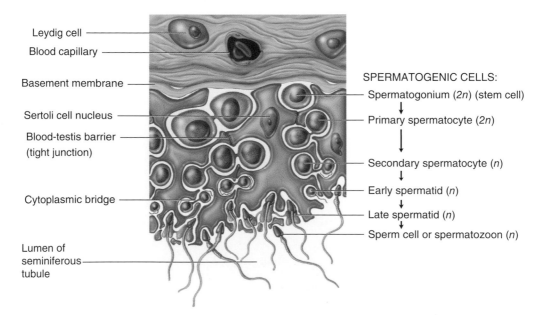

Figure 15.4   The stages of spermatogenesis.

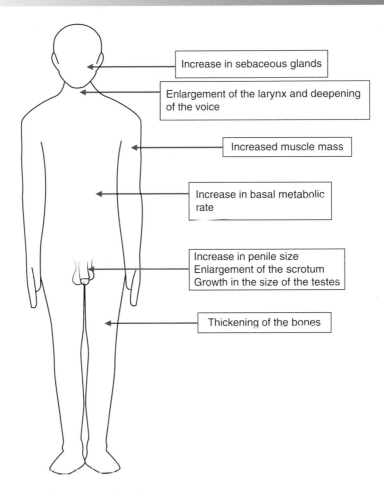

Figure 15.5   Some male changes related to testosterone.

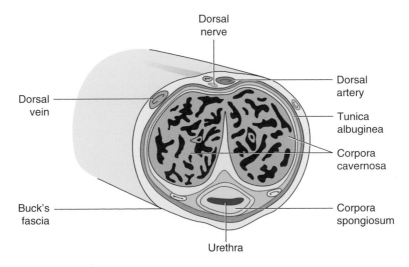

Figure 15.6   The penis – erectile tissue.

So far

An overview of the function of the organs of the male reproductive system:

Organ	Function
Penis	Made up of the corpora cavernosum, which when engorged causes the penis to become rigid and erect. The foreskin, where present provides protection to the glans penis.
Scrotum	This is a protective loose sac that is divided into two compartments for the internal organs: testes, epididymis, and vas deferens; temperature regulation of the testes.
Testes	Production of spermatozoa (seminiferous tubules) and testosterone.
Vas Deference	This cord-like structure transports sperm from the testes and epididymis into the urethra.
Spermatic cord	Offers protection to the vas deferens, internal and external spermatic arteries, artery of the vas, venous pampiniform plexus, lymph vessels, and nerves.
Prostate gland	Produces some of the seminal fluid; as well as a thin, white fluid that mixes with seminal fluid to neutralise the urethra and vagina to maintain sperm viability.
Seminal vesicles	Manufactures most of the seminal fluid

Assessing needs

The importance of a detailed health history and a physical examination cannot be underestimated. The nurse has to be able to differentiate normal from abnormal findings and must have an understanding of function and locations of the organs involved.

As the male reproductive system has a dual role (in conjunction with the urinary system), this will mean that the nurse will have to gather data concerning reproductive and elimination functions. Many diagnostic procedures will be the same in order to evaluate both. The nurse is required to undertake an assessment of the male reproductive system and an assessment of the man's needs in a variety of clinical situations, with the aim of making a diagnosis, planning care, and evaluating care interventions.

6Cs

Assessment of needs must be undertaken with the best interests of the man at heart, with compassion and respect at all times.

The nurse should remember that assessment of the reproductive system could reveal personal and private information. Inform the man that the information gathered will remain confidential and if this information is to be shared with others, this will only occur with his consent. The interview will focus on questions associated with the issues in Table 15.1.

Subjective data includes information about hygiene, safe sex practices, and habits that may create risks for reproductive system disorders. The assessment stage of the nursing process is linked with the findings from diagnostic tests, a health history where subjective data is collected, and a physical assessment enabling the nurse to collect objective data.

Table 15.1 The focus of the interview.

- Illnesses
- Signs and symptoms
- Sexual health problems
- Sexual activity
- Fertility
- Sexually acquired infections.

The initial interaction with the man should be undertaken in a non-threatening way. His health history and his current medications are reviewed. A complete assessment of the male reproductive system includes a detailed review of the man's history, as there are many conditions that can present as complaints of pain related to the reproductive structures. Pain as a result of a kidney stone may radiate along the spermatic cord and present as testicular pain. The man who informs the nurse that he is having difficulty starting the urinary stream and is also complaining of perineal tenderness could be displaying signs and symptoms of prostatitis or benign prostatic hypertrophy. Urethral pain may be a result of prostatitis, sexually acquired infection or recent instrumentation using a cystoscope.

6Cs

When the nurse respects the man, they must also respect the choices that the man makes, and this includes choices regarding his sexuality and sexual activity. At all times the nurse must act in a non-judgemental manner.

If a man complains of a swelling in the scrotum this could suggest an inguinal hernia. Details of any previous treatment for diseases related to the male reproductive tract or complaints should be discussed, including surgery as an adult or as a child.

269

Erectile dysfunction is a condition that cannot be seen or felt during a physical examination and because of this it is important that this issue be discussed with the man (if appropriate). Enquire, respectfully, about his relationship(s) as well as his level of sexual satisfaction. If the patient has diabetes, hypertension, or depression and he is taking any medication for these conditions, then he may have erectile problems, but he might be too embarrassed to broach the subject. The nurse can say, for example, 'Often having diabetes can cause erectile dysfunction. How are things for you, have you encountered any problems with getting an erection?' Use of a questionnaire may also help the man to discuss any problems he may have in a more open manner. The nurse asks the questions in such a way as 'This is what we ask everyone', in a matter-of-fact way.

Take note

When caring for men with erectile dysfunction some men may not be aware of the cause and this has the potential to increase anxiety. The man may think he is less than a man. Adopting a non-judgemental approach is key as the cause may be blamed on unconnected factors, for example age, medications, illness, or sexual partner.

So far

The health interview is an additional method for assessing and determining problems. There may be a number of situations whereby the health interview can be undertaken, such as during a health screening. It may focus on a chief complaint, or it can occur as part of an in-depth holistic health assessment.

Cultural considerations

Using a holistic approach, the nurse should consider issues from a psychological, social, and cultural perspective. The words used when carrying out the health interview should be given careful consideration; the nurse should choose words that the man can understand and try not to be offended or embarrassed by the words that he is using.

The physical examination

When history taking is complete, the nurse then examines the man. Permission must be sought prior to beginning the examination. Genital examination should be performed last in order to reduce embarrassment and to permit time for the man to become comfortable with the overall interaction. Always offer a chaperone and document the outcome of the offer made (Royal College of Nursing 2006). If appropriate, determine if the man wants his partner to accompany him during the examination.

Take note

The nurse should greet the patient appropriately with an introduction that includes the nurse's name and title. Enquire as to what the patient would prefer to be called. An introduction such as this can help to reduce anxiety, especially when the encounter is related to the man's sexual and reproductive health. The man must be offered a chaperone.

Ensure that the examination room is warm, private, and free from distraction. Place an 'Occupied', Room being used', or 'Do not disturb' sign on the outside of the door and, to reassure the man, inform him that you have done this. Ensure that you have all the equipment that you may need already available in the room. Doing this can prevent you from having to stop the examination and go in and out to bring back items of equipment, adding to the anxiety the man may be experiencing as well as prolonging the time that it takes to perform the examination. Usually, only examination gloves and water-soluble lubricant are required. However, a stethoscope and torch may be needed if the nurse is to examine the scrotum. The stethoscope can be used to listen for bowel sounds if there is a concern that there may be a hernia. The torch is used to transilluminate the scrotum during an evaluation for a hydrocele.

To alleviate any anxiety the man may have, the nurse should offer him explanations for the procedures that are to be undertaken. It may help to provide diagrammatic representations and the use of an anatomical model of the genitalia, pointing out to him those aspects of his anatomy that are to be examined.

Before the examination ask the man to empty his bladder, but always check if a urine specimen is required prior to this. A gown is usually worn after the man has been asked to remove his clothing or a drape is used to cover his genitals; he may keep his underwear on until examination of the genitalia is required. The man may be asked to sit, stand, or lay down (supine) for the examination. Only expose those body parts that are being examined, respecting the man's dignity.

The method of assessment should be adapted to meet the circumstances. Assessment is undertaken as part of a holistic evaluation or this may be specifically focused if the problem is known or suspected. If the examination is part of a total physical assessment. The reproductive and urinary systems are assessed. After taking a history, each symptom that has been identified is assessed.

Inspection

Penis

With the patient in the supine position, the nurse should only expose the genitalia, ensuring that the legs and the chest/abdomen are covered.

The patient's hair distribution pattern is examined, in the adult hair is usually abundant in the pubic area, coarser than the hair on other parts of the body, curlier, in the older man the hair may be grey and sparse. Does this correlate with the man's age? The suprapubic area is inspected for any rashes, lesions, folliculitis, scarring, nodules, bulges, or scratch marks (from a parasite), part the hair if it is full during the examination. Inspect the inguinal/groin area, when the patient coughs or bears down there should be no bulges or masses, the presence of a bulge or a mass could indicate a hernia.

The rate at which the penis grows is progressive. Size will vary from man to man and the average flaccid penis measures 4–10 cm; the erect penis is 7–13 cm, in the older man it is retracted, small, with some surface vascularities. Gomella (2015) suggests that an abnormally small penis could be indicative of a clitoris, Klinefelter's, or Down syndrome. The colour is usually darker than the skin on other parts of the body. Penile skin should be smooth and hairless and cylindrical in shape.

The foreskin

In the circumcised man the glans penis is exposed, in uncircumcised males the foreskin is retracted. An unretractable prepuce could indicate phimosis, and referral to a urologist may be required. On inspection, any drainage, lesions, scars, rash, or swelling should be noted. If there is smegma present this is normal. After inspection the nurse must always replace the foreskin back over the glans. Those men who were circumcised as children could have a much lower chance of getting penile cancer than those who were not; it is suggested that circumcision as an infant can prevent this cancer. The same protective effect, however, is not seen if circumcision is done as an adult (America Cancer Society 2018).

The glans penis

In the uncircumcised male the foreskin must be retracted in order to inspect the glans penis. The nurse notes any lesions, drainage, warts, scars, rash, skin texture, colour, or swelling. Balanitis (inflammation of the glans) may be caused by a fungal infection, balanoposthitis is inflammation of the glans and prepuce. If the nurse notes that the urethral meatus is located on the dorsal surface it is known as epispadias, if located on the ventral surface this is hypospadias. These are congenital disorders and can be located anywhere on the ventral surface, from the tip of the penis to the penoscrotal junction.

271

The urethral meatus

In order to inspect the urethral meatus, the nurse gently compresses the glans between the index finger, opening the meatus for inspection. Patients who have a sexually acquired infection (SAI) can present with dysuria and penile discharge, but asymptomatic patients may also have an SAI. It is important that the nurse discuss issues of sexuality during the examination, particularly if there is a possibility that the man may have an SAI. Questions should be asked in a non-judgemental manner regarding sex and sexuality.

The scrotal sac

The scrotal sac hangs between the thighs and is anterior to the anus. This is a supporting structure that is suspended from the root of the penis. Externally, the scrotum usually appears as a single sac of skin, separated into two portions by a ridge in the middle called the raphe. Internally the scrotum is divided into two sacs separated by a scrotal septum (see Figure 15.7).

The scrotum helps to control the temperature of the testes. The most favourable temperature for sperm production is approximately 2–3° below core body temperature. However, too low a temperature can also impact on spermatogenesis.

A number of mechanisms come into play when the position of the testes is adjusted in the scrotum in relation to the body. When the temperature of the testes is too low (if the ambient temperature falls), the scrotum will react in a way that it contracts causing the testes to move up closer to the body. Equally, if the testicular temperature is too high, the scrotum will relax. This allows the testes to descend, moving them further away from the body, exposing surface area and providing a faster dispersion of heat.

The penis

The urethra lies within the penis. The penis provides a route for the elimination of ejaculate and urine via the urethral orifice located at the end of the penis. The glans penis is the enlarged part of the penis. The cylindrical penis is made up of three columns of erectile tissue.

The bulbous glans penis is located at the end of the corpus spongiosum and is covered with a thin layer of skin allowing for erection. In a man who is uncircumcised the skin at the glans folds over on itself and forms the prepuce or foreskin. Where the foreskin is attached underneath the penis this is

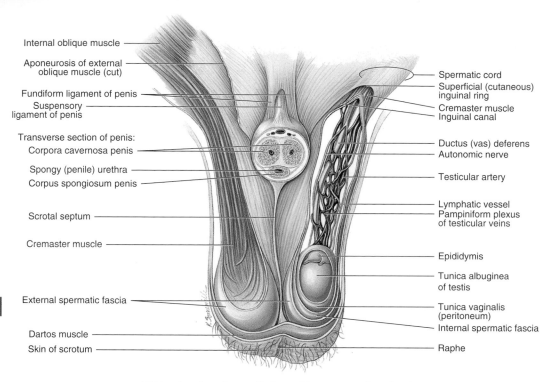

Internal oblique muscle

Aponeurosis of external
oblique muscle (cut)

Fundiform ligament of penis

Suspensory
ligament of penis

Transverse section of penis:
Corpora cavernosa penis

Spongy (penile) urethra
Corpus spongiosum penis

Scrotal septum

Cremaster muscle

External spermatic fascia

Dartos muscle
Skin of scrotum

Spermatic cord
Superficial (cutaneous)
inguinal ring
Cremaster muscle
Inguinal canal

Ductus (vas) deferens
Autonomic nerve

Testicular artery

Lymphatic vessel
Pampiniform plexus
of testicular veins

Epididymis

Tunica albuginea
of testis

Tunica vaginalis
(peritoneum)
Internal spermatic fascia

Raphe

Anterior view of scrotum and testes and transverse section of penis

Figure 15.7   The scrotum and testes.

272

known as the frenulum. The urethral meatus lies at the end of the urinary tract, at the tip of the glans
(see Figure 15.8).

Review

Genital piercings have been documented throughout human history. Genital piercings are defined as
developing a tract under the skin with a large bore needle, creating an opening into the anatomical
region for decorative ornaments such as jewellery.

Erectile physiology

Achieving and sustaining an erection requires a range of complex neurophysiological actions.
Erection occurs as blood rapidly flows into the penis, becoming trapped in its spongy chambers.
Three systems are directly involved in a penile erection, the spongy corpora cavernosa, autonomic
innervation of the penis, and the blood supply of the penis.

As ejaculation approaches, penile rigidity increases even more. Smooth muscles in the prostate,
vas deferens and seminal vesicles repeatedly contract, ejecting the seminal plasma and spermatozoa
into the urethra. Emission is facilitated by α-adrenergic sympathetic fibres travelling through the
hypogastric nerve. Ejaculation is dependent upon the smooth muscles of the urethra and the action
of the striated bulbocavernosus and ischiocavernosus muscles.

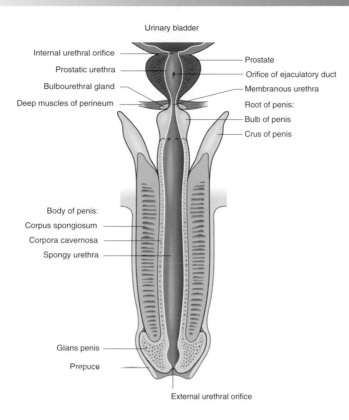

Urinary bladder

Internal urethral orifice

Prostatic urethra

Bulbourethral gland

Deep muscles of perineum

Prostate

Orifice of ejaculatory duct

Membranous urethra

Root of penis:

Bulb of penis

Crus of penis

Body of penis:

Corpus spongiosum

Corpora cavernosa

Spongy urethra

Glans penis

Prepuce

External urethral orifice

Figure 15.8 The penis.

273

Take note

Semen analysis involves more than just sperm count. In addition to sperm count, semen analysis is also concerned with the sperm's mobility, forward progression or velocity, its size and shape, the total volume produced, as well as its ability to go from a gel consistency when ejaculated to a more liquid state.

The prostate gland

The function of the prostate gland is not fully understood. The prostate is a glandular and muscular organ surrounding the beginning of the urethra, attached by a connective tissue sheath posterior to the symphysis pubis. Its measurements are about $2.5 \times 3.5 \times 4.5$ cm.

The median lobe of the prostate increases in size, and this can cause urinary outflow obstruction, often commonly occurring in older men. The anterior aspect of the prostate is composed chiefly of fibromuscular tissue. The glandular tissue of the prostate is situated at the sides of the urethra and immediately behind it. This glandular tissue is further divided into central and peripheral zones. The peripheral zone is larger than the central zone.

Review

What does benign prostatic hypertrophy mean? How would you explain this to a man who has been given this diagnosis?

All the muscular tissues in the vas deferens, prostate, prostatic urethra, and seminal vesicles are involved in ejaculation. Of the volume of the seminal fluid, 15% is made up of prostatic secretions. These secretions assist in semen liquefaction.

Take note

The fluid ejaculated by the man is not sperm, it is semen. The sperm is contained in the white fluid called seminal fluid. Pre-ejaculate contains sperm.

So far

The skills required to undertake an assessment of the male reproductive system include inspection and palpation. Effective verbal and non-verbal communication are key requisites.

The patient history

A detailed and systematic history and examination are key in the assessment of all patients presenting with reproductive/genitourinary symptoms. The nurse must undertake the assessment in the context of the age of the person, the gender and past medical and surgical history of the patient. Urinary symptoms may not be related to a urological abnormality – they may have other causes, for example frequency of micturition in anxiety or urinary symptoms caused by neurological disease. This dual role this will result in data collection about reproductive and elimination functions. Similar diagnostic procedures will be required to assess both the reproductive organs and the urinary system. The nurse will be required to undertake an assessment of the male reproductive system and an assessment of the man's needs in a number of care settings, with the aim of making a diagnosis, planning care, and evaluating care interventions. Assessment of needs has to be undertaken with the man's best interests at the heart of all that is done, and this needs to be compassionate and respectful at all times.

Ensuring privacy and comfort whilst obtaining a health history, meeting, and greeting the patient in an affable manner can establish a sense of confidence and rapport. The skilled practitioner is able to undertake the assessment in a skilled and sensitive manner. If the nurse is comfortable in discussing the man's issues then the man will reciprocate and be willing to discuss his problems. Let the patient describe the complaint or problem they are having. It may be necessary and may also appropriate to enquire about the person's sexual and psychosexual history.

Gathering subjective data will include information concerning urinary symptoms, hygiene, safe sex practices, and habits that could result in risks for reproductive system disorders. The assessment phase of the nursing process is associated with the findings from diagnostic tests, the health history where subjective data has been collected, and a physical assessment allowing the nurse to collect objective data. The history of urine symptoms should cover any pain during micturition, changes in voiding pattern, the colour of the urine, and the output. Urinary symptoms include genital or pelvic pain, genitalia swelling, sexual dysfunction, or issues concerning infertility (see Box 15.1).

In order to assess the patient's risk-taking behaviour the nurse must enquire about sexual health and preferences and practices. Ask the man about any health problems he is having, establish onset, characteristics and course, severity, aggravating and alleviating factors, and any related symptoms, noting timing and circumstances (see Table 15.2).

Box 15.1 Issues to include as part of the history-taking phase

- Is there any dysuria?
- Is there any discharge?
- Is there frequency of micturition?
- Is there any nocturia?
- Is there any terminal dribbling of micturition?
- Is there hesitancy of micturition?
- How full is the patient's urinary stream?
- Have the symptoms developed gradually or did they come on suddenly (timescale)?
- Is there any incontinence or urgency of micturition?
- Impact of symptoms of lifestyle and sexual activity
- Issues with fertility

Source: Adapted Young et al. (2018).

Review

Define the following terms:

Anuria	
Dysuria	
Nocturia	
Haematuria	
Oligura	
Polyuria	
Strangury	
Hydrocele	
Suprapubic	
Varicocele	
Spermatocele	
Orchiectomy	
Orchidoplexy	
Phimosis	
Paraphimosis	
Priaprism	
Urinary frequency	
Urinary urgency	
Urinary hesitancy	

Urodynamic studies

Urodynamic studies are able to test how well the bladder, sphincters and urethra can hold and release urine (see Box 15.2). There are many types of urodynamic tests, some are invasive and some are non-invasive. A patient may have more than one test performed depending on their symptoms.

Table 15.2   Some questions to ask in relation to the male reproductive system.

- When did you first notice you were having problems with your erection?
- Tell me about changes in your urine stream after your prostatectomy.
- Have you ever had problems with your penis, testicles, prostate gland? If so, how was the problem treated?
- Have you ever had surgery on your penis, testicles, prostate gland? What and when and how are you now?
- Do you now or have you ever had a discharge from your penis? What was this?
- When you urinate, have you noticed any changes, for example a burning sensation, frequency when passing urine, needing to pass urine urgently, difficulty commencing the stream, size of the stream, dribbling, or getting up at night more often than usual?
- Describe any pain in the groin area, testicles, penis, or scrotum. Where is it? Do you feel it in other parts of the body? How long does it last? What makes it worse or relieves it?
- Has this condition impacted on your relationships with others?
- Has this condition interfered with your ability to work?
- Are you currently in a sexual relationship? Has this condition affected your usual sexual activity?
- Has this problem affected your relationship with your sexual partner(s)?
- Do you use any medications to assist sexual ability? If so, what are these?

Ask the person about long-term illnesses, for example diabetes, chronic kidney disease, cardiovascular disease, multiple sclerosis, trauma, or thyroid disease (including autoimmune disease). These conditions and their treatments may result in erectile dysfunction. The following medications can cause difficulties with sexual functioning:

- Antidepressants
- Antihypertensives
- Antispasmodics
- Tranquillisers
- Sedatives
- H_2-receptor antagonists.
- Mental health problems, for example depression, may contribute to erectile dysfunction
- Mumps as a child can lead to infertility in later life
- Men who have had undescended testes and those with a family history of testicular cancer are more at risk for testicular cancer
- Ask about any neonatal surgery, type, and outcome
- Ask about lifestyle including social history; ask about alcohol use, use of tobacco or street drugs, these can impact or may affect sexual function
- Ask about sexual preference and sexual activity

Other questions regarding sexuality should include:

- Number of sexual partners
- Type of sexual activity
- History of premature ejaculation
- Erectile dysfunction (and other sexual problems)
- History of sexual trauma
- Use of condom or other contraceptives
- Current level of sexual satisfaction.

Box 15.2 Urodynamic studies

Urodynamic studies assess the function of the bladder and urethra and can be of value in the assessment and diagnosis of patients presenting with lower urinary tract symptoms (LUTS). Urodynamic tests include:

- Cystometry
- Uroflowmetry
- Pressure flow studies
- Electromyography
- Video-urodynamics

These tests can offer objective information concerning the normal and abnormal function of the urinary tract and a much better understanding of the cause of LUTS.

Urinary flow rate (also called uroflowmetry)

Uroflowmetry may be helpful in the assessment of voiding function for a number of urological conditions. This is a non-invasive test measuring the rate of flow of voided urine. Uroflowmetry measures how much urine is passed and how fast. It is done in two parts. By measuring the average and top rates of urine flow, this test can show a blockage such as an enlarged prostate.

It can be used to suggest the presence of bladder outlet obstruction or a poorly performing detrusor muscle.

Uroflowmetry is undertaken by using a flow meter to measure the quantity of urine voided per unit of time. This is expressed in millilitres per second (mL/s).

The patient is asked to void normally. They may sit or stand, with a comfortably full bladder.

A flow rate that is based on a voided volume of less than 150 mL is inadequate for reliable understanding.

Those men aged under 40 years usually have maximum flow rates over 25 mL/s. Flow rates decline with age and men aged over 60 years, with no urinary obstruction, will typically have maximum flow rate of over 15 mL/s.

6Cs

The NMC (2018) requires nurses to ensure that those who are recipients of care receive care with respect, that their rights are upheld, and that any discriminatory attitudes and behaviours towards those receiving care are challenged. The nurse must also respect the choices that people make. The nurse has to act in a non-judgemental way at all times.

So far

The most common complaints associated with the male reproductive systems are dysuria, changes in voiding pattern, alterations in urinary output, urethral discharge, erectile dysfunction, concerns with fertility and scrotal or inguinal masses. Once the history is taken, the nurse can then go on to gathering objective data through the physical examination.

Physical examination

Often there can be associated systemic upset or clinical signs related to urological disease. After the full history has been obtained. a physical examination is required. Inspection and palpation are needed in order to perform a physical examination.

6Cs

If the nurse is comfortable during the physical examination the patient is more likely to take cues from the nurse and also be more comfortable during this intimate procedure.

Table 15.3   The mnemonic SPACESPIT, features to note regarding lumps or swellings.

S	Size
P	Position
A	Attachments
C	Consistency
E	Edge
S	Surface and shape
P	Pulsation (thrills and bruits)
I	Inflammation • Redness • Tenderness • Warmth
T	Transillumination

As with any physical examination, the nurse must ensure that the room where the examination is to take place is private, warm, and free from distraction. Place an 'Engaged' notification on the door of the examination room, and let the man know you have done this. Explain to the man what is going to be done, for example, 'I am going to carry out an examination of your genitals and this requires me to undertake an examination of your penis, testicles and the surrounding area', provide a rationale for the proposed actions and confirm patient details. The nurse must gain the man's consent.

Wash hands and don gloves prior to the examination. Afford the patient privacy as he undresses and puts on a gown. The man should stand, exposing the lower aspect from the abdomen to mid thighs. He will be asked to lie down later in the examination. If need be, the nurse should offer physical support to the man as he is being examined, assistance with lying and standing and ensuring his comfort.

Gather all the equipment that is likely to be required in the room; this avoids having to go in and out to retrieve pieces of equipment. A moveable light source will be required.

A structured, sequential approach is required when examining the patient, ensuring that there are no omissions during the procedure. This is an intimate examination examining the penis and testes and as such, to reiterate, extra attention should be paid to the communication aspect to ensure the patient feels as comfortable as possible.

When meeting the patient observe the skin: Does the person appear pale? Is the skin dry? Do they appear dehydrated (lips dry and crusted, sunken eyes)? Request a urine specimen from the man (see Chapter 13).

With the man lying down, inspect the groin, skin creases, the perineum and the scrotal skin for rash, redness, bruising, swelling (see Table 15.3), and the presence of scars in the inguinal region that may indicate orchidopexy. Are there any obvious masses, signs of lymphadenopathy? Take note of hair distribution.

The Penis

When examining the penis, observe the shaft and note the position of the urethral opening. Palpate the shaft of the penis and determine the presence of fibrous plaques or other lesions. If the man is uncircumcised the foreskin should be retracted and observed for any red patches or vesicles and phimosis. The nurse must ensure the foreskin is drawn forward after examination so as to prevent paraphimosis. To assess the urethra, gently compress the tip of the glans, which will open the urethral meatus. This should be smooth and pink. If there is any discharge from the urethra then a urethral swab will be required.

Box 15.3 Transillumination

All masses and swellings should be transilluminated. Light will not transmit through a solid tumour, whilst a hydrocele will glow a soft red colour. This is a painless non-invasive test and requires no specific preparation.

The lights in the room may be dimmed for the procedure. The bright end of a torch is gently placed against the scrotal swelling. Cysts filled with fluid will permit the transmission of light and the scrotum will glow a bright red.

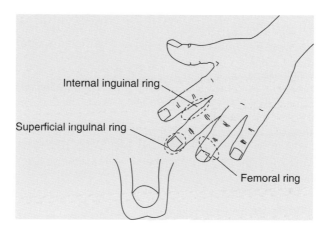

Figure 15.9   Palpating for an inguinal hernia.

The scrotum

Request that the patient hold their penis out of the way to permit easier inspection of the scrotum. Inspect the scrotum from the front, sides, and the posterior aspect by lifting the scrotum and undertake an inspection of the perineum.

If the dartos muscle is contracted it will not be possible to palpate the contents of the scrotal sac properly. This may be due to anxiety or cold. Palpate the testes to establish if they are able to move freely in the sac. They should feel smooth, firm, and rubbery.

A varicocele is dilation of the veins of the pampiniform plexus. It is often described as feeling like a 'bag of worms'. A hydrocele is a collection of fluid in the tunica vaginalis. A varicocele may be idiopathic or secondary to inflammation or tumour. Thorough examination of any male with a scrotal mass includes transillumination (see Box 15.3).

The testes are palpated; epididymides and spermatic cords. They should be smooth and non-tender, no swelling and no induration. Ask the patient to report any pain during the examination

To palpate for the presence of an inguinal hernia, with the patient standing, sit opposite and place two fingers over the inguinal ring and ask the patient to bear down (the Valsalva manoeuvre) (see Figure 15.9). If there is a hernia present this will feel and appear as a bulge.

A rectal examination is a key element of the genitourinary examination (see Box 15.4). It is an intimate and sometimes uncomfortable physical examination which should be undertaken appropriately for detection of disease and for patient comfort (Steggall 2008). The findings must be accurately and correctly recorded.

279

Box 15.4 Rectal examination

Explain the reasons for the examination and gain verbal consent. Explain that the examination may be uncomfortable, but it should not be painful. There may a feeling of rectal fullness and the desire to defecate.

Equipment required:

- Gloves
- Lubricant
- Good light source
- Tissues

Patient position:

- Position the patient comfortably in the left lateral position with the hips and knees flexed with the buttocks at the edge of the couch. The patient may need assistance to assume this position
- Gently separate the buttocks, exposing the anal verge and natal cleft.
- Assess the skin and anal margin, it should be unbroken with no protruding masses
- Apply lubrication to the gloved examining index finger, pressing the finger against the posterior anal margin (6 o'clock position, posterior).
- Slip the finger into the anal canal, with the fingertip directed posteriorly following the sacral curve.
- Gently rotate the finger through 180°, palpating the walls of the rectum. With the finger then rotated in the 12 o'clock position (anterior), the anterior wall can be palpated. The prostate gland will be felt anteriorly.

Examination of the prostate gland (felt anteriorly):

- Normal size is 3.5 cm wide, protruding about 1 cm into the lumen of the rectum.
- Consistency: it is normally rubbery and firm, with a smooth surface and a palpable sulcus between right and left lobes.
- There should not be any tenderness.
- There should be no nodularity.
- Prostatic massage may enable prostatic fluid to be examined at the urethral meatus.

These findings may suggest prostate cancer (the mnemonic PAINS):

P	Prostate cancer
A	Asymmetry
I	Irregular
N	Nodules
S	Stony (hard) and fixed

When the examining finger is removed, check the tip of the glove (for stool, blood). Provide the patent with a tissue to clean himself.

So far

The subjective and objective data collected helps the nurse make a diagnosis. The diagnosis can be confirmed with the use of tests and other diagnostic investigations if needed.

Take note

When undertaking a rectal examination in the elderly patient it may be uncomfortable to assume the left lateral position. The nurse should help the man to find a comfortable position that will permit satisfactory examination. It should also be taken into account that hearing difficulties can hinder explanations, so a little more time may be needed to ensure that the procedure and the reasons for it are understood.

When the examination is completed thank the patient and allow time for him to get dressed. Dispose of gloves, wash hands, record and report the findings, and adhere to local policy and procedure.

Howard Samuda (Son)

Howard is at the walk-in centre with scrotal pain. Howard is alone.
You are required to take a focused history and undertake a physical examination.
You must consider:

- Infection prevention and control factors (handwashing, wearing of gloves, and safe disposal)
- Consent and introduction
- A chaperone
- Patient position (standing/supine)
- Promotion of dignity
- Explanation of procedure
- The use of open-ended questioning
- To what depth is the examination taken (do you inspect the penis, the perineum, do you palpate the lower abdomen)? What would be appropriate in this case?
- Explore the symptoms at presentation
- Acute or chronic
- Any precipitating events such as trauma (a blow to the scrotum)
- Sexual history, past medical history, history of neonatal surgery
- Social and drug history
- How do you close the interaction?
- Propose further tests and investigations
- How would you summarise your findings?
- Howard is clearly very embarrassed. How might you alleviate his embarrassment?
- Howard is in pain

Pain is such a common complaint and the responses have to be completely and concisely documented, the use of this mnemonic may help:

W	Words...that describe the pain
I	Intensity...on a scale of 1–10
L	Location...what is the specific location of the pain?
D	Duration...how long has the pain lasted/intermittent or continuous?
A	Aggravating/Alleviating factors ... what makes the pain worse or what makes the pain better?

During the consultation, Howard informs the nurse that he has a new boyfriend. He has only been going out with him for the last six weeks and they have had sexual activity. Howard explains that Paolo, his new boyfriend, has recently been treated for chlamydia but he has told him that it has all cleared up now and the clinic said he had a 'clean card'.
Suggest a differential diagnosis. This may include, for example, testicular torsion epididymo-orchitis, testicular cancer, or sexually acquired infection.

Conclusion

The male reproduction system is closely related to the male urinary system. Understanding the anatomy and physiology will allow the nurse to make a holistic patient-centred assessment of needs. Disorders of the reproductive system can also have an impact on other body systems, impacting negatively on quality of life, health, and wellbeing.

Many men are reluctant to talk about problems concerning the reproductive system. Assessment of the male reproductive system is an intimate activity and the nurse has to be aware of not only the patient's feelings but also their own. A skilled practitioner can put the patient at ease and carry out the assessment in an effective and efficient way.

References

America Cancer Society (2018) Risk cancer for penile cancer. www.cancer.org/cancer/penile-cancer/causes-risks-prevention/risk-factors.html (accessed September 2018).

Gomella, L.G. (2015). *The 5-Minute Urology Consult*, 2e. Philadelphia: Wolters Kluwer Health.

Heffner, L.J. and Schust, D.J. (2014). *The Reproductive System at a Glance*, 4e. Oxford: Wiley.

Marieb, E.N. and Hoehn, K. (2016). *Human Anatomy and Physiology*, 10e. San Francisco: Pearson Benjamin Cummings.

Nursing and Midwifery Council (2018). The Code. Professional Standards of Practice and Behaviour for Nurses, Midwives and Nursing Associates. https://www.nmc.org.uk/globalassets/sitedocuments/nmc-publications/nmc-code.pdf last accessed 8 May 2019.

Royal College of Nursing (2006). *Chaperoning: The Role of the Nurse and the Rights of the Patient; Guidance for Nursing Staff*. London: RCN.

Steggall, M.J. (2008). Digital rectal examination. *Nursing Standard* **22** (47): 46–48.

Tortora, G.J. and Derrikson, B.H. (2014). *Principles of Anatomy and Physiology*, 14e. New Jersey: Wiley.

Waugh, A. and Grant, A. (2018). *Ross and Wilson's Anatomy and Physiology in Health and Illness*, 13e. Edinburgh: Elsevier.

Young, O., Duncan, C., Dundas, K., and Laird, A. (2018). The reproductive system. In: *Macleod's Clinical Examination*, 14e (ed. J.A. Innes, A.R. Dover and K. Fairhurst), 211–236. Edinburgh: Elsevier.

Chapter 16

Assessing the female reproductive system

Aim

This chapter introduces the reader to the assessment of the female reproductive system and the care required for those women who experience problems related to this system.

Learning outcomes

By the end of the chapter the reader will be able to:

1. Provide a brief overview of the female reproductive system and its functions
2. Discuss a number of conditions that might affect the female reproductive system
3. Outline the various ways in which the nurse may undertake an assessment of the female reproductive system
4. Describe care planning that is related to the female reproductive system

Introduction

The female reproductive system is considered in this chapter. Chapter 15 addresses the male reproductive system. It has been acknowledged that whilst these two systems are different, some issues concern both systems. The female reproductive system encompasses the urinary and reproductive organs.

Reproduction of the human species is a complex activity that requires a series of integrated anatomical and physiological events. The physiological and anatomical aspects of the reproductive tract are predominately associated with procreation. The psychological and social aspects of reproduction are also important, as too is the pleasure that is often provided by the reproductive organs. Ill health in relation to the reproductive tract can result in loss of life, acute and chronic illness, as well as physical and emotional distress.

How an individual decides to express themselves is a key component of reproductive health and this is often associated with attitudes (the person's attitudes as well as the nurse's attitudes). Social norms and cultural upbringing also impact on an individual's reproductive health; sexuality and sexual health are closely linked to reproductive health. This chapter provides an overview of the assessment of the female reproductive tract.

The nurse must use a framework, a systematic approach to guide assessment, diagnosis, planning, implementation, and the evaluation of care required. When a systematic approach is applied, the physical, psychological, and cultural needs of the woman and her family (if appropriate) are taken into consideration.

Fundamentals of Assessment and Care Planning for Nurses, First Edition. Ian Peate.
© 2020 John Wiley & Sons Ltd. Published 2020 by John Wiley & Sons Ltd.

The female reproductive system

Collectively the external female genitalia are referred to as the vulva. They include the mons pubis, the labia, the clitoris, the vaginal and urethral openings, and glands (see Figure 16.1). There are three key functions associated with the external genitalia:

1. Allowing sperm to enter the body
2. Protecting the internal genital organs from infectious organisms
3. The provision of sexual pleasure

The mons veneris

The mon veneris (ls called the mons pubis) is the pad of elevated fatty tissue that covers the pubic bone and is situated inferior to the abdomen and superior to the labia. During puberty, the amount of fat increases and after the menopause this decreases. The mons protects the pubic bone from the impact of sexual intercourse. The mons is covered with coarse pubic hair during puberty and after puberty this then decreases.

Labia majora

The outer lips of the vulva are the labia majora and they are made of two symmetrical pads of fatty tissue that wrap around the vulva, extending from the mons veneris to the perineum. They offer protection to the urethral and vaginal openings. These labia are usually covered with pubic hair. They contain a number of sweat and oil glands. The scent (pheromones) from these glands may have a role to play in sexual arousal.

Labia minora

The inner lips of the vulva are called the labia minora. They are composed of thin stretches of tissue within the labia majora, folding and protecting the vagina, urethra, and the clitoris. The labia minora are thin, delicate folds of fat-free, hairless skin that are positioned between the labia majora. The labia minora contain a core of spongy tissue. Within this there are a number of small blood vessels but there is no fat. The appearance of the labia minora varies from woman to woman, from tiny lips that are hidden between the labia majora to larger lips that can protrude. Internally the surface is comprised of thin skin and has a pink colour associated with mucous membranes, with a number of sensory nerve endings. The inner and outer labia are very responsive to touch and pressure.

Clitoris

This is a small white aspect of oval tissue located at the top of the labia minora and the clitoral hood. The clitoris is a small body of spongy tissue that is sexually sensitive. Externally it is only the tip or glans of the clitoris that is visible, the organ is elongated and branches into two forks, the crura, this

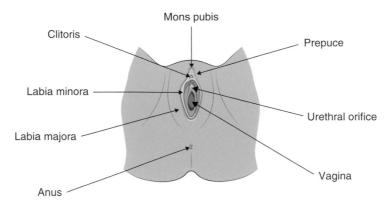

Female External Genitalia

Clitoris
Mons pubis
Prepuce
Labia minora
Urethral orifice
Labia majora
Vagina
Anus

Figure 16.1   The external female genitalia.

then extends downwards along the edge of the vaginal opening towards the perineum. The clitoris is approximately 3 cm in length, size varies. The external tip of the clitoris or the clitoral glans is protected by the prepuce, (also called the clitoral hood), this is a covering of tissue that corresponds to the foreskin of the male penis. The clitoris may extend and the hood will retract, making the clitoral glans more accessible during sexual excitement. The clitoris is an erectile organ; usually hidden by the labia when in the flaccid state, it will, as does the penis, enlarge upon tactile stimulation; it does not, however, lengthen significantly. It is highly sensitive and very important in the sexual arousal of a woman. There are variations in size; in some women the clitoral glans may be very small, in others the woman may have a large clitoris and the hood may not completely cover it. The clitoris is suspended by a suspensory ligament.

The urethra

The external urethral orifice is situated 2 to 3 cm posterior to the clitoris and immediately anterior to the vaginal orifice. The openings of the ducts of the paraurethral glands (also called Skene's glands) are located either side of the vaginal orifice. The urethra is not related to sex or reproduction, it is where urine is excreted when it passes from the urinary bladder.

Hymen

The hymen is pinkish and often shaped like a crescent, though there may be many other variations. It is a thin membrane located at the lower end of the vagina. In nearly all young women, there is a large gap in the membrane, it does not block off the vagina completely. This is important, because the gap in the hymen permits menstrual blood flow when the girl menstruates. The hymen is the traditional representation of virginity. As it is a very thin membrane, it can be torn by vigorous exercise, the insertion of a tampon, masturbation, or the use of sex toys such as dildos.

285

Blood supply

Arterial supply of the female external genitalia

The rich arterial supply to the vulva comes from two external pudendal arteries as well as one internal pudendal artery located on either side. The internal pudendal artery supplies the skin, sex organs, and the perineal muscles. The labial arteries are branches of the internal pudendal artery, and this is the same for the dorsal and deep arteries of the clitoris.

Venous drainage of the female external genitalia

The labial veins are offshoots of the internal pudendal veins and venae comitantes of the internal pudendal artery.

Lymph drainage

Within the vulva there are a number of very rich networks of lymphatic channels. Most lymph vessels in the vulva pass to the superficial inguinal lymph nodes and deep inguinal nodes.

Nerve supply

The nerves that supply the vulva are branches of, the ilioinguinal nerve, the genital branch of the genitofemoral nerve, the perineal branch of the femoral cutaneous nerve, and the perineal nerve.

The internal female reproductive organs that are located in the bony pelvis comprise the ovaries, the Fallopian tubes, the uterus, and the vagina (see Figure 16.2).

Review

What does the surgical procedure tubal ligation involve?

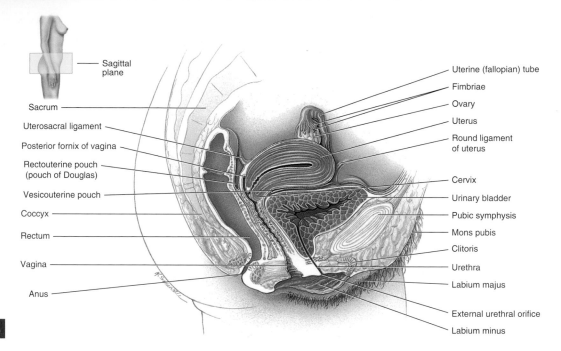

Sagittal plane
Sacrum
Uterosacral ligament
Posterior fornix of vagina
Rectouterine pouch (pouch of Douglas)
Vesicouterine pouch
Coccyx
Rectum
Vagina
Anus

Uterine (fallopian) tube
Fimbriae
Ovary
Uterus
Round ligament of uterus
Cervix
Urinary bladder
Pubic symphysis
Mons pubis
Clitoris
Urethra
Labium majus
External urethral orifice
Labium minus

Figure 16.2   The female reproductive system.

The ovaries

The paired ovaries are the primary reproductive organs. These glands also produce female sex hormones. In the adult woman they are flat, almond-shaped structures positioned on each side of the uterus below the ends of the Fallopian tubes. They are held in position by ligaments that attach them to the uterus. They are also attached to the broad ligament that attaches them to the pelvic wall. The ovaries act as a storage space for the female germ cells and also the production of the female hormones oestrogen and progesterone. A woman's total number of ova (singular ovum) is present at her birth. When a girl reaches puberty she usually ovulates each month.

The ovary is made up of a number of small structures called ovarian follicles. The follicles contain an immature ovum (an oocyte). Follicles are stimulated each month by two hormones, follicle-stimulating hormone (FSH) and luteinising hormone (LH), which stimulate the follicles to mature. The developing follicles are enclosed in layers of follicle cells. Mature follicles are called Graafian follicles.

The ovarian cortex

Located deep and close to the tunica albuginea is the ovarian cortex, which contains the ovarian follicles, surrounded by dense, irregular connective tissue. These follicles contain oocytes in various stages of development and a number of cells that nourish the developing oocyte. As the follicle grows it will secrete oestrogen.

Graafian follicles

The Graafian follicles make oestrogen, promoting the growth of the endometrium. Each month in the woman who is menstruating, one or two of the mature follicles (the Graafian follicles) will release an oocyte. This is known as ovulation. The large ruptured follicle becomes a new structure; the corpus luteum, the fragments of a mature follicle.

Corpus luteum

The corpus luteum produces oestrogen and progesterone that supports the endometrium until conception or until the cycle starts again. The corpus luteum will gradually disintegrate, leaving a scar on the outer aspect of the ovary (the corpus albicans). The outer ovary is enclosed in a fibrous capsule called the tunica albuginea, which is composed of cuboidal epithelium. The inner ovary is divided into parts.

The ovarian medulla

Within the ovarian medulla are the blood vessels, nerves, and lymphatic tissues that are surrounded by loose connective tissue.

Figure 16.3 shows the developmental sequences associated with the maturation of an ovum.

Oogenesis

This is related to the development of relatively undifferentiated germ cells called oogonia, which are fixed in numbers between two and four million diploid (2n) stem cells during foetal development. All of the ova are ultimately derived from these clones, developing into larger primary oocytes. The meiotic phase is not completed until puberty. FSH and LH are released by the anterior pituitary gland, which stimulates primordial follicles monthly after puberty and until menopause; usually only one will attain maturity as needed for ovulation (see Figure 16.4).

Female sex hormones

The ovaries repeatedly produce the hormones oestrogens, progesterone, and androgens. Oestrogens are necessary for the development and maintenance of secondary sex characteristics together with a number of other hormones, preparing the female reproductive organ to prepare for the growth of a foetus and also having a key role to play in the usual structure of the skin and blood vessels. They help to reduce the rate of bone resorption, enhance increased high-density lipoproteins, decrease cholesterol levels and increase blood clotting.

The menstrual cycle is controlled by hormones. In each cycle, rising levels of the hormone oestrogen causes the ovary to develop and for ovulation to occur. The endometrium of the uterus begins to thicken.

The length of the menstrual cycle varies from woman to woman. However, the average is to menstruate every 28 days (Waugh and Grant 2018). A regular cycle may be longer or shorter than this; from 21 to 40 days are normal. The menstrual cycle begins from the time of the first day of a woman's period to the day before her next period.

In the second half of the cycle progesterone helps prepare the uterus for implantation of a developing embryo. The ovum travels down the Fallopian tubes and if pregnancy does not occur, the egg is reabsorbed into the body. The levels of oestrogen and progesterone fall and the uterine lining comes away and leaves the body as a period (the menstrual flow). The time taken from the release of an egg to the start of a period is approximately 10–16 days.

The uterus

This is a hollow muscular organ situated in the pelvic cavity, located posteriorly and superiorly to the urinary bladder and anteriorly to the rectum, and is approximately 7.5 cm long. The fundus of the uterus is a thick muscular region above the Fallopian tubes; the body is joined to the cervix by the isthmus (see Figure 16.5). The cervix is the narrowest aspect of the uterus opening into the vagina. The uterus also has three layers; the uterine wall has three distinct layers (see Table 16.1).

The fallopian tubes

The two Fallopian tubes are delicate, thin cylindrical structures approximately 8–14 cm long, they are attached to the uterus at one end supported by the broad ligaments. The lateral ends of the Fallopian tubes are open and are made of projections known as fimbriae that are draped over the ovary (see Figure 16.5). The fimbriae pick up the ovum after discharge from the ovary, the fimbriae are composed of smooth muscle that are lined with ciliated mucous-producing epithelial cells, moving the ovum along the tubes towards the uterus. Fertilisation of the ovum usually occurs in the outer portion of the Fallopian tubes.

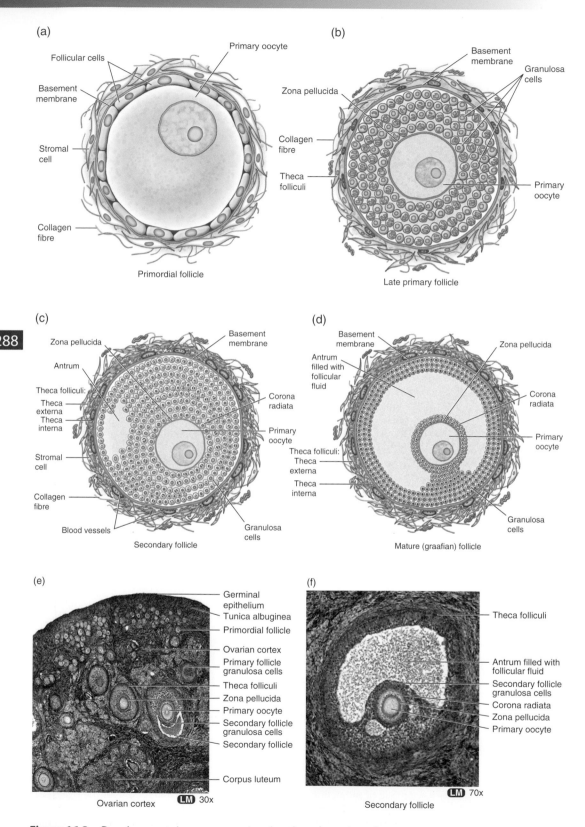

Figure 16.3 Developmental sequences related to the maturation of an ovum.

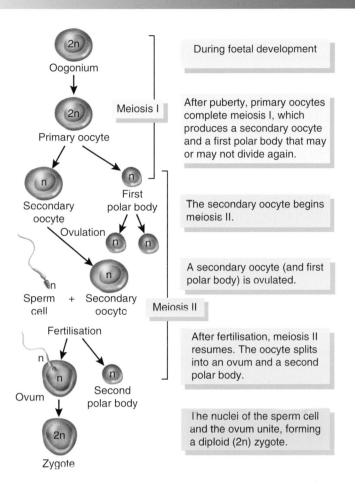

Figure 16.4   Oogenesis.

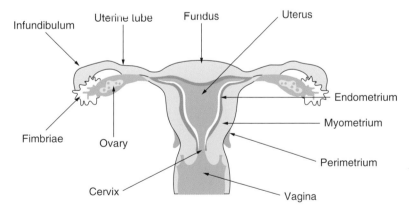

Figure 16.5   The uterus and associated structures.

The vagina

This is a tubular, fibromuscular structure that is approximately 8–10 cm in length and receives the penis during sexual intercourse, an organ of sexual response. The vaginal canal permits the menstrual flow to leave the body and is the passage for the birth of the child. It is located posterior to the urinary bladder and urethra and anterior to the rectum. The upper aspect contains the uterine cervix.

Table 16.1   The three distinct layers of the uterus.

Layer	Description
Perimetrium	A serous membrane enveloping the uterus. This is the outer layer, it provides support to the uterus and is located within the pelvis. The perimetrium is also known as the parietal peritoneum.
Metrometrium	The middle layer of the uterus is made up of smooth muscle. During pregnancy and childbirth the uterus is required to stretch, and this muscular layer allows this to happen. The muscle contacts during labour. Postnatally this muscular layer will forcefully contract to force out the placenta.
Endometrium	This is the inner layer of the uterus with a mucus lining. The outer aspect is continuous with the vagina and the Fallopian tubes. During menstruation the endometrium is shed, sloughing away from the inner layer; this is the menstrual period occurring as a result of hormonal changes. During the menstrual period the endometrium thickens and becomes rich with blood vessels and glandular tissue until the next period occurs and the cycle begins again.

The vaginal walls are made of membranous folds of rugae that are composed of mucous-secreting stratified squamous epithelial cells.

The vaginal walls are usually moist with a pH that ranges from 4.9 to 3.5 (Waugh and Grant 2018). Oestrogen is responsible for the growth of vaginal mucosal cells, causing them to thicken and develop, increasing glycogen content, which results in a slight acidifying of vaginal fluid.

The cervix

The cervix forms a pathway between the uterus and the vagina. The uterine opening of the cervix is known as the internal os and the vaginal opening is known as the external os. The area between these openings is the endocervical canal and this acts as a channel for the discharge of menstrual fluid, the opening for sperm and the delivery of the infant during birth.

The breasts

The breasts are a part of the female external reproductive system. Both men and women have breasts. Women, however, have more breast tissue than men.

Function

The key function of the breast is to produce, store, and release milk to feed a baby. Milk is produced in lobules located throughout the breast after they have been stimulated by hormones produced in the woman's body after she has given birth. The milk is transported to the nipple by the ducts and from the nipple to the baby during breast-feeding.

Review

A woman wishes to breast feed her baby. She has a nipple piercing. What advice might you offer her?

Structure

The structure of the female breast is complex. Within it there are fat and connective tissue and also lobes, lobules, ducts, and lymph nodes (see Figure 16.6). The breast lies over a muscle of the chest known as the pectoral muscle.

The female breast covers a large area, extending from just below the clavicle to the axilla and across to the sternum (see Figure 16.7). The breast is a mass of glandular, fatty, and connective tissue.

Lobules and ducts

Each breast houses a number of lobules (sections) that branch out from the nipple, the lobules are the glands responsible for the production of milk. A lobule holds very small, hollow alveoli that are linked by a network of thin ducts. During breast-feeding, the ducts carry milk from the alveoli towards

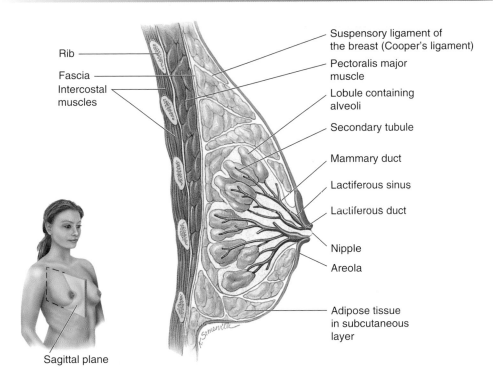

Figure 16.6   The breast.

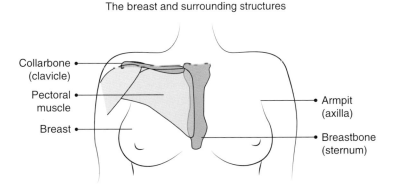

Figure 16.7   The breast and surrounding structures.

the breast areola. From the areola, the ducts join together into larger ducts which then terminate at the nipple. The areola is the circular area around the nipple, containing small sweat glands which secrete moisture that acts as a lubricant during breast-feeding. The nipple is the area found at the centre of the areola where the milk emerges.

Fat, ligaments, and connective tissue

The spaces around the lobules and ducts are filled with fat, ligaments, and connective tissue. The amount of fat in the breast will determine their size; the fat gives the breast its shape. In all women, the actual milk-producing structures are nearly the same. Cyclic changes in hormone levels will have an impact on breast tissue. Younger women usually have denser, less fatty breast tissue than older women who have gone through the menopause. Ligaments provide support to the breast, running from the skin through the breast and attaching themselves to muscles on the chest (Tortora and Derrickson 2012; McLafferty et al. 2014).

Nerve supply

There are several major nerves in the breast area. These include nerves in the chest and arm. There are also sensory nerves in the skin of the chest and axilla. Branches from the 4th, 5th, and 6th thoracic nerves supply the breasts.

Arteries and capillaries

Arterial blood supply comes from the thoracic branches of the axillary arteries and the internal mammary and intercostal arteries. Venous drainage of the breast is primarily undertaken by the axillary vein. The subclavian, intercostal, and internal thoracic veins will also aid in returning blood to the heart.

Lymph nodes and lymph ducts

The lymphatic system is a network of lymph nodes and lymph ducts that assist in fighting infection. Axillary lymph nodes are located above the clavicle, behind the sternum as well as in other parts of the body. Lymph circulates throughout body tissues, picking up fats, bacteria, and other unwanted materials and filtering them out through the lymphatic system. Breast lymph nodes include supraclavicular nodes above the clavicle, infraclavicular (or subclavicular) nodes below the clavicle, axillary nodes in the axilla, and internal mammary nodes situated inside the chest around the sternum.

There are around 30–50 lymph nodes in the axilla. This number will vary from woman to woman. The axillary lymph nodes are divided into three levels depending on how close they are to the pectoral muscle on the chest:

- Level I (low axilla) – in the lower or bottom part of the axilla, along the outside border of the pectoral muscle
- Level II (mid axilla) – in the middle aspect of the axilla, under the pectoral muscle
- Level III (high axilla) – below and near the centre of the clavicle, above the breast area and along the inside border of the pectoral muscle

Breast development

Breast tissue changes at different times during a woman's life. Changes occur during puberty, during the menstrual cycle, during pregnancy, and after menopause. Female breasts do not begin growing until puberty and at this time are responding to hormonal changes, mainly due to increases in oestrogen and progesterone as they begin to develop. During puberty, breast ducts and milk glands grow. The breast skin stretches as the breasts grow and this creates a rounded appearance. Young women tend to have more glandular tissue than older women; most of the glandular and ductal tissue in older women will be replaced with fatty tissue and the breasts will become less dense. Ligaments lose their elasticity as the women ages and this can cause the breasts to sag. A woman's two breasts are rarely the same size, with one breast being slightly larger or smaller, higher or lower, or shaped differently than the other.

Hormones and the breast

The principal female hormone is oestrogen. This hormone affects female sexual characteristics such as breast development and is necessary for reproduction. The ovaries make up most of the oestrogen in a woman's body. However, a small amount is made by the adrenal glands. Progesterone (the other female sex hormone) is made in the ovaries, it is progesterone that prepares the uterus for pregnancy and the breasts for producing milk for breast-feeding (lactation). Each month breast tissue is exposed to cycles of oestrogen and progesterone throughout a woman's childbearing years, during the first part of the menstrual cycle oestrogen stimulates the growth of the milk ducts. Progesterone takes over in the second part stimulating the lobules. Post menopause, the monthly cycle ends. The adrenal glands, however, will continue to produce oestrogen and a woman retains her sexual characteristics.

So far

The female reproductive system is complex. It is essential for sexual reproduction as well as other important issues, and the nurse must take this into consideration when caring for women – for example, the psychological and social features of reproduction, as well as the pleasure often provided by the reproductive organs. The female reproductive organs have been outlined along with their key functions.

The patient history

A comprehensive health assessment of the female reproductive system will include gathering subjective and objective data. Before you begin talking with the patient, the nurse should clarify goals for the interview. A gynaecological history requires the nurse to ask questions relevant to the female reproductive system. Some of these questions are highly personal and therefore effective communication skills and a respectful approach are absolutely essential.

Take note

The nurse practises in a holistic manner, by respecting individual choice, offering support, and promoting the health, wellbeing, and dignity of women.

Taking a gynaecological history requires asking a lot of questions that are not part of what might be considered the 'standard' history-taking format and as such it is important to understand what information you are expected to gain.

Take note

Addressing sensitive topics

- It is most important never to be judgemental. The privileged role of the nurse is to learn about the patient and to assist the patient in achieving better health. If the nurse shows condemnation of behaviours or elements in the health history, this will only interfere with this goal.
- Take time to explain why certain information is needed. Doing this can help the patient feel less anxious. For example, think about saying, 'Because there are some sexual practices that can put people at risk for certain conditions, I ask all patients the following questions.'
- For sensitive topics, use open questions and allow the patient to elaborate.
- Be consciously aware of the discomfort that you are feeling. Failing to acknowledge your discomfort could lead you to avoid the issue altogether.

6Cs

The nurse should introduce themselves to the patient. State your name and what your role is, and confirm patient identification. You should also explain to the patient why there is a need to take the history, and gain the patient's consent. The patient should be made comfortable and reassurance given that the consultation is private and the data that is collected will only be shared with the patient's permission.

Box 16.1 Some components of the health history: the female reproductive system

- Menstrual cycle history, onset, length, amount of flow, cramps, bloating, pre-menstrual syndrome, age of first period, age of menopause. If the presentation condition is cyclical, this may be related to the menstrual cycle (intermenstrual, post-menopausal bleeding).
- Abnormal vaginal bleeding: does bleeding occur after sexual intercourse?
- Any pregnancies – and if so, how many live births, miscarriages or abortions any complications, mode of delivery, birth weights. Antenatal, perinatal, postnatal complications.
- Current list of medications (including use of hormone replacement therapy) and reason for taking them. Also ask the patient about over-the-counter medications, vitamins, and herbal supplements.
- Symptoms of vaginitis, discharge, itching, irritation, dysuria, light bleeding or spotting
- Problems with urinary function, frequency, urgency, nocturia, haematuria, difficult controlling flow of urine
- Bowel problems, constipation/straining, urgency of stool, faecal incontinence, flatus, a feeling of incomplete evacuation, the need to apply digital pressure to the perineum or posterior vaginal wall to enable defaecation, the need for digital evacuation to pass a stool.
- Sexual history: is the patient sexually active, any difficulties with the physical act of intercourse
- Sexual health history (contact with a partner who may have had sexually acquired infection)
- Current or previous sexual abuse or physical abuse
- Contraceptive history (clarify type, questions, or concerns)
- Past surgical history (including female genital mutilation, Caesarean section)
- Long-term conditions (include physical and mental health conditions)
- Genetic disorders (for example, possible familial inheritance BRCA gene)
- Any breast tenderness, lumps, discharge, or concerns? Does the patient perform monthly self-breast examinations?
- Does the patient have regular smear tests?
- Social history, smoking, alcohol and recreational drug use, weight, home situation, occupation

Source: Adapted Jarvis (2015).

Take note

In order to promote the rights, options, and wishes of all women, the nurse is required to be confident and competent as well as understanding the importance of working in partnership with women to address women's needs in all care settings.

It is important to ask questions about the woman's past health history, this will provide information about the patient's childhood illnesses and immunisations, accidents or traumatic injuries, hospitalisation, surgery, psychiatric or mental illnesses, allergies, chronic illnesses, history of menstrual cycle, how many pregnancies, and how many births. As well as gathering data about the patient's general health, the nurse asks about past history and experiences specific to the woman's health (see Box 16.1).

Take note

The information that is obtained during the physical examination will help the nurse to narrow the list of possible diagnoses to explain the patient's symptoms and to refine plans for additional testing and treatment.

Cultural considerations

As far back as (1996) Harlow and Campbell noted that a person's ethnicity has strong influences on the duration and heaviness of bleeding during menses. In this early study, Black girls tended to have longer menses than white girls of the same age, with heavier menstrual blood flow.

So far

A focused approach to gathering subjective data during the history taking phase is required. The data gathered at this stage can provide direction for collecting primary data during the physical examination. A sensitive and respectful approach is required throughout. It is important to listen to the patient and each response that she makes so that you can ask additional questions as indicated.

Physical examination

The skills required to competently and confidently undertake an assessment of the female reproductive system are refined over the years. The nurse must employ a non-judgemental approach. Questions should be asked using open-ended questions, allowing the woman to elaborate. There is also a place for closed-ended questions, i.e. 'Did the episode come suddenly or not?' (acute or chronic). Physical assessment is undertaken in an environment that promotes patient comfort, cooperation, and participation.

Take note

Assumptions should never be made about aspects of the patient's background such as marital status or sexual orientation.

Griffiths (2015) suggest that an abdominal examination should take place before any examination of the female reproductive system occurs. Gynaecological examination is not something most women will enjoy. However, it is a necessity, and assessing the women's reproductive system can be difficult as it is complex and its functions can have an impact psychosocially. A pelvic examination should not be carried out unless this is symptomatically indicated (Griffiths 2015). There are some women who feel so intimidated by the examination that they delay it until something is obviously wrong, or they may avoid the examination altogether, fearing physical discomfort, embarrassment, a negative diagnosis, or questions and queries about past sexual trauma. The woman should be assured that information provided and results of the examination will remain confidential and that information will only be disclosed with her permission.

Assessment of the breasts

Breasts are a secondary reproductive characteristic; this means that reproduction can occur without them. In contemporary culture the breasts have an important role to play in sexual health as they are visible. Size and shape may be seen by some as a measure of sexuality, attractiveness, and femininity.

Breast assessment is carried out in an environment that enhances patient comfort, cooperation, and participation. A chaperone must be present. The gynaecological assessment (if appropriate) will begin with an examination of the breasts. The goal is to assess breast health, including the breasts' lymphatic system and changes related with puberty, pregnancy, and the menopause. The nurse can offer to teach the woman how to perform breast self-examine if she does not already do this.

All findings are documented and reported in line with local policy and procedure noting all masses, location, size, shape, texture, mobility, and any overlying skin changes. If the woman has

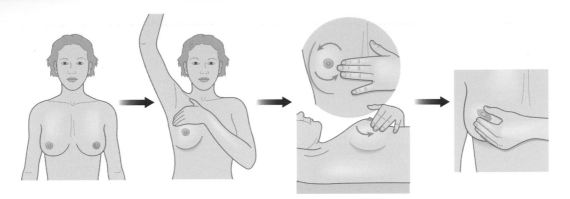

Figure 16.8 Breast examination.

had a mastectomy, a routine assessment of the unaffected side is performed. Inspect and palpate the surrounding tissue, lymph nodes and axilla for lumps, redness, swelling, tenderness, and any lesions. For women who have had breast surgery, examine in the same sequence, paying specific attention to scars.

With the woman seated, wash your hands and explain the procedure. Inspect each breast visually, taking note of any nipple retraction or deviation, skin dimpling, erythema, oedema, peau d'orange (this is oedema with skin pitting), induration, or asymmetry. Ask the woman to raise her arms above her head, lowering them and shrugging her shoulders forward, this may bring an otherwise unnoticed abnormality into sight. With the woman supine and with one hand under her head (lifting the breast slightly), palpate the ipsilateral axilla and breast. Palpate in a smooth, gentle back-and-forth or circular motion with the palmar surfaces of the three middle fingers, using light and deep but gentle palpation. In a systematic manner, palpate first the axilla and then the entire breast lightly, using deeper palpation to assess full tissue thickness. Explain to the woman what you are doing. Gently compress each nipple, discovering any masses or discharges that are not attributable to pregnancy or postpartum changes. See Figure 16.8.

Assessment of the organs of the female reproductive system

The organs of the female reproductive system cannot usually be felt on palpation. Physical assessment of the reproductive system begins with inspection and palpation of the external genitalia. A speculum is used to visualise the inner vagina and cervix and when the collection of specimens is required.

Prior to undertaking the examination, ask the patient to empty her bladder (a urine specimen may be required). An empty bladder promotes comfort and can make the examination easier; a full bladder can make palpation uncomfortable for the woman. Provide the woman with a gown. She should be asked to remove her clothing from the waist down and to remove any sanitary protection (Young et al. 2018); she can leave her socks and shoes on for comfort. A chaperone will be required and privacy must be afforded. The usual position to undertake the examination is with the woman in the lithotomy position with her knees flexed and apart. The nurse may need to help the woman to assume this position. In some instances of assessment of the female genitalia, the woman may be asked to stand, or to lie in the left lateral position, for example when assessing for pelvic organ prolapse.

Equipment

The equipment needed will depend on the purpose of the examination. The equipment should be readily available in the room, ensuring that the examination proceeds without unnecessary pauses or interruptions. The equipment cited in Box 16.2 should be available to examine the genitalia.

Box 16.2 Equipment needed for genital examination

- A flexible light source
- Vaginal speculae
- Alcoholic hand rub
- Disposable examination gloves
- Water-soluble lubricant
- Several types of sampling devices (for example, wooden or plastic spatula, cytobrush, cervix brush)
- Glass slides, slide container
- Pencil for marking slides
- Fixative solution
- Specimen forms and bag
- Tissue paper
- Clinical waste container

Explain to the woman what the examination entails; verbal consent must be obtained. Wash hands and don gloves. With the woman in the lithotomy position, examine her external genitalia:

- Skin colour
- Hair distribution
- Labia and clitoris (oedema, lesions)
- Urethral opening (stricture, inflammation)
- Vaginal opening (malodourous discharge, inflammation, lesions)
- Palpate the vagina (tenderness, oedema, discharge, Bartholin's glands)

Document and report the findings after you have inspected the external genitalia.

Box 16.3 provides information for passing a vaginal speculum

The Papanicolaou smear test is used in most cases to undertake cervical screening. A sample of cells are taken from the cervix at the junction between the endocervix and the ectocervix in an area known as the transformational zone (see Figure 16.9).

Review

What does cervical cancer CIN IV mean?

Digital bimanual palpation

The bimanual examination enables the examiner to palpate the uterus and ovaries externally and internally concurrently. Griffiths (2015) notes that if ectopic pregnancy is suspected, a vaginal examination should not be undertaken as there is a possibility that rupture of the tubal pregnancy can occur. As with any examination, the examiner must be competent and confident in performing the examination.

Wash hands. Standing, explain to the woman the steps in the examination. Explain the examination can be stopped or paused at any time. The nurse uses gloved fingers and a water-soluble lubricant to gently insert the first two fingers of the dominant hand into the vagina, asking the woman to take deep breaths as this is done. Inside the opening (the introitus), the fingers are slowly and gently advanced along the vaginal canal vertically and the vaginal wall is palpated. Place the other hand above the symphysis pubis, gently pushing down towards the pelvis. Examine the cervix, uterus, and adnexa. As you are doing this, note any irregularities, such as masses or abnormal tenderness. Slowly

Box 16.3 Passing a vaginal speculum

Passing a vaginal speculum

An experienced practitioner is required to pass a vaginal speculum. This procedure should only be undertaken by a practitioner who has been deemed competent to carry it out. Observing a skilled practitioner insert a vaginal speculum can help to enhance learning and skill acquisition.

The speculum can be metal or single-use plastic. If using a metal speculum, running it under warm water prior to insertion will warm it up, and also provide lubrication. If using a plastic speculum, a water-soluble jelly can be used as lubricant; apply the gel only to the side of the blades and not the tip, as this can interfere with sample or swab results. Local policy and procedure must be adhered to at all times.

Standing at the foot of the bed, explain to the woman what you intend to do and that she will feel internal pressure and possibly some slight, transient discomfort. Ensure you have adjusted the light source so you can see clearly. To insert the speculum, spread the inner lips of the vulva with two fingers of the dominant hand, hold the blades (sometime called bills) of the speculum tightly together with the thumb and index finger of the other, and gently guide it into the vaginal canal, ask the woman to take some deep breaths.

Insert the speculum initially at a 90° angle, sideways initially, then asking the woman to take some deep breaths gently rotate it to 45° angle in the direction of the rectum. You can insert it with the handles up, or with the handles down.

Always apply pressure downward during insertion. Never apply pressure upward during insertion; pressing the urethra against the symphysis pubis causes pain or discomfort to the patient.

When the handles of the speculum are pinched together, they will open the blades, stretching the vaginal walls to reveal the cervix. Avoid catching the pubic hair, and with the handles held tightly together, the short handle slides down and the long handle slides up. Once the cervix is fully visualised, lock the speculum into place by the fixing mechanism, this can either be a screw or a ratchet.

Throughout the procedure, observe the woman for signs of pain or discomfort and reassure her that at any time you can stop or pause the procedure.

With the speculum locked, both hands are free to angle the lamp to illuminate the vaginal walls and the cervix and allow for procedures to be performed. Be aware of infection prevention and control practices when adjusting the lamp; use a paper towel when touching the lamp or request a colleague to assist you.

Once you have finished the procedure explain this to the woman. To remove the speculum, place the thumb of the dominant hand on the thumb rest, hold the handles and release the secured position by loosening the fixing mechanism. Gently apply pressure to the handles to ensure the cervix is not caught within the blades.

Ask the woman to take a deep breath and gently rotate clockwise. Take care to remove the blades at an oblique angle and avoid pulling pubic hair or pinching the labia. Offer the woman a paper tissue to clean herself, or you may be required to assist her. Ensure privacy for the patient to get dressed. Dispose of the equipment using local policy and procedure and document and report findings.

and gently remove the finger from the vagina. Provide the woman with tissues to clean herself; you may need to assist her with this. Dispose of the used materials and wash hands.

Document and report all examinations and outcomes according to local policy and procedure. Provide the woman with clear explanations of any findings as well as proposed next stages of care and treatment.

Basing care and treatment decisions on one diagnostic approach (i.e. digital bimanual examination) would be erroneous. Abnormal findings should always be followed up using further assessment that will involve other modes of assessment or diagnostic techniques.

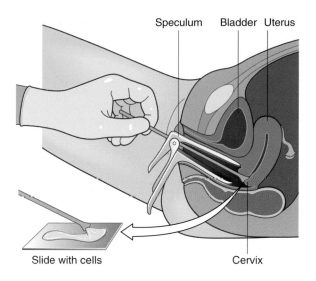

Speculum   Bladder Uterus

Slide with cells   Cervix

Figure 16.9   Cervical cell sampling.

Review

Define the following terms

Menses	
Menarche	
Amenorrhoea	
Oligomenorrhoea	
Menorrhagia	
Metrorrhagia	
Hypermenorrhoea	
Dysmenorrhoea	
Vulvodynia	
Libido	
Vaginitis	
Perimenopause	
Anovulation	
Climacteric	
Dyspareunia	
Hirsutism	
Hysteroscopy	

So far

There are several ways of undertaking an assessment of the female reproductive system; relying on one approach would be imprudent. Screening and diagnostic tests are available to help offer women care that is responsive and appropriate. The role of the nurse is varied and will include acquiring competence and confidence when carrying out several intimate examinations. The role also includes acting as the woman's advocate.

Kamina (Kam) Samuda

At the general practice. Kamina presents with a 2-year history of dysmenorrhoea. Her symptoms commenced when she was 14 years of age. This was 2 years after menarche. Kam's chief complaint was abdominal pain. The primary presenting symptoms included a four-month history of severe painful menstrual cramps accompanied by painful intercourse. Severe menstrual cramping and pain began four months ago when the oral contraceptives Kam was receiving were changed; the pain was so severe that she had several instances of absence from school. Kam takes naproxen 500 mg daily when cramps and pain begin with no relief. Painful cramping starts five to seven days before menses begin, with the worst pain experienced on the first day of flow; the pain disappears completely by the third day of flow.

Kam has had no children, no miscarriages and no termination of pregnancy. Her last normal menstrual period began six days ago. The physical examination undertaken by the practice nurse was unremarkable, with the exception of a dry vaginal vault. She had been treated conservatively by her general practice with over-the-counter non-steroidal anti-inflammatory drugs for her dysmenorrhoea with no relief. Her surgical history included abdominal surgery as a child to remove a gangrenous appendix with no subsequent problems. Kam also reported dyspareunia and vaginal dryness with penile thrusting for the past four months approximately one week before onset of her period. No history of sexually acquired infections, she has only ever been sexually active with her current boyfriend. Kamina reported no change in vaginal discharge with no itching, burning, or malodour.

Initial observations:

Looks well
> Temperature: 36.8 °C
> Pulse: 76 beats per minute
> Respirations: 18 breaths per minute
> Blood pressure: 120/60 mm/Hg
> Using the SOCRATES mnemonic, gather a history from Kam. What questions will you ask her and how will you ask them in order to gather data?

S	Site. Where is the pain	
O	Onset. When did the issue start? Did this come on suddenly or was it gradual?	
C	Character. Is the pain dull or sharp? Is it intermittent or continuous? Describe the pain.	
R	Radiation. Does the pain radiate to other places? Where is it felt?	
A	Associations. Are there any other symptoms associated with the presenting condition?	
T	Time. How long have you had the condition? Does the condition worsen, is it improving, does it fluctuate?	
E	Exacerbating or reliving factors. Does anything make the condition worse or better? Does sexual intercourse exacerbate the condition (dyspareunia)? Is there any pain associated with the menstrual period (dysmenorrhoea)?	
S	Severity. Use a pain scale to assess severity of pain.	

The diagnosis of dysmenorrhoea has been made. What else can be done to help Kam manage her condition?

Is there any other information required and are there any other tests that might need to be carried out?

Conclusion

The reproductive system is key to the survival of the species. Nurses are required to have a working knowledge of the female reproductive system if their aim is to provide care that is delivered in a sensitive, patient-centred manner as well as being safe and effective. Undertaking a patient health history has to be focused and the nurse needs to always remember the intimate nature associated with the assessment of this system. A physical examination can cause embarrassment and thus the nurse should care for the woman in an environment where she feels safe and comfortable.

The female reproductive system is complex; so too is the care offered. A nurse who is skilled in the understanding of assessment is required to adopt a sensitive approach to care. It is also a key requirement that the nurse understands and respects the individual and the holistic needs of the woman and if appropriate her family.

There are several conditions that affect the female reproductive system and thus the person's overall health and wellbeing. Being familiar with these conditions can assist the nurse to help the woman in a timely manner, ensuring a timely diagnosis, treatment, and, if appropriate, referral.

References

Griffiths, B. (2015). The genitourinary system. In: *Physical Examination Procedures and Non-Medical Prescribers: Evidence and Rationale*, 2e (ed. Z. Rawles, B. Griffith and T. Alexander), 55–69. London: CRC Press.

Harlow, S.D. and Campbell, B. (1996). Ethnic differences in the duration and amount of menstrual bleeding during the postmenarcheal period. *American Journal of Epidemiology* 144 (10): 980–988.

Jarvis, C. (2015). *Physical Examination and Health Assessment*, 7e. St Louis: Elsevier.

McLafferty, E., Johnstone, C., Hendry, C., and Farley, A. (2014). Male and female reproductive systems and associated conditions. *Nursing Standard* 28 (36): 37–44.

Tortora, G.J. and Derrickson, B.H. (2012). *Essentials of Anatomy and Physiology: International Student Version*, 9e. New Jersey: Wiley.

Waugh, A. and Grant, A. (2018). *Ross and Wilson's Anatomy and Physiology in Health and Illness*, 13e. Edinburgh: Elsevier.

Young, O., Duncan, C., Dundas, K., and Laird, A. (2018). The reproductive system. In: *Macleod's Clinical Examination*, 14e (ed. J.A. Innes, A.R. Dover and K. Fairhurst), 211–236. Edinburgh: Elsevier.

Chapter 17

Assessing the nervous system

Aim

This chapter introduces the reader to the assessment of the nervous system and the care required for those who experience problems related to this system.

Learning outcomes

By the end of the chapter the reader will be able to:

1. Provide a brief overview of the nervous system and its functions
2. Discuss a number of conditions that might affect the nervous system
3. Outline the various ways in which the nurse may undertake a focused assessment of the nervous system
4. Describe care planning that is related to the needs of a person with a disorder of the nervous system

Introduction

It is essential for the nurse to have a comprehensive understanding of the nervous system if assessment of needs, diagnosis, planning, care provision, and care evaluation is to be safe and effective. Like many body systems, the nervous system is complex, and so too is the assessment of needs. This chapter provides an overview only of the nervous system; the reader is advised to delve deeper into this fascinating system. Braine (2018) offer a comprehensive overview of the system.

The nervous system regulates, controls, and integrates all other body systems, playing a key role in the maintenance of homeostasis. The nurse will be required to care for patients with nervous system disorders in a wide variety of care settings. The NMC (2018) make it a requirement that all nurses ensure they prioritise the care of people, practise effectively, preserve safety and promote professionalism and trust. These requirements made by the NMC are equally important for those people and their families who may have a neurological disorder. Neurological diseases can have a substantial impact on an individual's physical and mental health, which can result in both physical disorder and disordered cognition. There are over 1000 neurological disorders that affect millions of people globally (Braine 2018).

Fundamentals of Assessment and Care Planning for Nurses, First Edition. Ian Peate.
© 2020 John Wiley & Sons Ltd. Published 2020 by John Wiley & Sons Ltd.

6 Cs

Those people with neurological disorders require a dignified approach to care delivery, as a number of neurological disorders result in personality, cognitive, and behavioural changes.

The nervous system

This nervous system receives, processes, and initiates actions through a complicated network of billions of specialised cells that are called neurones (nerves). It consists of two main subdivisions:

1. The central nervous system (CNS): brain and spinal cord
2. The peripheral nervous system (PNS): all nervous tissue outside the CNS

Figure 17.1 shows the main components of the nervous system.

Cells of the nervous system

Nervous tissue consists of two major classes of cells, the neurone and neuroglia cells. The neurone, the basic anatomical and functional unit of the nervous system, forms a complex processing network communicating with other neurones and cells within the brain and spinal cord. The neuroglia (also called 'glia') are the supporting cells in the CNS, offering protection, support, and nourishment to the neurones and maintaining homeostasis in the interstitial fluid that they bathe in.

303

Neurones

The majority of neurones consist of a cell body and two types of neuronal processes: dendrites and axon (see Figure 17.2). Neurones vary in shape and size, the longest extending from the brain to the toes. Cell bodies also vary in size. They are found in clusters in the PNS known as 'ganglia'. In the CNS

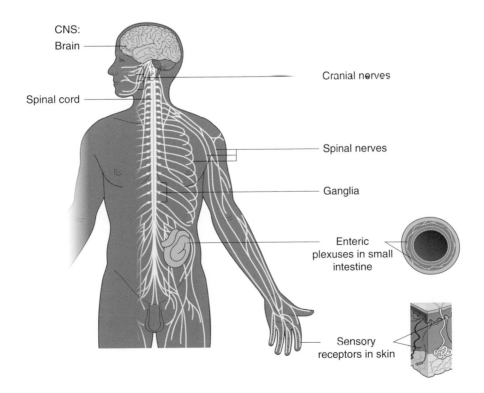

Figure 17.1 Main components of the nervous system.

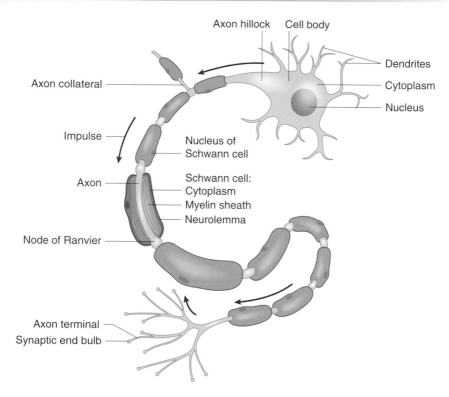

Figure 17.2   A typical motor neurone and Schwann cell.

these clusters are called 'a centre', and a centre with a discrete boundary is called a 'nucleus'. The dendrites emerge from the cell body, conducting impulses towards (afferent) the cell body from the synapses at the end of the dendrites. Synapses are junctions where a neurone meets another cell; in the CNS, this is another neurone but in the PNS, this may be a muscle (neuromuscular junction), gland, or organ. The axon (there is only one per neurone), a long process, conducts impulses away (efferent) from the cell body towards another neurone, muscle fibre, or a gland cell.

Axons may be insulated by a white lipid sheath known as 'myelin' (myelinated) or not (unmyelinated). The myelin sheath is formed by Schwann cells in the PNS and oligodendrocytes in the CNS. The myelin sheath contains gaps (bare segments) called nodes of Ranvier, allowing movement of ions between the axon and the extracellular fluid; this increases the speed of nerve impulse conduction. The cell bodies and dendrites comprise what is often called the 'grey matter' of the CNS.

Neuroglia cells

A number of different neuroglia cells are found in the CNS and PNS. Glia cells, once considered as just scaffolding for the neurones, are now known to play important roles in CNS functions, but they cannot conduct impulses (see Figure 17.3).

Synapses and neurotransmitters – how communication occurs within the CNS

Neurones communicate with precision through 'synaptic transmission'. When a neurone is stimulated, this results in an electrical reaction travelling down the axon to the terminal. Here it passes the message onto another neurone that is called the synapse. Synaptic transmission may occur in two ways:

1. Electrical transmission – the electrical charge is transmitted via a small gap. The message can flow both ways across the synapse. Usually found in the cardiac and smooth muscle for rapid transmission.

(a)

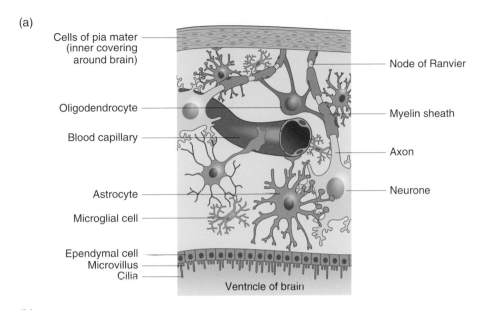

Cells of pia mater (inner covering around brain)

Node of Ranvier

Oligodendrocyte

Myelin sheath

Blood capillary

Axon

Astrocyte

Neurone

Microglial cell

Ependymal cell
Microvillus
Cilia

Ventricle of brain

(b)

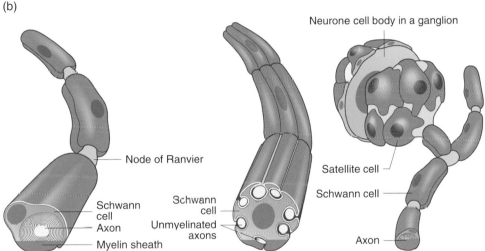

Neurone cell body in a ganglion

Node of Ranvier

Satellite cell

Schwann cell

Schwann
cell

Schwann
cell

Axon
Myelin sheath

Unmyelinated
axons

Axon

Figure 17.3   Neuroglia.

2. Chemical transmission (most synapses) requires chemicals to transmit the message, called 'neurotransmitters'; synthesised by the neurone and released into the gap between two neurons (the 'synaptic cleft'), they diffuse across the gap to activate the other neurone.

Some neurotransmitters modulate the effect of a particular neurotransmitter by prolonging, exciting, inhibiting or limiting their effect, known as 'neuromodulators'.

The central nervous system

The CNS is responsible for controlling and integrating the whole nervous system receiving information (input) about the changes in the internal and external environment and processes and interprets this information, providing signals that are manifested in sensory or motor outputs. The brain is the control centre of the nervous system also generating thoughts, emotions, and speech.

On average the brain weights 1400 g, it is a relatively small structure, making up about 2% of body weight in adults (Braine 2018). The brain is protected from the external environment by three barriers:

1. The skull
2. The meninges
3. The cerebral spinal fluid

There are four major parts associated with the brain:

1. The cerebral cortex
2. The diencephalon (thalamus, hypothalamus, and epithalamus)
3. The brain stem
4. The cerebellum

Table 17.1 summarises the general functions of the four regions and Figure 17.4 represents the brain.

Cerebral cortex (cerebrum)

The surface of the cerebral cortex (cerebrum) is folded into elevated ridges of tissue called 'gyri', separated by shallow grooves called 'sulci' or 'fissures' (deeper groves). Fissures further divide the surface of the cerebrum into the four lobes. The longitudinal fissure separates the two hemispheres, the transverse fissure separates the cerebrum from the cerebellum, and the lateral fissure separates the temporal lobe from the frontal and parietal lobes. The thick white matter is comprised of hundreds of millions of myelinated axons (fatty sheaths causing the white appearance) bundled into different tracts or pathways that run in three principal directions connecting the various grey matter areas (neurone cell bodies).

Each cerebral hemisphere is divided into frontal, parietal, temporal, and occipital lobes. The cortex can be divided up into areas that serve a single function; 'primary areas' (touch, vision, hearing, taste and smell and the production of movement). Clustered around these primary areas and associated with them, are areas known as association areas (cortex). Understanding these functional areas of the cortex is important, as selective damage to these regions may lead to neurological deficits.

The right side of the body is controlled by the left hemisphere of the cerebral cortex and vice versa, known as decussation. Each hemisphere has highly specialised regions that serve differing functions, lateralisation (see Table 17.2).

The limbic system

The limbic system is a highly complex system. It consists of the limbic lobe; although not a discrete lobe, it is made up of a number of cortical structures forming a ring of cortex spanning the frontal, temporal, and parietal lobes and subcortical areas interconnected with each other and with the hypothalamus.

Spinal cord

This is a long cylindrical segmented structure, beginning at the foramen magnum, terminating at the first lumbar vertebra. It receives sensory information from the limbs, trunk, and internal organs and somatic motor tracts that supply the skeletal muscles, visceral, smooth muscles, and glands. The spinal cord gives rise to 31 spinal nerves (part of the PNS) corresponding to each segment exiting the spinal cord between the vertebral bones of the spinal cord. The spinal cord does not reach the end of the vertebral column; as a result, the lumbar and sacral nerve roots travel inferiorly through the vertebral canal for some distance before exiting the vertebral column through their associated intervertebral foramina. This collection of descending nerve roots is called the 'cauda equina' (Figure 17.5).

Table 17.1   The general function of the four main parts of the brain.

Main part	Functions
Cerebral cortex	
<ul><li>Largest part of the brain</li><li>Divided into right and left hemispheres</li><li>Both hemispheres are connected internally by the corpus callosum</li><li>The right sends and receives information from the left side of the body and vice versa</li><li>Each hemisphere is divided into four lobes named after the bone that covers them</li><li>Hemispheres are composed of outer cerebral cortex grey matter, internal white matter, and nuclei deep within the white matter</li></ul>	<ul><li>Receives sensory (afferent) impulses</li><li>Initiates motor (efferent) impulses</li><li>Controls skeletal muscle activity</li><li>Contains the seat of consciousness</li><li>Processes sensory information</li><li>Responsible for many 'higher-order' functions, e.g. language and information processing</li><li>Governs intelligence, reasoning, learning, memory, and other complex behaviours</li></ul>
Diencephalon	
Provides a structural connection between the cerebrum and the brainstem, in particular the midbrain. Includes the following areas:<ul><li>Thalamus consists of small, paired egg-shaped nuclei approximately 3 cm in length, constituting 80% of the diencephalon</li><li>Hypothalamus, located below the thalamus and composed of several nuclei. A stalk-like infundibulum connects the pituitary gland to the hypothalamus</li><li>Epithalamus consists of the pineal gland</li><li>Subthalamus consists of two main cell groups: the subthalamic nuclei and the zona incerta</li></ul>	*Thalamus*<ul><li>Main synaptic relay centre, processes motor information</li><li>Receives and relays sensory information to and from the cerebral cortex</li></ul>*Hypothalamus*<ul><li>Main visceral control and vital for overall homeostasis</li><li>Regulates autonomic nervous system</li><li>Senses change in body temperature and regulates core body temperature</li><li>Regulates and produces hormones</li><li>Mediates emotional responses</li><li>Regulates water balance and thirst</li><li>Regulation of appetite</li><li>Regulation of sleep–wake cycle (circadian rhythm)</li><li>Part of the arousal/alerting mechanism</li></ul>
Brainstem	
Consists of the:<ul><li>Midbrain, composed of the paired bundles of axons called *cerebral peduncles*, several nuclei including the red nuclei and the substantia nigra, and is approximately 1 cm long</li><li>Medulla oblongata, containing all ascending and descending motor and sensory tracts and several nuclei and serves as site of crossing of nerve tracts (decussation)</li><li>Pons consists of bundles of ascending and descending fibres and nuclei</li></ul>Also extensive throughout the brainstem are a network of white and grey fibres called the *reticular formation*	*Midbrain*<ul><li>Conducts impulses from the motor areas in the cerebral cortex to the brainstem</li><li>Reflex centre for some visual activities, e.g. eye movement, light reflex, and accommodation and convergence reflex</li></ul>*Medulla oblongata*<ul><li>Controls voluntary movement of lower limbs and trunk</li><li>Cardiovascular centre controls heart rate and force of heartbeat</li><li>Rhythmicity area controls basic breathing rate</li><li>Controls reflexes for vomiting, coughing, swallowing, hiccupping, yawning and sneezing</li><li>Nuclei for several cranial nerves</li></ul>*Pons*<ul><li>Coordinates voluntary movements</li><li>Pneumotaxic and apneustic areas help control breathing</li><li>Nuclei for several cranial nerves</li></ul>
Cerebellum	
<ul><li>Second largest area and contains nearly half of all the neurones in the brain</li><li>Consists of two hemispheres and a central area (*vermis*) attached to the brainstem by three paired *peduncles*</li><li>Consists of an outer cortex of grey matter and an inner white matter called the *arbor vitae*</li><li>Incoming information is received from the cortex via the pons and outgoing information goes to the cortex via the thalamus</li></ul>	<ul><li>Balance</li><li>Muscle tension</li><li>Eye movement</li><li>Equilibrium of the trunk</li><li>Spinal nerve reflexes</li><li>Provides information necessary for balance, posture and coordinated muscle movement</li></ul>

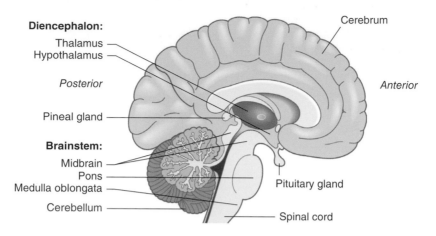

Figure 17.4   The brain.

Table 17.2   Key specific functions of key cerebral hemispheres.

Left-side dominance	General function	Right-side dominance
Words and letters	Vision	Geometric patterns Face recognition and facial emotional expression Visual imagery
Language sounds	Audition	Non-language sounds Music and artistic awareness
Complex movements	Touch	Tactile patterns (Braille)
Verbal memory	Movement	Spatial movement patterns
Speech (70–90%) Reading, writing Arithmetic and logical abilities	Language	Generating emotional content
	Spatial ability	Geometry Direction Distance Mental rotation of shapes

The meninges: the coverings of the brain and spinal cord

Three layers of connective tissue (the meninges) cover the brain and spinal cord. The cranial and spinal meninges are continuous and bear the same structure (see Figure 17.6):

- The dura mater is a pain-sensitive thick double outer fibrous membrane consisting of external periosteal layer and inner meningeal layer.
- The arachnoid mater is a middle thin avascular membrane which is attached tightly to the inner dural layer. The space between the arachnoid and pia is called the 'subarachnoid space'. The arachnoid contains specialised parts that protrude into venous sinuses and are responsible for the reabsorption of cerebrospinal fluid (CSF), known as arachnoid villi or granulations
- The pia mater is a thin inner transparent fibrous membrane, tightly attached to the surface of the brain parenchyma, following the contours of the gyri and sulci and the spinal cord.

CSF is a clear, colourless liquid that flows in the subarachnoid space in a unidirectional flow. Around 400–500 mL of CSF is produced per day. At any one time the total volume of CSF is 80–150 mL.

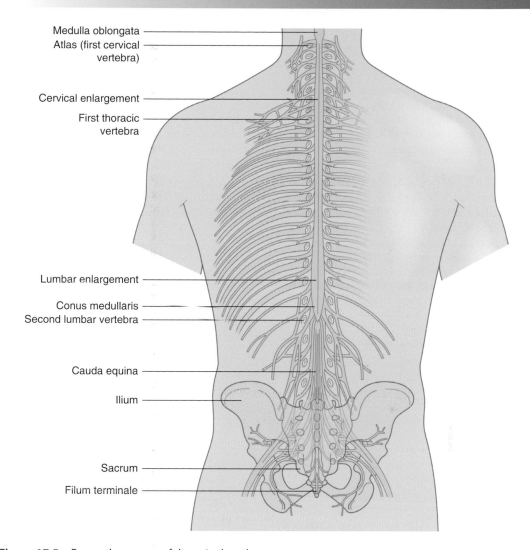

Figure 17.5 External anatomy of the spinal cord.

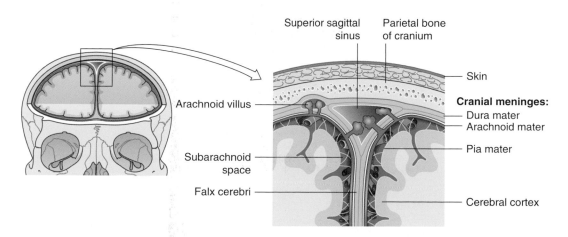

Figure 17.6 The coverings of the brain.

Approximately 30 mL is located in the chambers in the brain known as the 'ventricles', the remainder is in the subarachnoid space. It has three basic functions:

1. Mechanical protection – cushioning and protecting the delicate brain against impact, injury, the fluid acting as a buoyancy aid for the brain
2. Chemical protection – providing optimum chemical environment for accurate neuronal signalling
3. Circulation protection – a medium for carrying nutrients from the blood to the adjacent brain tissue and removing waste and potentially noxious substances, such as drugs

Blood–brain barrier

The blood–brain barrier (BBB), located at the interface between the capillary walls and the brain tissue, acts to isolate the brain from the rest of the body. It regulates the exchange of substances entering the brain in order to maintain optimum levels of, e.g. glucose, proteins and electrolytes, for normal brain activities. In addition, the BBB acts to filter and restrict diffusion and permeation of molecules in order to protect against harmful toxins and metabolites. The BBB is important as it limits most potential drugs that can be administered to treat brain disorders from penetrating the tight mesh of endothelial cells, and only allows the entry of small/fat (lipid) molecules, e.g. some viruses and toxins (carbon monoxide).

Blood supply

The CNS is one of the most metabolically active systems in the body and requires a blood system to meet these demands. A brief interruption of blood flow (seconds) to the brain can cause serious neurological disturbances and cell death in minutes.

Blood supply to the brain comes from two main sources: two internal carotids arising from the common carotid artery, and two vertebral arteries arising from the subclavian artery. Both sets of arteries give rise to pairs of arteries that supply the blood to both sides of the brain and are joined at the base of the brain to form the Circle of Willis, from which major arteries supplying the brain arise. Venous drainage of the brain – cerebral drainage – is dependent upon a system of valveless superficial and deep veins into three main dural sinuses, which then empty into the right and left internal jugular vein.

The blood supply of the spinal cord comes from the anterior spinal artery and paired posterior spinal arteries, arising from the vertebral artery.

The peripheral nervous system

This system links the CNS with the rest of the body. It is responsible for receiving and transmitting information from and about the external environment. The PNS includes the neuromuscular structures outside the skull and vertebral column; spinal nerves and cranial nerves, neuromuscular junction and receptors. Spinal nerves emerge from the spinal cord whilst cranial nerves emerge from the brain (see Figure 17.7).

The PNS provides input via the sensory neurones and output information via motor neurones to the CNS and can be further subdivided into the somatic nervous systems (SNS) (nerves that transmit information from the skeletal muscles), autonomic nervous system (ANS), and the enteric nervous system (ENS).

The spinal (peripheral) nerves contain motor and sensory fibres that can be myelinated or unmyelinated. Spinal nerves innervate a specific skin area called a dermatome, and each spinal nerve further divides into branches called rami. Some of these branches form complex clusters of nerves known as 'plexuses'; there are four: cervical, brachial lumbar and sacral. Ganglia are small clusters of nervous tissue, primarily neurone cell bodies, outside the CNS.

The nerves can be classified according to size, which is related to speed of conduction and if they are myelinated or unmyelinated. The PNS is divided into a sensory (afferent) division and a motor (efferent) division.

Autonomic nervous system

The ANS, a division of the PNS, is subdivided into enteric, sympathetic (SNS), and parasympathetic nervous system (PNS) and functions to control the internal environment of the body and the exchange between the internal and external environment. Working with the endocrine system, the

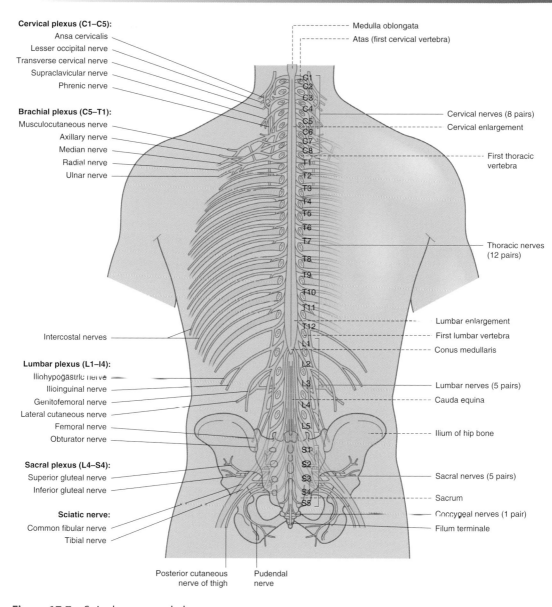

Cervical plexus (C1–C5):
Ansa cervicalis
Lesser occipital nerve
Transverse cervical nerve
Supraclavicular nerve
Phrenic nerve

Brachial plexus (C5–T1):
Musculocutaneous nerve
Axillary nerve
Median nerve
Radial nerve
Ulnar nerve

Intercostal nerves

Lumbar plexus (L1–I4):
Iliohypogastric nerve
Ilioinguinal nerve
Genitofemoral nerve
Lateral cutaneous nerve
Femoral nerve
Obturator nerve

Sacral plexus (L4–S4):
Superior gluteal nerve
Inferior gluteal nerve

Sciatic nerve:
Common fibular nerve
Tibial nerve

Posterior cutaneous nerve of thigh
Pudendal nerve

Medulla oblongata
Atas (first cervical vertebra)

C1
C2
C3
C4
C5
C6
C7
C8

Cervical nerves (8 pairs)
Cervical enlargement

First thoracic vertebra

T1
T2
T3
T4
T5
T6
T7
T8
T9
T10
T11
T12

Thoracic nerves (12 pairs)

L1
L2
L3
L4
L5

Lumbar enlargement
First lumbar vertebra
Conus medullaris

Lumbar nerves (5 pairs)
Cauda equina

Ilium of hip bone

S1
S2
S3
S4
S5

Sacral nerves (5 pairs)

Sacrum

Coccygeal nerves (1 pair)
Filum terminale

Figure 17.7 Spinal nerves and plexuses.

311

ANS regulates homeostasis and controls a range of functions and behaviours. The ENS found in the wall of the gut, is involved in coordinating the contractions of the gut musculature, resulting in gastrointestinal mobility (peristalsis).

The major sensory system consists of somatic, visual, auditory, vestibular, taste, and olfactory systems. The somatic sensory system includes sensations for pain, tactile sensation (touch, pressure, and vibration), temperature, perception of the joint position, and movement. Information is gathered from the environment via peripheral sensory nerve receptors and specialised sensory cells. Sensory receptors are grouped into different classes, depending upon structure location and function. Sensation is relayed via somatosensory pathways (spinothalamic), somatosensory area, via the brain stem and thalamus, to the primary somatosensory area in the cerebral cortex located in the parietal lobe and the cerebellum. Each area receives sensory information from different parts of the body as depicted in Figure 17.8.

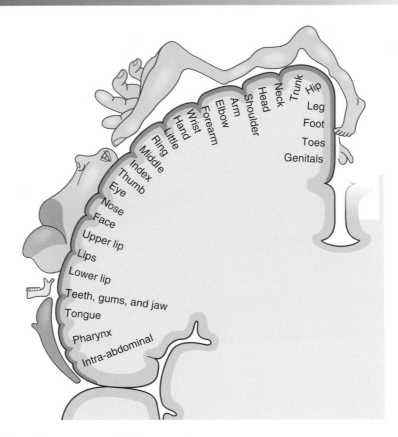

Figure 17.8   Somatic sensory map in the cerebral cortex.

The cranial nerves

There are 12 pairs of cranial nerves (I–XII). All emerge from the brain, apart from the IXth cranial nerve, which emerges from the spinal cord and the PNS. The numbers specify the order, anterior to posterior, in which the nerves arise from the brain. In Table 17.3 the major functions of each cranial nerve is described and in Figure 17.9 the origins of the cranial nerves are shown.

So far

The neurological system is both complex and challenging. An overview of the organisation, structure and functions of the central and PNS has been presented. The different cells that make up the nervous system were described along with their functions. The 12 pairs of cranial nerves have been described.

If there is a disruption to any of the processes associated with the neurological system, there is potential that the rest of the body will also be impacted.

The patient history

Key to understanding the needs of people with neurological conditions is the gathering of a comprehensive patient history. A detailed and systematic history and a focused examination are essential during the assessment stage. Appropriate questioning will help focus and give structure to the assessment. The nurse combines the steps of the neurological history with the steps taken during the complete physical examination.

The neurological history and the physical examination permit the nurse to determine various areas of the brain or the nervous system that may be dysfunctional. Specific signs and symptoms demonstrated by the patient are associated with specific areas of the brain.

Table 17.3 The cranial nerves and their major functions.

Number	Name	Classification	Major function
I	Olfactory	Special sensory	Sense of smell
II	Optic	Special sensory	Conducts impulses for vision from retina to occipital cortex (acuity and field of vision)
II[a]	Oculomotor	Motor	Eye movements Eyelid elevation Pupillary constriction
IV[a]	Trochlear		Downward/inward eye movements
VI[a]	Abducens		Lateral eye movements
V	Trigeminal, three branches: • Ophthalmic • Maxillary • Mandibular	Mixed • Motor • Sensory	*Sensory* Facial sensation of: • Cornea • Face • Mouth • Jaw *Motor* • Chewing
VII	Facial	Mixed • Motor • Sensory	*Sensory* • Sensation of the face • Lacrimal gland secretion of tears • Salivary gland secretion of saliva • Taste: anterior two-thirds of the tongue *Motor* • Control of facial expression
VIII	Known as acoustic or vestibular-cochlear	Special sensory	Conducts impulses from the ear to the auditory temporal lobe: hearing Equilibrium
IX	Glossopharyngeal	Mixed • Motor • Sensory	*Sensory* • Coordination of swallowing and gag reflex • Sensations to pharynx • Taste: posterior third of the tongue • Regulation of blood pressure via chemoreceptors in the carotid sinus *Motor* • Salivation and assists in swallowing
X	Vagus	Mixed • Motor • Sensory	*Sensory* • Sensation to mucosa of pharynx, soft palate, tonsils, viscera of the thorax and abdomen *Motor* • Controls swallowing, phonation and movement of the soft palate and uvula • Motility and secretion of gastrointestinal organs • Decreased heart rate
XI	Spinal accessory	Motor	Movement of the head and neck via sternocleidomastoid muscles, upper trapezius
XII	Hypoglossal	Motor	Movement of the tongue facilitating speech, manipulation of food and swallowing

[a]These three cranial nerves are usually grouped together because they are concerned with eye movement.

313

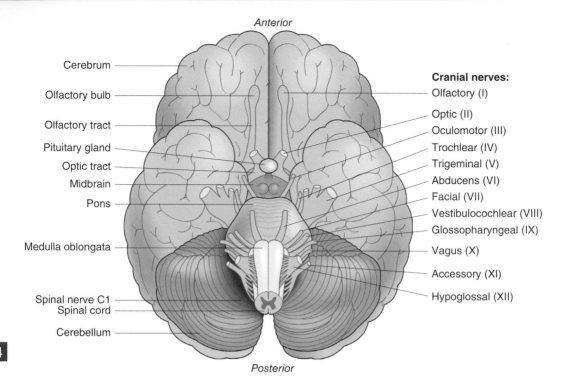

Figure 17.9   The origins of the cranial nerves.

Whilst it may seem rather overwhelming at first, the myriad ways in which the neurological system can be assessed by some of the tests used are basic and uncomplicated. Speaking with a patient will enable the nurse to assess orientation, and assessing motor function occurs when the patient is up and walking.

Davenport and Manji (2018) suggest that common neurological symptoms include headache, numbness, disturbance/loss of consciousness, and memory loss. Other symptoms include dizziness, faintness, and disturbance in balance or gait. There are some symptoms, for example loss of consciousness or amnesia, that will require an additional witness to give a history (obtain a collateral history). The International Headache Society categorises headache syndromes into primary and secondary. See Table 17.4 for an overview of headache.

Take note

All of the below are warning signs that require further investigations by a specialist.

- Change in characteristics of headache, i.e. increased frequency, severity, or associated symptoms
- New onset of headache, in particular those less than 10 and over 50 years of age
- New onset of headache in those with pre-existing cancer, HIV infection, or head injury
- Progressive headache that has become worse over weeks or longer
- Stubborn morning headache with nausea
- Headache that is associated with postural changes, physical exertion, coughing, or Valsalva
- Thunderclap headache (intense, sudden onset)

Source: British Association for the Study of Headache (2010), Scottish Intercollegiate Guideline Network (2008).

Table 17.4 Primary and secondary headache.

Primary headaches	
Migraine	Unilateral, throbbing, and disproportionately disabling. Often accompanied with nausea. Migraine can occur with or without a warning sign (an aura). If there is an aura, the most common manifestations are visual symptoms, such as flickering lights, spots or zig-zag lines, fortification spectra (images that can float in vison), or blind spots.
Tension-type headaches	The most common type of headaches. They can be both episodic and chronic. They are bilateral, pressing or tightening in kind, mild-to-moderate in intensity, and no nausea. They are not provoked by any physical activity; however, there may be pericranial tenderness and sensitivity to light or noise
Cluster headaches	Characterised by attacks of severe unilateral pain in a trigeminal distribution (affecting the face). They occur in clusters after a remission period of months or years. Often, they begin during sleep and can wake the patient, as the pain is so severe. They are associated with watering of the eye (on the same side of the body), conjunctival redness, rhinorrhoea (runny nose), nasal blockage and ptosis (drooping of the eyelid).
Primary thunder clap headache	A high-intensity headache of sudden onset reaching maximum intensity in under a minute and lasting from 1 hour to 10 days. Generally, primary thunderclap headache is not recurrent; however, it may recur in the first week after onset. Thunderclap headache is often linked to serious vascular intracranial disorders, particularly sub arachnoid haemorrhage
Secondary headache	
Head and neck trauma	A variety of types of headache may follow head and neck trauma, tension-type headaches are the most common. These are classified as: ● Acute and chronic post-traumatic headache. ● Acute and chronic headache attributed to whiplash injury. ● Headache attributed to traumatic intracranial haematoma. ● Headache attributed to other head and/or neck trauma. ● Post-craniotomy headache.
Cranial or cervical vascular disorder	These headaches are usually rapid, acute onset, with the presence of neurological symptoms and the rapid remission of symptoms. Classified as: ● Ischaemic stroke or transient ischaemic attack ● Vasculitis or temporal arteritis ● Subarachnoid haemorrhage Non-vascular intracranial disorder: ● Intrathecal injection ● Epileptic seizure ● High or low cerebral spinal fluid pressure
Substance use or its withdrawal	Includes toxins and environmental pollutants, food allergies, caffeine, and alcohol as well as therapeutic substances (i.e. analgesia) and drugs of misuse.
Infection	Intracranial infection HIV/AIDS Chronic post-infection headache
Non-traumatic disorders	Disorder of the neck Disorder of the eyes Disorder of the ears Sinusitis Disorder of the teeth, jaws, or related structures
Cranial neuralgia	Trigeminal neuralgia

Source: Adapted from International Headache Society (2018).

When obtaining a history, the nurse should use the patient's own words when documenting the chief complaint or the reason(s) they are seeking information. Those people with neurological conditions may find it difficult to express or describe their symptoms. Try to clarify what they mean when describing symptoms, different patients have different ways of describing neurological symptoms, such as 'unconscious', 'blacked out', or 'had a turn'. Clarify what it is that you are being told.

6Cs

Having experienced neurological symptoms, the patient (and their family) may be very anxious and alarmed by what they are experiencing or what they have seen. They will need reassurance from the nurse in the form of listening and acknowledging what it is that they are telling you.

Ask about onset and frequency of the problem the person is experiencing; discuss patterns occurring over time:

- When did the symptoms begin or did the witness recognise that there was a change in the patient? When was the patient last well? What was the person's mental/physical state after the event?
- Are the symptoms persistent or occasional?
- If the symptoms occur occasionally, how long do they last?
- If they are persistent, then are they getting any worse, getting better, or staying the same?
- Determine information about onset: was it gradual or sudden?
- Was/is there any loss of balance when standing or waking?
- With headache, for example, where is the headache, does it radiate?

Discover if there were any factors that triggered the presenting complaint, anything that exacerbated the condition, or any relieving factors. Ask what the patient was doing when the symptoms began. Precipitating factors: Is there anything that makes the symptoms better or worse, for example straining at stool or physical exercise? Do the symptoms come on at a particular time of day? Does menstruation make things better or worse? Are there any associated symptoms, such as nausea, vomiting, headache, photophobia, phonophobia? Does anything relieve the symptoms?

See Table 17.5 for an overview of other elements of the history-taking process. The nurse should recall that effective history taking is essential in reducing the differential diagnosis. A collateral history may need to be provided by someone who witnessed the episode and is often required to gain accurate details. If the patient is unconscious, the witness may be able to provide details about what happened during and after the episode

Take note

Do not position the unconscious person on their back, as their tongue may slide back, occluding the airway, and if there is any vomit this will not be able to drain out.

There are a number of neurological conditions that have manifestations in systems other than the neurological system. Where possible, the nurse should undertake a comprehensive review of systems. Table 17.6 provides an outline of some common manifestations of neurological problems.

Review

What specific aspects of medication management might need to be considered for some patients who are receiving treatment for their multiple sclerosis?

Table 17.5   Some components of the neurological system history.

Element of the history-taking process	Ask about:
Past history	Birth history and a developmental history A history of syncope (temporary loss of consciousness) – determine type of syncope, any triggers, frequency, and when last event occurred Epilepsy/febrile seizures – frequency, treatment, and last event Vascular disease (cardiovascular syncope) – hypertension, hypercholesterolaemia, coronary artery disease, arrhythmia Parkinson's/diabetes, orthostatic hypotension can cause temporary loss of consciousness Any past head trauma, this can increase the risk of seizures A malfunctioning pacemaker can result in cardiovascular syncope Recent surgery can increase a risk of pulmonary embolism
Drug history	Drugs prescribed, over-the-counter, complementary, and recreational can cause neurological symptoms, for example: • Anticonvulsants establish if patient has been taking these as prescribed • Beta-blockers can cause bradycardia/hypotension • Short-acting benzodiazepines may result in seizures on withdrawal • Consider compliance, inadequate administration of insulin in diabetes may lead to hypoglycaemia
Family history	Determine health history of family members Is there a history of neurological disease in the family? Any cardiovascular disease Epilepsy Diabetes Multiple sclerosis (not an inherited condition, though there is genetic risk it may be inherited)
Social history	Alcohol is the most common neurological toxin, ask how many units a week and determine type/volume/strength of alcohol Smoking, how many cigarettes a day? How many years has the person smoked for? Diet – a poor diet along with vitamin deficiency can impact negatively on neurological function It is important to understand the patient's level of functional independence, about care needs, as this will influence how the person will be cared for. Understanding how the patient performs their activities of living will allow the nurse to consider if there are any actual or potential risks posed by further episodes of impaired neurological status
Occupational history	Check what the person's job is and what is involved in their job Exposure to some occupational toxins can result in damage to the neurological system

Source: Adapted from Davenport and Manji (2018), Rhoads and Wiggins Petersen (2018).

So far

History taking is a skilled activity and when taking a neurological history the nurse needs to ensure that the activity is undertaken in a systematic manner but in response to the patient needs and condition.

The history may be taken from the patient or there may need to be collateral history, for example from a family member or eye witness. The history will inform the physical examination, subsequent imaging (i.e. neuroimaging), and other tests as well as making a diagnosis and subsequent treatment and care.

Physical examination

The examination (as with the examination of other systems) begins when the nurse first meets the patient and continues for the duration of the examination. Only a practitioner who has been trained and considered competent in how to assess and document neurological observations can undertake a neurological system assessment.

Table 17.6 Some common manifestations of neurological problems.

System	Sign or symptoms	Potential associated condition
General	Fever, chills	Meningitis, encephalitis
	Sleeplessness	Parkinson's
	Fatigue	Multiple sclerosis, myasthenia gravis
	Dizziness	Ménière's disease
Skin	Petechial or purpuric rash	Meningitis
Eye	Visual disturbance/difficulty	Cerebrovascular accident, ruptured intracranial aneurysm or arteriovenous malformation, encephalitis, multiple sclerosis, brain tumour, migraine.
	Tearing or redness of eye	Cluster headaches (see Table 17.4)
Respiratory	Respiratory anomalies	Guillain-Barré syndrome
Cardiovascular	Bruits, thrills	Cerebrovascular accident
Gastrointestinal	Nausea vomiting	Cerebral and spinal abscesses, ruptured intracranial aneurysm or arteriovenous malformation, brain tumour, migraine
Genitourinary	Urinary dysfunction	Multiple sclerosis, brain tumour
Musculoskeletal	Back ache	Spinal abscesses
	Nuchal rigidity (inability to flex the neck forward)	Meningitis
	Weakness	Cerebrovascular accident
Mental health	Depression	Parkinson's Multiple sclerosis

Source: Adapted from Rhoads and Wiggins Petersen (2018).

Box 17.1 Equipment required in order to undertake a neurological systems assessment

- Pen torch
- Ophthalmoscope
- Tongue depressor
- Tuning fork
- Sterile needles
- Cotton wisp
- Reflex hammer (tendon hammer)
- Aromatic substances
- Solutions for tasting
- Snellen chart (eye chart)

As the patient walks in, take note of how the patient speaks when you greet them, their behaviour (demeanour), posture, and gait. You are required to ensure the patient is comfortable; the room should be warm and well lit. The equipment needed to undertake a physical examination of the neurological system is detailed in Box 17.1.

A comprehensive physical examination of the neurological system is vast. An initial assessment of the patient may reveal the need to undertake a detailed assessment. The physical examination should be conducted in an orderly, symmetrical fashion; this ensures that all areas are assessed. Each side of the body should be compared with the other side, allowing the nurse to detect any abnormalities or deficiencies. Rhoads and Wiggins Petersen (2018) suggest that a complete assessment of the neurological system requires an assessment of:

- Mental status
- Sensation
- Cranial nerves
- Motor function
- Cerebellar function
- Reflexes

Assessment of mental status

Mental state assessment can be undertaken using the Mini Mental State Examination (MMSE). This is a common tool that uses a set of questions for screening cognitive function (de Boer et al. 2014). The MMSE measures orientation, registration (immediate memory), short-term memory (but not long-term memory), and language functioning.

The MMSE is not a suitable tool for making a diagnosis. However, Sallam and Amr (2013) suggest it can be used to indicate the presence of cognitive impairment, for example in a person with suspected dementia or following a head injury. The MMSE should be used in determining cognitive impairment as opposed to the use of informal questioning or an overall impression of a patient's orientation. Other approaches to mental status assessment can include screening for cognitive impairment and screening for depression in the primary care setting.

319

Review

What advice and support could you offer a patient who is experiencing post-stroke depression?

Cultural consideration

When interpreting test scores arrived at using the MMSE, allowance may need to be made for education and ethnicity.

Source: Spering et al. (2012).

The General Practitioner Assessment of Cognition (GPCOG) Score (Brodaty et al. 2002) is an alternative to the MMSE. This tool was designed as a GP screening tool for dementia and is a valid, efficient, well-accepted instrument for dementia screening in primary care. There are two components: a cognitive assessment that is undertaken with the patient and an informant questionnaire, this is only considered necessary if the results of the cognitive section are ambiguous.

Assessing the cranial nerves

The cranial nerves transmit motor or sensory messages, some transmit both predominately between the brain and brain stem and the head and neck. Explain to the patient the rationale for undertaking an assessment of the cranial nerves and what their role is in assessment. Wash hands prior to carrying out the assessment and have all equipment required available in the room. See Table 17.7 for details of assessing the cranial nerves.

After the assessment is complete, thank the patient and explain what is to happen next and how the results of the assessment will be provided. Wash hands and dispose of used items using local policy and procedure. Document and report findings.

Table 17.7 Assessing the cranial nerves (in the conscious patient).

Number	Name	Major function	Assessment
I	Olfactory	Sense of smell	Ensure the patient's nostrils are patent. Test the patient's recognition of familiar odours (an aromatic substance). Test each nostril independently
II	Optic	Conducts impulses for vision from retina on occipital cortex (acuity and field of vision)	Evaluate visual acuity and visual fields using a Snellen chart The optic disc should be examined using the ophthalmoscope
III	Oculomotor	Eye movements Eyelid elevation Pupillary constriction	These three cranial nerves are usually grouped together because they are concerned with eye movement. Inspect and compare both eyes Check cross lateral eye movements (gaze). Abnormalities associated with nerve damage include, ptosis, or pupillary inequality. Ensure the pupils constrict when a light is shone into them (assessing accommodation). Ask the patient to follow your finger as you bring it towards the bridge of his nose. Note the convergence of the eyes and pupillary constriction.
IV	Trochlear	Downward/inward eye movements	
VI	Abducens	Lateral eye movements	
V	Trigeminal – three branches: • Ophthalmic • Maxillary • Mandibular	Sensory facial sensation of: • Cornea • Face • Mouth • Jaw Motor: • Chewing	Using a cotton wisp in order to assess the sensory aspect, determine the patient's ability to feel light touch on the face. With the eyes closed, check sensation on the forehead, cheek, and jaw. With a sterile needle, test pain perception on the same three areas, asking the patient to describe and compare the sensations. In order to test the motor component, request the patient clench the teeth and simultaneously palpate the temporal and masseter muscles
VII	Facial	Sensory • Sensation of the face • Lachrymal glands – secretion of tears • Salivary glands – secretion of saliva • Sensory-taste – anterior two-thirds of the tongue Motor • Control of facial expression	Assess the sensory aspect by placing items with various tastes on the anterior part (sour, bitter, sweet). After each taste the patient rinses the mouth. Assess the motor component by observing the face for symmetry and rest and when the patient smiles, ask the patient to raise the eyebrows and frown. Note strength and symmetry.
VIII	Known as: acoustic or vestibular-cochlear	Conducts impulses from the ear to the auditory temporal lobe – hearing Equilibrium	Assess hearing acuity, ask the patient to cover one ear stand on the opposite side and whisper a few words – can the patient repeat what was said? Do the same with the second ear. A tuning fork can be used to give a very crude assessment of hearing. To test the vestibular component, observe the patient for nystagmus, disturb balance and report of dizziness vertigo, nausea.

Table 17.7   (Continued)

Number	Name	Major function	Assessment
IX	Glossopharyngeal	Sensory • Coordination of swallowing and gag reflex • Sensations to pharynx • Taste posterior third of the tongue • Regulation of blood pressure via chemoreceptors in the carotids sinus Motor • Salivation and assists in swallowing	These nerves are tested together. Using a tongue depressor, test gag reflex by touching the tip towards the posterior pharynx, ask the patient to say 'ah'. Phonation should be clear. Observe for symmetrical upwards movement of the soft palate and uvula and also for the mid-line position of the uvula.
X	Vagus	Sensory • Sensation to mucosa of pharynx, soft palate, tonsils, viscera of the thorax and abdomen Motor • Controls swallowing, phonation, and movement of the soft palate and uvula • Motility and secretion of gastrointestinal organs • Decreased heart rate	
XI	Spinal accessory	Movement of the head and neck via sternocleidomastoid muscles, upper trapezius	When assessing this nerve, ask the patient to shrug the shoulders up and try to push them down. Ask the patient to push the head forwards against your hand. Both these movements should be very difficult to resist.
XII	Hypoglossal	Movement of the tongue facilitating speech, manipulation of food and swallowing	Ask the patient to protrude the tongue note any deviation, the tongue should be midline and no tremors. Check the tongue for symmetry

Source: Adapted from Blumenfeld (2010), Braine (2018), and Rhoads and Wiggins Petersen (2018).

321

Take note

Sluggish or suddenly dilated unequal pupils are an indication that the oculomotor cranial nerve is being compressed due to raised intracranial pressure or local compression such as an expanding aneurysm. Such a discovery requires urgent medical attention.

Assessing altered states of consciousness

The exact understanding of consciousness is unknown; however, it can be seen as having two main components: arousal and awareness. Both rely upon a complex network of activating pathways. Consciousness is a state of general awareness of oneself as well as the environment. Consciousness is the most sensitive indicator of any change neurologically and although it is difficult to measure by directly observing how a patient responds to certain stimuli, there are ways which it can be appraised.

Altered states of consciousness arise as a result of damage to neural pathways and coma is caused by disordered arousal, as opposed to impairment of the content of consciousness. Braine (2018)

Table 17.8 Some common terms used to describe the assessment of level of consciousness (LOC).

Term	Characteristics
Full consciousness	Alert; oriented to time, place, and person; understands spoken and written words
Confusion	Unable to think rapidly and clearly in a logical and coherent way; easily bewildered, poor memory and short attention span; misinterprets stimuli; impaired judgement, can respond to simple orders
Disorientation	Not aware of or not oriented to time, place or person
Obtundation	Lethargic, somnolent; responsive to verbal or tactile stimuli but will quickly drift back to sleep
Stupor	Generally unresponsive; may be briefly aroused by vigorous, repeated, or painful stimuli
Semi-comatose	Does not move spontaneously; is unresponsive to stimuli, although vigorous or painful stimuli may result in stirring, moaning, or withdrawal from the stimuli but without arousal
Coma	Lack of arousal; will not stir or moan in response to any stimulus; may exhibit non-purposeful response (slight movement) of area stimulated; no eye opening and no verbal response
Deep coma	Complete lack of arousal and is unresponsive to any kind of stimulus, including pain; absence of reflexes
Vegetative state one month	Wakefulness without awareness of self or surroundings; eyes are open or closed, there is evidence of sleep–wake cycle on electroencephalogram (EEG). If the vegetative state duration is longer than one month, this is termed persistent vegetative state
Minimal consciousness state	Awareness is partial and inconsistent; there may be purposeful movements; eyes may be open or closed and there is evidence of sleep–wake cycle on EEG. May also be referred to as post-coma unresponsiveness or minimally responsive state
Locked-in syndrome	Pseudocoma is not a disorder of consciousness, as the patient is fully conscious and has preserved cognitive function, but there is impairment of voluntary motor function. In complete locked-in syndrome there are no motor movements

Source: Adapted from Braine (2018).

noted that there are some common terms used to describe the assessment of level of consciousness (LOC). See Table 17.8 for an overview of some patient characteristics and disorders of consciousness. It is important to ensure that the terms being used are defined and used in a consistent manner. Regular neurological assessments can identify trends and any changes in LOC and specific signs and neurological function are essential for early detection; even subtle changes may be clinically important.

The Glasgow Coma Scale (Teasdale and Jennett 1974) is a universal assessment instrument, developed in 1974 by neurosurgeons Dr Brian Jennett and Dr Graham Teasdale in Glasgow. It has been adopted internationally in more than 80 countries as a standardised tool for assessment of conscious level (Teasdale 2014). The Glasgow Coma Scale provides an indication of the initial severity of trauma to the brain and its subsequent changes over time. The Glasgow Coma Scale does not diagnose the cause of the altered state of consciousness, it is a scoring system to grade the best possible central (brain) response. The Glasgow Coma Scale is divided into three subscales, with each subscale given a score that is added together to give an overall score of between 3 and 15. The three key areas of the Glasgow Coma Scale are:

- Eye opening (1–4)
- Verbal response (1–5)
- Motor response (1–6)

Table 17.9 An overview of the Glasgow Coma Scale.

Feature	Response	Score
Best eye response (record C if unable to open eyes, e.g. from orbital swelling or facial fractures)	Opens spontaneous	4
	Open to verbal commands	3
	Open to pain	2
	No eye opening	1
Best verbal response (Record 'ET' if the person has an endotracheal or 'T' for a tracheostomy tube in place and record 'D' if the person is dysphasic)	Oriented to questions	5
	Disoriented/confused	4
	Inappropriate words	3
	Incomprehensible sounds	2
	No verbal response	1
Best motor response (Record best upper arm response)	To verbal commands obeys	6
	To painful stimuli localises pain	5
	Withdrawal from pain	4
	Flexion to pain	3
	Extension to pain	2
	No response to pain	1

Source: Teasdale and Jennett (1974).

Take note

The Glasgow Coma Scale provides a baseline against which changes can be evaluated and is used to score the neurological examination and to quantify the patient's neurological condition. The Glasgow Coma Scale does not diagnose the cause of the altered state of consciousness.

The Glasgow Coma Scale is the universal gold standard means of assessing consciousness (see Table 17.9). Initially developed to assess the head injury patient, it is now used to assess a range of patients with neurological problems.

Take note

The Glasgow Coma Scale score may be affected if:

- Eyes are closed due to severe swelling (oedema)
- The verbal and motor responses may be absent or reduced as a result of:
  - Intubation
  - Muscle relaxants
  - Sedation or other drugs such as alcohol and recreational drugs

Neurological assessment using the Glasgow Coma Scale

The highest possible score using the Glasgow Coma Scale is a 15, this reflects an individual who is fully alert, aware, and oriented, and the lowest possible score is a 3 and reflects an unconscious individual.

Prior to undertaking assessment, explain the procedure to the patient (and if appropriate family). Ascertain the patient's acuity of hearing and check the patient's notes for any medical condition that might impact the accuracy of the Glasgow Coma Scale, such as a previous stroke that can affect the movement of the patient's arms. Check the neurological observation chart for the previous Glasgow Coma Scale score so a comparison can be made. Wash hands, and ensure the Glasgow Coma Scale and pen torch are close to hand so as to avoid interruption of the assessment process.

Ascertain if the patient opens their eyes without the need to speak or to touch them; if the patient does, then the score for this is 4E. If the patient does not open their eyes spontaneously, speak to them. Start off with a normal volume and if needed increase volume if necessary. If they now open their eyes, then the score will be 3E.

If the patient does not open their eyes to speech, adhering to local policy and procedure, you may be required to administer a painful stimulus, such as a trapezius squeeze (using the thumb and two fingers grasp the trapezius muscle where the neck meets the shoulder and twist). Or apply supra-orbital pressure (in order to do this, locate the notch on the supra-orbital margin and apply pressure to it). If there is any doubt in distinguishing between flexion to a painful stimulus and localisation to pain, supra-orbital notch pressure should be used. If supra-orbital notch pressure is contraindicated, for example as a result of bruising or swelling in this region, then fingernail pressure could be used (Scottish Intercollegiate Guidelines Network n.d.). If the patient opens their eyes to a painful stimulus then record the score as 2E. If the patient does not respond, the score is recorded 1E.

Assessing the motor function of the patient during a neurological assessment needs to be individualised, as the techniques employed are dependent on the patient's condition. If, for example, the patient is conscious, then the nurse makes the assessment by observing the patient's motor response to commands such as squeeze my hands. If the patient is unconscious or unable to provide accurate responses, motor function may only be able to be assessed by observation. There are two types of limb movement: flexion (bending or flexing) and extension (straightening or extension).

The nurse also takes note of the strength and tone of the patient's limbs, whether they are experiencing any weakness, and whether these effects are unilateral or bilateral. Limb strength can be described as either being of normal power, mild weakness, severe weakness, extension, or no response, and a score is given to each. This assessment focuses on the arms and legs and will determine if there is any improvement or deterioration in function. However, it must be noted that lower limb function can impact on spinal function. In some patients this can then impact on assessment findings (Koutoukidis et al. 2017).

It is essential to consider the patient's temperature and other vital signs as part of the neurological assessment. Temperature, for example, can be raised as a result of infection; however, a patient who has sustained a severe head injury may have localised damage impacting on the temperature-regulating centre in the hypothalamus.

Cushing's triad or reflex is described by Waterhouse (2004) as a classic set of clinical and physiological signs and symptoms which indicate that intracranial pressure is dangerously high and the patient is in danger of cerebral herniation that will rapidly lead to the death. The reflex is a very late sign and is characterised by hypertension, bradycardia, and respiratory irregularity.

During assessment abnormalities may have been detected. Common abnormalities include loss of consciousness, cranial nerve defect, abnormal muscle movements, and gait abnormality. When the assessment is complete the nurse should ensure that the patient is comfortable. Wash hands. The findings must be recorded and reported using local policy and procedure.

So far

A neurological assessment is undertaken to assess the function and integrity of the nervous system and should be conducted in a systematic way. An initial assessment will provide a baseline against which subsequent assessments can be compared.

Early diagnosis, based on clinical history, the examination, laboratory findings, and imaging, is important in facilitating the exclusion of alternative diagnoses and early implementation of treatment.

The physical examination must be structured around the patient's needs and their condition. It is informed by the subjective data (the patient history or the findings from a collateral history). The nurse undertakes a number of non-invasive assessment processes such as assessment of LOC using the Glasgow Coma Scale to gather objective data.

Judith Higgins (Aunt)

Judith came to the GP surgery with her sister Shahine. The GP observed Mrs Higgins as she entered the surgery and took note of her demeanour, gait, posture and manner, she shook hands with Mrs Higgins and noted a slight tremor. The GP asked Mrs Higgins what it was that brought her to the surgery and she replied, 'her sister was in charge'. The GP asked Mrs Higgins if it was OK for Shahine to stay during the consultation and Mrs Higgins replied she had no idea and would have preferred to have stayed on holiday. Mrs Higgins was agitated and seemed to be argumentative. The GP was aware of potential difficulties and considered the 7 Ds associated with communication difficulties:

Problem	Discussion
Deafness	Nerve or conductive deafness
Dysphasia	Usually due to a cerebrovascular accident, sometimes may be feature of dementia
Dysarthria	Cerebrovascular accident, motor neurone disease, Parkinson's
Dysphonia	Parkinson's
Dementia	Global impairment of cognitive function
Delirium	Impaired attention, disturbance of arousal and perceptual disturbances
Depression	Can mimic dementia or delirium

(Source: Elder and MacDonald 2018).

The GP checked that Mrs Higgins could hear clearly and engaged with Mrs Higgins a little more and her responses were hesitant and inconsistent. The GP had to rely on a collateral history from Shahine (never ignoring what Mrs Higgins was telling her). The GP determined:

- Mrs Higgin's normal cognitive state and whether the change was abrupt or gradual in onset
- If there were any symptoms of common infections such as urinary tract infection, chest infection, or if Mrs Higgins had a pyrexia
- What Mrs Higgin's current drug regimen was, if Mrs Higgins was concordant, and if there had been any recent changes in medication (including complementary and over-the-counter medicines)

The GP took a history from Mrs Higgins and Shahine, asking about any concerns and the impact Mrs Higgins' condition was having on her activities of living, the timescale of onset, and deterioration, so as to differentiate dementia from other conditions with similar features.

The GP undertook an assessment of cognition using the GPCOG. Familiarise yourself with this tool or another, for example:

- Mini Mental State Examination
- The 6-item Cognitive Impairment Test (6-CIT)
- The 7-Minute Screen

Make notes about the pros and cons of using a standardised cognitive assessment tool.

What might be a differential diagnoses for Mrs Higgins?

With an assessment of cognition undertaken and a diagnosis being made, health, and social care practitioners can now, with Mrs Higgins and her family, work to ensure that her care plan is patient-centred and that it clearly identifies the aims/goals of care as well as describing strategies that will be needed to make an evaluation of interventions.

Are there any safeguarding issues in this scenario (actual or potential)? If there are any issues, who might the nurse liaise with? What is your local policy and procedure for raising concerns?

Conclusion

This chapter has provided an overview of the organisation, structure, and functions of the neurological system. Those patients with neurological conditions have complex needs and detailed and accurate assessment of consciousness, neurological function and other body systems the principles of which have been outlined including clinical, non-invasive, and invasive assessment techniques and tools, such as the Glasgow Coma Scale. Nurses play a key role at the heart of a multidisciplinary team in helping patients maintain function and independence as far as possible and also offering support to families. In order to care for people with a neurological condition it is paramount that the nurse has insight and understanding as well as having excellent, effective communication skills as they offer physical, psychological, and emotional support to patients and their families. Care is not only complex but it is also challenging and requires the acquisition and development of a wide range of skills and experience.

References

Blumenfeld, H. (2010). *Neuroanatomy Through Clinical Cases*, 2e. Oxford: Oxford University Press.

de Boer, C., Mattace-Raso, F., van der Steen, J., and Pel, J.J. (2014). Mini-mental state examination subscores indicate Visuomotor deficits in Alzheimer's disease patients: a cross-sectional study in a Dutch population. *Geriatrics and Gerontology International* 14 (4): 880–885. https://doi.org/10.1111/ggi.12183.

Braine, M. (2018). The person with a neurological disorder. In: *Nursing Practice, Knowledge and Care*, 2e (ed. I. Peate and K. Wild), 797–849. Oxford: Wiley.

British Association for the Study of Headache (2010). *Guidelines for all Healthcare Professionals in the Diagnosis and Management of Migraine, Tension-Type Headache, Cluster Headache, Medication-Overuse Headache*, 3e. BASH.

Brodaty, H., Pond, D., Kemp, N.M. et al. (2002). The GPCOG: a new screening test for dementia designed for general practice. *Journal of American Geriatrics Society* 50 (3): 530–534.

Davenport, R. and Manji, H. (2018). The nervous system. In: *Macleod's Clinical Examination*, 14e (ed. J.A. Innes, A.R. Dover and K. Fairhurst), 119–150. Edinburgh: Elsevier.

Elder, A. and MacDonald, E. (2018). The frail elderly patient. In: *Macleod's Clinical Examination*, 14e (ed. J.A. Innes, A.R. Dover and K. Fairhurst), 329–338. Edinburgh: Elsevier.

International Headache Society (2018). The international classification of headache disorders, 3rd edition. *Cephalalgia* 38 (1): 1–211. https://doi.org/10.1177/0333102417738202.

Koutoukidis, G., Stainton, K., and Hughson, J. (2017). *Tabbner's Nursing Care: Theory and Practice*, 7e. Sydney: Elsevier.

Nursing and Midwifery Council (2018). The Code. Professional Standards of Practice and Behaviour for Nurses, Midwives and Nursing Associates. https://www.nmc.org.uk/globalassets/sitedocuments/nmc-publications/nmc-code.pdf last accessed 8 May 2019.

Rhoads, J. and Wiggins Petersen, S. (2018). *Advanced Health Assessment and Diagnostic Reasoning*, 3e. Burlington: Jones and Bartlett.

Sallam, K. and Amr, M. (2013). The use of the mini-mental state examination and the clock-drawing test for dementia in a tertiary hospital. *Journal of Clinical Diagnosis Res* 7 (3): 484–488. https://doi.org/10.7860/JCDR/2013/4203.2803.

Scottish Intercollegiate Guideline Network (2008). *Diagnosis and Management of Headache in Adults: A National Clinical Guideline 107*. Edinburgh: Scottish Intercollegiate Guidelines Network.

Scottish Intercollegiate Guideline Network (n.d.) Annexe 3. Neurological assessment using the Glasgow Coma Scale. www.sign.ac.uk/assets/sign110_annex3.pdf (accessed October 2018).

Spering, C.C., Hobson, V., Lucas, J.A. et al. (2012). Diagnostic accuracy of the MMSE in detecting probable and possible Alzheimer's disease in ethnically diverse highly educated individuals: an analysis of the NACC database. *Journal of Gerontolology Series A Biological Sciences and Medical Sciences* 67 (8): 890–896. https://doi.org/10.1093/gerona/gls006.

Teasdale, G. (2014). Forty years on – updating the Glasgow Coma Scale. *Nursing Times* 110 (42): 12–16.

Teasdale, G. and Jennett, B. (1974). Assessment of coma and impaired consciousness. A practical scale. *Lancet* 110 (42): 12–16.

Waterhouse, C. (2004). The Glasgow Coma Scale and other neurological observations. *Nursing Standard* 19 (33): 56–64.

Chapter 18

Assessing the endocrine system

Aim

This chapter introduces the reader to the assessment of the endocrine system and the care required for those who experience problems related to this system.

Learning outcomes

By the end of the chapter the reader will be able to:

1. Provide a brief overview of the endocrine system and its functions
2. Discuss a number of conditions that might affect the endocrine system
3. Outline the various ways in which the nurse may undertake an assessment of the endocrine system
4. Describe care planning related to the endocrine system

Introduction

Every cell in the body is influenced by the endocrine system. The endocrine system acts in order to maintain equilibrium at the cellular level and is a key system in supporting homeostasis. When abnormalities associated with endocrine occur, this can result in illness or death. Effective treatment is often associated with the manipulation of a hormone(s), either by reducing or increasing production or by secretion from the associated endocrine gland(s). A prerequisite in order to accurately assess and treat endocrine disorders demands a thorough understanding of the endocrine system and how it functions. The endocrine system is made up of endocrine glands. Endocrine glands produce hormones, and these chemicals control a number of body functions.

This chapter provides an overview of the anatomy and physiology of the endocrine system. Discussion is made concerning history taking and the physical examination required to undertake a full assessment of patient needs in order to make a diagnosis, plan care, provide care, and evaluate interventions.

The endocrine system

The endocrine system is made up of glands that produce and secrete hormones, regulating the activity of cells or organs. These hormones regulate metabolism and sexual development and function. The hormones are released into the bloodstream and can affect one or several organs throughout the body.

Endocrine glands are groups of secretory cells scattered throughout the body surrounded by a large network of capillaries; this rich blood supply facilitates diffusion of hormones. This arrangement of blood vessels and hormone-producing cells ensures that the hormones enter the blood rapidly

Table 18.1   Nervous system versus endocrine system.

	Nervous system	Neurological system
Speed of action	Seconds	Minutes to hours even days
Duration of action	Seconds to minutes	Minutes to days
Methods of transmitting messages	Electrical	Chemical
Transportation methods	Neurones	Hormones

Source: Clare (2017).

and are then transported throughout the body (Marieb and Hoehn 2016). In general, endocrine glands are ductless, vascular, and most of them usually contain intracellular vacuoles or granules that store hormones. Exocrine glands, however, for example the salivary glands, the mammary glands, sweat glands, and those glands located within the gastrointestinal tract (such as mucus glands), are typically much less vascular, with a duct or lumen to a membrane surface.

There are two main body systems responsible for maintaining homeostasis the nervous system and the endocrine system, in Table 18.1 the differences between these two systems are depicted. The purpose of each hormone varies but their common primary role is to maintain homeostasis (that is, keeping a normal physiological balance in the body).

Endocrine-releasing organs can be divided into three main categories:

1. Endocrine glands – the sole function of these organs is the production and release of hormones. The pituitary, thyroid, parathyroid and adrenal glands are examples.
2. Organs that are not pure glands but contain relatively large areas of hormone-producing tissue, include the pancreas, the hypothalamus and the gonads.
3. Other tissues and organs also produce hormones – areas of hormone-producing cells are found in the wall of the small intestine, the stomach, the kidneys and the heart.

Figure 18.1 provides details of the location of the endocrine glands. Each of these organs will typically have a rich vascular (blood vessel) network and the hormone-producing cells within them are arranged into cords and branching networks around this supply (Marieb and Hoehn 2016).

The pituitary gland and the hypothalamus

The hypothalamus is an aspect of the brain that has a number of functions, it is one of the most important components of the nervous system. The pituitary gland is approximately 1 cm in diameter (the size of a pea) and is cone-shaped (Waugh and Grant 2018). It rests in the hypophyseal fossa, a depression in the sphenoid bone under the hypothalamus. The gland is connected to the hypothalamus by a slender stalk known as the infundibulum (see Figure 18.2).

The pituitary gland and the hypothalamus work as a unit, controlling most of the other endocrine glands. Within the gland there are two distinct areas:

1. The anterior lobe (adenohypophysis), composed of glandular epithelium arising for the pharynx
2. The posterior lobe (neurohypophysis), made of a down growth of nervous tissue from the brain

Arterial blood supply is from the internal carotid artery, with venous drainage (containing hormones) leaving the gland via short veins that enter the venous sinuses between the layers in the dura mater. The activity of the adenohypophysis is controlled by the release of hormones from the hypothalamus. The neurohypophysis is controlled by nerve stimulation.

The pineal gland

The pineal gland secretes the hormone melatonin when sleeping. This influences circadian rhythm (this is roughly a 24-hour cycle in the physiological processes). The pinealocytes synthesise melatonin directly into the cerebrospinal fluid, which then takes it into the blood. Secretion of the hormone is controlled by daylight, with levels fluctuating throughout the day and the seasons.

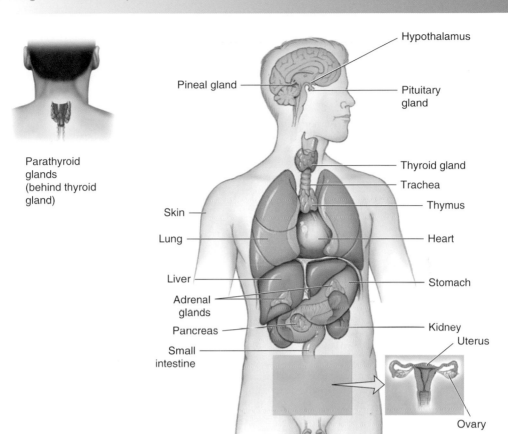

Figure 18.1 Location of the endocrine organs.

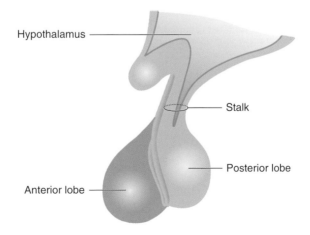

Figure 18.2 The hypothalamus and pituitary gland.

The anterior pituitary lobe

Anterior pituitary lobe (influenced by the hypothalamus) is supplied by arterial blood that has passed through the hypothalamus; blood is transported away from the gland via pituitary portal system. The anterior pituitary lobe secretes various hormones (see Table 18.2). The anterior pituitary lobe is larger

Table 18.2   Hormones released by the hypothalamus and anterior pituitary gland (Clare 2017).

Hypothalamus	Anterior pituitary gland	Target organ or tissues	Action
Growth hormone releasing factor (GHRF)	Growth hormone (GH)	Various (particularly bone)	Stimulates the growth of body cells
Growth hormone release inhibiting factor (GHRIF)	Growth hormone (inhibits release)	Various	
Thyroid-releasing hormone (TRH)	Thyroid-stimulating hormone (TSH)	Thyroid gland	Stimulates thyroid hormone release
Corticotrophin-releasing hormones (CRH)	Adrenocorticotropic hormone (ACTH)	Adrenal cortex	Stimulates the release of corticosteroid
Prolactin-releasing hormone (PRH)	Prolactin	Breasts	Stimulates the production of milk
Prolactin-inhibiting hormone	Prolactin (inhibits release)	Breasts	
Gonadotropin-releasing hormone (GRH)	Follicle-stimulating hormone Luteinising hormone	Gonads	Numerous reproductive functions

than the posterior lobe, made up of three parts; this partially surrounds the posterior lobe and infundibulum. This lobe is made up of glandular tissue producing and releasing hormones. There are no direct nerve connections with the anterior pituitary and the hypothalamus. Control of the anterior pituitary occurs when releasing and inhibiting factors in the form of hormones are released by the hypothalamus. Hormones usually produce one of the flowing changes:

- Modifications in cell membrane permeability and/or the cells electrical state by causing the ion channels in the cell membrane to open or close
- Synthesis of proteins or regulatory molecules, for example enzymes within the cell
- Activation or deactivation of enzymes
- Producing secretory activity
- Stimulation of mitosis

Growth hormone (GH) stimulates the growth of bones, muscles, and other organs by promoting protein synthesis. This hormone significantly affects the appearance of an individual as GH influences height.

Thyroid-stimulating hormone (TSH) causes the glandular cells of the thyroid to secrete thyroid hormone. If there is a hypersecretion of TSH, the thyroid gland enlarges, secreting excessive amounts of thyroid hormone.

Adrenocorticotropic hormone (ACTH) reacts with receptor sites located in the cortex of the adrenal gland, stimulating the secretion of cortical hormones.

Gonadotropic hormones react with receptor sites in the gonads, regulating the development, growth, and function of the testes or ovaries.

Prolactin is a hormone that encourages the development of glandular tissue in the female breast during pregnancy and stimulates the production of milk after the child is born.

The posterior pituitary lobe

The posterior pituitary is mainly composed of nerve fibres (nerve bundle) originating in hypothalamus; the supporting nerve cells are called pituicytes. The hypothalamic-hypophyseal tract links the posterior pituitary and the hypothalamus (this is the nerve bundle). The posterior pituitary releases two hormones, they arrive directly from the hypothalamus:

1. Oxytocin
2. Antidiuretic hormone (ADH)

Oxytocin is responsible for the contraction of the smooth muscle in the wall of the uterus. It also stimulates the discharge of milk from the lactating breast; this is called the 'let down' response and occurs in response to suckling when milk is released. The role of this hormone in males and non-lactating females is unclear; oxytocin in men and women is believed to play a role in sexual arousal and orgasm.

The key role of ADH (vasopressin) is to reduce urinary output. ADH promotes the reabsorption of water by acting on the distal convoluted tubules and collecting ducts of the nephrons of the kidneys that result in an increased permeability to water. The result is that less water is lost as urine as reabsorption of water from the glomerular filtrate is increased. The amount of ADH secreted is controlled by the osmotic pressure of circulating blood to the osmoreceptors located in the hypothalamus. This mechanism conserves water for the body. Insufficient amounts of ADH cause excessive water loss in the urine.

When there is a high concentration of ADH, for example after excessive blood loss or severe dehydration, smooth muscle contracts and vasoconstriction in small arteries occurs. This results in the pressor effect, where systemic blood pressure is elevated.

The thyroid gland

The thyroid gland is located in the neck, anterior to the larynx and the trachea situated at the level of the 5th, 6th, and 7th cervical vertebrae and the 1st thoracic vertebra. This is a butterfly-shaped gland (see Figure 18.3), with two lobes on either side of the thyroid cartilage and the upper incomplete cartilaginous rings of the trachea of a fibrous capsule, weighing around 25 g.

The gland is brownish red in colour. Situated in front of the trachea is the narrow isthmus joining the left and right lobes. Each lobe is cone-shaped, measuring approximately 5 cm long and 3 cm wide. The upper aspects of the lobe are known as the upper poles and the lower ends are the lower poles. The lobes are composed of hollow, spherical-shaped follicles surrounded by capillaries.

The blood supply to this gland is extensive (it is said to be a highly vascular gland). The arterial blood supply comes from the superior and inferior thyroid arteries. Venous return is by the thyroid veins draining into the internal jugular vein.

Principal innervation originates from the autonomic nervous system. Parasympathetic fibres come from the vagus nerves; sympathetic fibres are distributed from the superior, middle, and inferior ganglia of the sympathetic trunk. These small nerves enter the gland accompanied by the blood vessels. Autonomic nervous regulation of the glandular secretion is not fully understood.

331

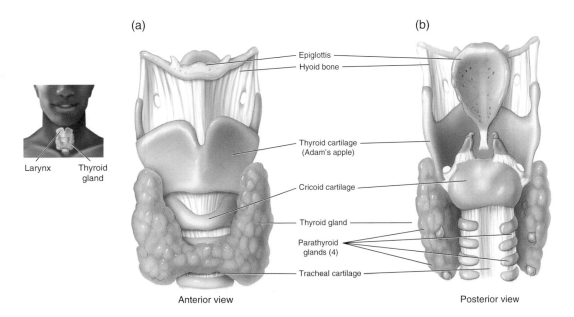

(a)   (b)

Epiglottis
Hyoid bone

Larynx   Thyroid
           gland

Thyroid cartilage
(Adam's apple)

Cricoid cartilage

Thyroid gland

Parathyroid
glands (4)

Tracheal cartilage

Anterior view   Posterior view

Figure 18.3   The location of the thyroid and para thyroid gland.

Table 18.3 Some effects associated with an abnormal secretion of thyroid hormones (Clare 2017).

Increased secretion of T_3 and T_4 (hyperthyroidism)	Decreased secretion of T_3 and T_4 (hypothyroidism)
Increased basal metabolic rate	Decreased basal metabolic rate
Weight loss (despite good/increased appetite)	Weight gain (despite anorexia)
Tachycardia, palpitations, arrhythmia	Bradycardia
Excitability, nervousness, irritability	Tiredness, depression
Tremor	Numbness in the hands
Hair loss	Lifeless hair
Changes in menstruation patterns	Irregular menstrual periods
Goitre	Deep voice
Diarrhoea	Constipation
Exophthalmos	Feeling cold

Lying against the posterior surfaces of each lobe are the parathyroid glands embedded in the thyroid tissues. The recurrent laryngeal nerve passes upwards and close to the lobes of the gland.

A single layer of epithelial cells comprises the follicles, and these form a cavity containing thyroglobulin molecules that are attached to iodine molecules. The thyroid hormones are formed by these molecules. This gland releases two types of thyroid hormone, thyroxine (T_4) and triiodothyronine (T_3).

Iodine is essential for the synthesis of these hormones. Dietary iodine is concentrated by the thyroid gland, in the follicle cells, changing it into iodine. TSH simulates thyroid hormone production. The primary hormone released by the thyroid gland is T_4 converted into T_3 by the target cells. Thyroid hormones are required for normal growth and development. When there is deficiency of iodine, TSH is secreted in excess, causing proliferation of thyroid gland cells accompanied by an enlargement of the gland. Table 18.3 outlines common effects associated with abnormal thyroid hormone secretion. Most of the cells in the body are affected by thyroid hormone, there is an increase in basal metabolic rate and production of heat.

The regulation of thyroid hormone secretion is via a negative-feedback mechanism involving the amount of circulating hormone, hypothalamus, and adenohypophysis (see Figure 18.4).

The parafollicular cells of the thyroid gland secrete calcitonin. Calcitonin combats the action of the parathyroid glands by reducing the levels of calcium in the blood. If blood calcium becomes too high, calcitonin is secreted until calcium ion levels decrease to normal.

Parathyroid glands

Four small masses of epithelial tissue embedded in the connective tissue capsule on the posterior surface of the thyroid glands are the parathyroid glands which secrete parathyroid hormone (Figure 18.3). They are responsible for the creation and secretion of parathyroid hormone. Parathyroid hormone is the most important regulator of blood calcium level. The key target cells are those in the bones and the kidneys. The hormone increases intestinal calcium absorption, stimulation of renal calcium absorption, and the stimulation of osteoclast activity and thus the reabsorption of calcium from the bones. The hormone is secreted in response to low blood calcium levels and its effect is to increase those levels.

Hypoparathyroidism leads to increased nerve excitability. The low blood calcium levels trigger spontaneous and continuous nerve impulses, which then stimulate muscle contraction. Calcium is also needed for the formation of clotting factors in the blood, which is monitored by cells in the gland. When there is a reduction in blood calcium levels, this leads to an increase in the formation and secretion of parathyroid hormone.

The adrenal glands

The adrenal glands are located one each near the upper portion of each kidney (see Figure 18.5). Each gland has an outer cortex and an inner medulla. The cortex and medulla, like the anterior and posterior lobes of the pituitary gland, secrete different hormones (see Figure 18.6). The adrenal cortex is essential to life; the medulla may be removed with no life-threatening effects.

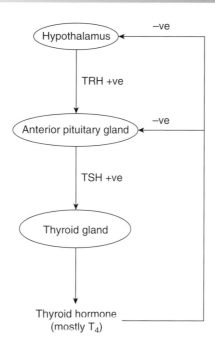

Figure 18.4 Negative feedback control of thyroid hormone production.

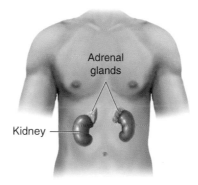

Figure 18.5 The position of the adrenal glands.

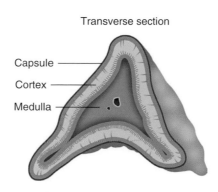

Figure 18.6 Cross-section of an adrenal gland.

The hypothalamus influences both aspects of the adrenal gland but uses different mechanisms. The adrenal cortex is regulated by negative feedback involving the hypothalamus and ACTH; the medulla is regulated by nerve impulses from the hypothalamus.

Hormones of the adrenal cortex

The adrenal cortex consists of three different regions. Each region produces a different group or type of hormone. All cortical hormones are steroid.

The outermost region secretes mineralocorticoids. Aldosterone is the chief mineralocorticoid, conserving sodium ions and water in the body. The middle region of the adrenal cortex secretes glucocorticoids. The key glucocorticoid is cortisol, increasing levels of blood glucose.

The third group of steroids is the gonadocorticoids (sex hormones), secreted by the innermost region. Male hormones (androgens) and female hormones (oestrogens) are secreted in minimal amounts in both sexes by the adrenal cortex, and their effect is often masked by hormones from the testes and ovaries.

Review

Write notes on:

Mineralocorticoids	
Glucocorticoids	
Gonadocorticoids	

Hormones of the adrenal medulla

The adrenal medulla secretes two hormones, epinephrine and norepinephrine, secreted in response to stimulation by sympathetic nerves, predominantly during stressful situations. A lack of hormones from the adrenal medulla will have no significant effects. Hypersecretion causes prolonged or continual sympathetic responses.

The pancreas

The pancreas is located in the epigastric and left hypochondriac regions of the abdomen. The head of the pancreas lies close to the first part of the small intestine – the duodenum and the body behind the stomach – anf the tail extends out towards the spleen. It is about 12 to 15 cm in length and weighs approximately 60 g. The pancreas is a pale grey, elongated gland (Figure 18.7).

Blood supply comes from the splenic and mesenteric arteries, these arteries drain the pancreas where this drainage joins and forms the portal vein. The pancreas is innervated by the parasympathetic and sympathetic nervous systems. The secretion of insulin and glucagon is stimulated by the nervous system.

This gland has endocrine and exocrine functions. Most of the tissue within the pancreas is made up of exocrine tissue and the associated ducts.

The exocrine pancreas

The exocrine pancreas is made up of a number of lobules composed of acini secreting digestive enzymes, carried through a duct to the duodenum. The function of the exocrine pancreas is to produce pancreatic juice that is rich in enzymes whose responsibility is to digest carbohydrates, protein, and fats.

The endocrine pancreas

The endocrine portion scattered throughout the exocrine tissue consists of the pancreatic islets (the islets of Langerhans). The islets are the endocrine cells of the pancreas, secreting insulin and

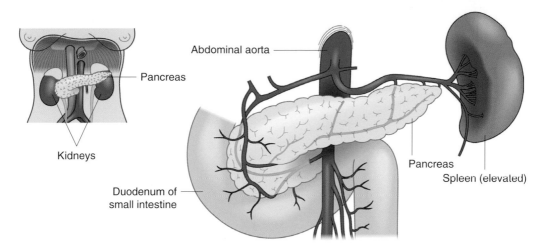

Figure 18.7   The pancreas.

glucagon. The islets, have no ducts; hormones are diffused directly into the blood. There are three key cell types in the islets, each producing a different hormone:

1. Alpha cells secreting glucagon
2. Beta cells secreting insulin – these are the most abundant of the three cell types
3. Delta cells secrete somatostatin

335

All three cell types are specifically placed within the islets' beta cells, located in the central aspect of the islet, surrounded by the alpha and delta cells. As the islets are highly vascularised, they enable the transportation of the hormones into the blood to occur at speed.

Insulin

This hormone is responsible for a number of things (including its effect on protein and mineral and lipid metabolism); one of the most well-known responsibilities is its ability to reduce blood glucose levels. Insulin facilitates the movement of glucose into muscle, adipose, and other tissues (the brain and the liver do not require insulin for the uptake of glucose). Insulin stimulates the liver to store glucose as glycogen.

Insulin synthesis is in response (principally) to a rise in blood glucose levels and an increase in blood amino acids and fatty acids also have a stimulating effect. When blood glucose levels fall, there is a matching drop in insulin production and secretion, glycogen synthesis in the liver is reduced and enzymes responsible for the breakdown of glycogen are activated.

Glucagon

This hormone is also responsible for the maintenance of normal blood glucose. Glucagon has the opposite effects on blood glucose to insulin (see Figure 18.8). Glucagon increases blood glucose levels by simulating the conversion of glycogen to glucose in the liver and skeletal muscles. Low blood sugar levels, exercise, and decreased somatostatin and insulin stimulate the secretion of glucagon.

Somatostatin

Inhibits the release of insulin and glycogen. When released it has effects locally. The exact way this hormone functions is unknown.

The gonads

The gonads are the primary reproductive organs; the testes in the male and the ovaries in the female. These organs are responsible for producing the sperm and ova and also secrete hormones, and as such are considered endocrine glands.

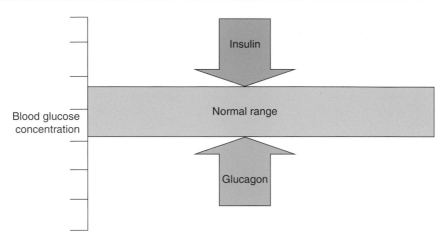

Figure 18.8   The effects of insulin and glucagon on blood glucose concentrations.

The ovaries

Chapter 16 discusses the functions of the female reproductive system. The ovaries produce two groups of female sex hormones – the oestrogens and progesterone. These are steroid hormones contributing to the development and function of the female reproductive organs and sex characteristics. At the onset of puberty oestrogens promote breast development, fat distribution, and maturation of reproductive organs such as the uterus and vagina.

Progesterone causes the uterine lining to thicken in preparation for pregnancy. Progesterone and oestrogens are responsible for the changes occurring in the uterus during the female menstrual cycle.

The testes

Chapter 15 discusses the functions of the male reproductive system. Male sex hormones are called androgens. The main androgen is testosterone, secreted by the testes; the adrenal cortex also produces a small amount. Testosterone production starts during foetal development, continuing for a short time after birth, almost ceases during childhood and then at puberty resumes. It is responsible for the growth and development of the male reproductive structures, increased skeletal and muscular growth, enlargement of the larynx accompanied by voice changes, growth and distribution of body hair, and increased male sexual drive.

The secretion of testosterone is regulated by a negative-feedback system involving the release of hormones from the hypothalamus and gonadotropins from the anterior pituitary.

Other endocrine glands

In addition to the major endocrine glands discussed in this chapter, other organs have some hormonal activity as part of their function. These include the thymus, stomach, small intestines, heart, and placenta (see Table 18.4).

The patient history

Dover and Zammitt (2018) and Bevan (2013) note that as hormones circulate throughout the body signs and symptoms are often non-specific and can affect a number of body systems. When undertaking a focused endocrine assessment, the nurse should begin with a thorough history of the patient's chief complaints. It is important to obtain information about any experienced signs or symptoms of endocrine disease or disorders. Jarvis (2015) notes that endocrine disorders and diseases manifest according to which endocrine hormone is being overproduced and secreted, or underproduced. In order to ascertain the nature of symptoms the nurse must have an understanding of the functions of the endocrine hormones. In addition, the nurse needs to listen carefully to what the patient is saying. See Table 18.5, outlining common clinical features seen in endocrine disease.

Table 18.4 Other endocrine glands.

Organ	Description
Thymus gland	Thymosin, a hormone produced by the thymus gland, has an important role in the development of the immune system.
Stomach	The lining of the stomach, the gastric mucosa, produces gastrin when food is present in the stomach. This stimulates the production of hydrochloric acid and the enzyme pepsin, used in the digestion of food.
Small intestine	The mucosa of the small intestine secretes secretin and cholecystokinin. Secretin promotes the pancreas to produce a fluid that neutralises stomach acid. Cholecystokinin stimulates contraction of the gallbladder, releasing bile, and stimulates the pancreas to secrete digestive enzymes.
Heart	The heart also acts as an endocrine organ as well as pumping blood. Special cells in the wall of the atria produce atrial natriuretic hormone or atriopeptin.
Placenta	The placenta develops as a source of nourishment and gas exchange for the developing foetus. It also serves as a temporary endocrine gland. One hormone it secretes is human chorionic gonadotropin, which signals the woman's ovaries to secrete hormones to maintain the uterine lining so that it does not degenerate and slough off in menstruation.

Review

Define the following terms:

Hypogonadism

Hyperthyroidism

Cushing's syndrome

Graves' disease

Hyperparathyroidism

Hypothyroidism

Goitre

Hashimoto's

Thyroiditis

Phaeochromocytoma

Acromegaly

Diabetes mellitus

Diabetes insipidus

Polycystic ovary syndrome

Resistant hypertension

337

When collecting secondary data through the health history the nurse must focus on the chief complaint. Determine onset, location, quality and severity, signs and symptoms, and the history of the present illness. As abnormalities associated with the endocrine system may impact on metabolic function, the patient may be restless and agitated. They may also have a short attention span. See Table 18.6 for assessment activity that is related to the patient's chief complaint of fatigue.

Take note

Make sure that you get properly informed consent and document it before carrying out any action.

Source: NMC (2018).

Table 18.5   Some common clinical features in endocrine disease.

Sign, symptom, or problem	Differential diagnoses
Tiredness	Hypothyroidism, hyperthyroidism, diabetes mellitus, hypopituitarism
Weight gain	Hypothyroidism, polycystic ovary syndrome (PCOS), Cushing's syndrome
Weight loss	Hyperthyroidism, diabetes mellitus, adrenal insufficiency
Diarrhoea	Hyperthyroidism, gastrin-producing tumour, carcinoid
Diffuse neck swelling	Simple goitre, Graves' disease, Hashimoto's thyroiditis
Polyuria (excessive thirst)	Diabetes mellitus, diabetes insipidus, hyperparathyroidism, Conn's syndrome
Hirsutism	Idiopathic, PCOS, congenital adrenal hyperplasia
Funny turns or spells	Hypoglycaemia, phaeochromocytoma, neuroendocrine tumour
Sweating (diaphoresis)	Hyperthyroidism, hypogonadism, acromegaly, phaeochromocytoma
Flushing	Hypogonadism, carcinoid syndrome
Resistant hypertension	Conn's syndrome, Cushing's syndrome, phaeochromocytoma, acromegaly
Amenorrhoea/oligomenorrhoea	PCOS, hyperprolactinaemia, thyroid dysfunction
Erective dysfunction	Primary or secondary hypogonadism, diabetes mellitus, medication-induced (such as beta-blockers)
Muscle weakness (myalgia)	Cushing's syndrome, hyperthyroidism, hyperparathyroidism, osteomalacia
Bone fragility and fractures	Hypogonadism, hyperthyroidism, Cushing's syndrome, primary hyperparathyroidism

Source: Adapted Bevan (2013), Dover and Zammitt (2018), Rhoads and Wiggins Petersen (2018).

Table 18.6   Assessment activity with regard to fatigue.

Determine	Ask about	Considerations
Onset	Was onset sudden or gradual?	Sudden onset may be related to hypoglycaemia. More gradual onset hyperthyroidism, hypothyroidism, hypoparathyroidism, hypopituitarism. Addison's disease and Cushing's syndrome
Duration	How long has the patient been experiencing fatigue? Does the fatigue occur daily or does it fluctuate? Ask the patient if the fatigue is associated with any specific activity. Is there any insomnia? Does the patient have sleep apnoea?	In thyrotoxicosis and Graves' disease, constant fatigue may be a key feature. When the body is unable to utilise glucose as in diabetes mellitus, fatigue can be experienced
Quality and severity	Does the fatigue interfere with the patient's ability to perform the activities of living? Are there any personality changes, anger outbursts, irritability?	Those with hyperthyroidism will often report that the fatigue prevents them from carrying out their activities of living
Signs and symptoms	Is there any weight gain or loss, excessive diaphoresis, palpitations, anorexia, nausea or vomiting, depression, irritability heat or cold intolerance?	These associated signs and symptoms could point to an endocrine disorder
Activities/ factors that alleviate	Does the patient take any prescribed, over-the-counter herbal remedies? Does the patient engage in any self-help treatments such as yoga in order to address the fatigue?	Understanding alleviating factors can help the nurse help the patient. Are the alleviating factors effective?

Source: Adapted de Wit et al. (2017), Rhoads and Wiggins Petersen (2018), Waugh and Grant (2018).

Ask the patient about the past medical history; the past medical history is a key feature of the history-taking process. Ascertain if the patent has had any surgery, when, and what for. Also ask about the outcome of the surgery. Has the patient been hospitalised, and if so what for? As a dysfunction of the endocrine system can impact on any of the body systems, comprehensive details about the past medical history have to be gathered.

When asking about family history the nurse is seeking information about the medical status of family members; parents, siblings and children. Establish if there have been any deaths in the family, and gather information about the relation of the deceased to the patient, age, and cause of death. There are a number of diseases that are genetic/familial. Patients often have a family history of endocrine disorders, so ask the patient about a history of congenital birth defects in the family.

Take note

For some people accessing health care can be difficult. They may be afraid as a result of their past experiences or the past experience of their family or friends, or due to the condition they are presenting with. Fear and anxiety can impact on obtaining a comprehensive health history and the nurse needs to develop their skills in order to offer care that acknowledges any fear or apprehensions.

Obtaining information about the patient's social history is important, as endocrine disorders can impact negatively on a patient's social health and wellbeing. What is the patient's occupation (past or present)? Ask if the patient is or has been exposed to toxic substances or radiation. Where does the patient live? Living in an iodine-deficient area can impact on a person's health and wellbeing. Is the patient allergic to anything in the environment?

Cultural considerations

Not all groups adapt or integrate into the mainstream culture. These groups may instead wish to retain the unique features associated with their culture. This has led to an increase in visibility and a greater respect of different groups.

The nurse must strive to work with people in a sensitive and appropriate manner to ensure that any response is culturally sensitive. In doing this the nurse, with the patient at the centre of all that is done, can work together to devise a culturally responsive plan of care. A skilled nurse can conduct a culturally competent assessment that will enable care delivery to incorporate and respect the patient's values, beliefs, and practices, aligning care delivery to the principles enshrined in The Code (NMC 2018).

When the data is gathered, the nurse must ask if the patient has any questions. The nurse should thank the patient and explain the need for a physical examination. The data is documented and reported according to local policy.

So far

When assessing the endocrine system, it is usual to perform a problem-focused assessment in order to identify any potential endocrine abnormalities, noting that a dysfunction with the endocrine system can impact negatively on other body systems. As with any physical assessment, a systematic and structured approach is advocated.

At all times when obtaining a patient history, the nurse must be respectful and undertake the assessment in a culturally sensitive manner. Privacy is a must and the nurse needs to be aware of their own posture, body language, and tone of voice (as well as the patient's) whilst interviewing the patient.

Physical examination

Thyroid disease and diabetes mellitus and some reproductive disorders are mostly forms of endocrine disease, endocrine disorders are uncommon. Careful observation of the patient is needed in order to make a diagnosis as the nurse moves from non-specific symptoms to the recognition of specific features (Bevan 2013). Physical examination techniques that are used in a focused endocrine assessment are the same techniques used in a general examination: inspection, percussion, auscultation, and palpation, although Rhoads and Wiggins Petersen (2018) note that assessment may be a challenge due to the locations of most of the glands (excepting the thyroid and the testes). The nurse must be skilled in making an assessment of the patient with an endocrine disorder. It can take time and much supervised practice to become competent and confident in inspection, palpation, and auscultation.

When meeting and greeting the patient, observe the person's appearance, height, weight, fat distribution, and muscle mass in relation to age. Explain to the patient the purpose of the examination and what will be done, and that the examination can be halted or stopped at any time.

Does the patient have prominent forehead, jaw, round or puffy face; or is there a dull or flat face expression? Are there any signs of exophthalmos? Inspect the lower half of the neck. Observe the skin: note the colour, areas of hypo- or hyperpigmentation; are there any fungal skin infections, evidence of slow wound healing, any petechiae, skin infections or foot ulcers.

Weigh the patient and note any significant changes in weight loss or weight gain. If the endocrine system is malfunctioning then there is a possibility that there will be disruption in metabolism. With the patient sitting in front of you, check facial features, facial expression (facies). In endocrine disorders changes can occur with facial features (see Table 18.7).

6 Cs

Psychological aspects are important components of endocrine conditions that nurses have to be aware of. They relate to all phases of illness. Disorders of the endocrine system can bring with them altered body image, changes in physical appearance, impaired sexual functioning, and a decrease in activity level.

Inspect the hands for dry skin and sweating. Assess for peripheral tremor: take a piece of paper and ask the patient to stretch their arms out in front of them, place a piece of paper over the back of the hands, and note any tremor. Take the patient's pulse, noting the rate and rhythm.

Table 18.7 Facial changes that can occur in endocrine disorders.

Disorder	Facial manifestations
Hyperthyroidism (thyrotoxicosis)	Exophthalmos Retracted eye lid Lid lag (delayed descent of upper lid in a downward gaze) Thin face due to weight loss Goitre
Hypothyroidism (myxoedema)	Periorbital oedema Dry skin Puffy face Coarse hair
Acromegaly	Prominent brow Nose and lip tissues enlarged Prognathism (prominent jaw)
Cushing's syndrome	Facial flushing Moon face Acne Hirsutism Dorsocervical fat pad (buffalo hump)

Review

Nurses are required to take personal responsibility for good record keeping. Clarify the issues of delegating record keeping and countersigning records where you are working. What is local policy and procedure?

Assessing the thyroid Gland

Assessment of the thyroid gland is an important part of the overall assessment of the person with endocrine disorders. Inspection and palpation are key elements of the physical assessment process, and auscultation is also included as part of the physical examination. A stethoscope and a glass of water is the equipment required for the examination.

Inspection

When inspecting the trachea and thyroid, explain to the patient what you are going to do. The trachea should be midline and on either side the space should be symmetrical, as should be the neck muscles. There should be no visible thyroid enlargement and no lumps. Thyroid enlargement or a tumour can displace the trachea, causing deviation. Observe the patient swallowing: offer them a glass of water and look for upward movement of the thyroid, size, and symmetry

Palpation

Explain to the patient what the next stage of the examination entails and wash hands. The nurse gently palpates the cervical lymph nodes, anterior and posterior cervical chain, and the submental nodes. Determine the position of the trachea, palpating the isthmus of the thyroid gland, taking note of its size, shape, outline, presence of nodules, and tenderness. Note any palpable thrill. The thyroid gland can be palpated from the anterior and posterior perspectives.

Auscultation

Placing a stethoscope over an enlarged thyroid (or if nodules are suspected) will enable the nurse to assess each lobe of the thyroid gland. A thyroid bruit may be heard; this is a continuous sound heard over the thyroid mass (Williams et al. 2014). A thyroid bruit is heard in Graves' disease as a result of a proliferation of blood supply to gland as it enlarges.

Review

What is the local policy where you are working as regards infection prevention and control and the use of a stethoscope?

After the examination has been completed thank the patient. Wash your hands, document, and report findings adhering to local policy and procedure.

Together, the health history and the physical examination will determine what diagnostic tests are required in order to determine the patient's diagnosis. Diagnostic testing can include blood test, ultrasound, fine needle biopsy, radioactive iodine uptake, urine testing, and MRI and CT scans.

So far

Unlike other disorders of the body, endocrine system disorders affect more than one anatomical site or organ. Most endocrine disorders do not present as a single visible or palpable abnormality. The exception to this is the thyroid and the testes, the other endocrine glands cannot be felt. Diagnoses rely on astute observations that are complemented by the taking of a careful history. A structured sequential approach is required that can lead to other laboratory and radiological testing and evaluation.

Shahine Samuda (Mother)

Shahine was being seen by the clinical nurse specialist (CNS) in the dermatology department, she had a red rash and bruising to her arms and legs. The CNS explained to Shahine that he wanted to make a referral to the endocrinologist because the signs and symptoms appeared to suggest that Shahine may have an endocrine disorder.

In the endocrinology clinic Shahine told the nurse that she was 'so tired all of the time, but despite this excessive tiredness I just could not sleep, I am so irritable and short-tempered with people, I can feel my heart pounding in the centre of my chest, as if it is about to explode, sometimes I am short of breath'. Shahine explained that she was getting 'a bit down with it all', she doesn't even have the energy to go swimming or enjoy her salsa classes.

A health history was taken. Shahine explained that she had been experiencing the symptoms for about two months. She fatigued very easily, had insomnia, palpitations, and an increase in perspiration. 'I have lost my "get up and go", I have no energy' and 'I sweat so much these days.' She informed the nurse that there has been 'some changes in how her eyes look, not in eyesight, but how they look, they seem to be droopy' and 'the skin nurse has already had a look at my arms, legs, and the bruises'. The eyes are 'stinging, burning' but that has been going on for about four or five months, 'I am due to see the eye doctor next month'.

There is no past or current health history of diabetes, cardiovascular disease, mental health issues, or cancer. Shahine was in hospital a few months back for a varicose vein operation.

One of Shahine's aunts was diagnosed with hyperthyroidism (she died six years ago).

The nurse found her pulse to be 98 beats per minute, irregular and bounding, blood pressure 142/92 mm/Hg, respirations 18 breaths per minute and temperature 36 °C.

With the history above, use the mnemonic OLDCARTS to help you systematically assess the needs of Shahine.

- **O**nset – when did it start?
- **L**ocation/Radiation – where is it located?
- **D**uration – how long has this gone on?
- **C**haracter – does it change with any specific activities? Does the patient use any descriptive words to describe the quality of the symptom?
- **A**ggravating factors – what makes it worse?
- **R**eliving factors – what makes it better?
- **T**iming – is it constant, cyclic, or does it come and go?
- **S**everity – how bothersome, disruptive is the problem?

What might the diagnosis be?
What else might you require to make a definitive diagnosis?
What might be the plan of care for Shahine?
How will you evaluate care interventions delivered?

Conclusion

The anatomy and physiology of the endocrine system has been discussed. There are a number of hormones the endocrine system produces, and each of these hormones has very different effects and affects various cells and organs. The major bodily processes that hormones influence or regulate are reproduction, growth and development, defence mechanisms against stressors, levels of electrolytes, water and nutrients, and cellular metabolism and energy. This system has a wide and varied role in the maintenance of normal body functioning and works to ensure homeostasis. Disorders of any of the endocrine organs can result in a number of signs and symptoms and could even lead to a life-threatening crisis. The nurse has a key role to play in detecting endocrine conditions, the monitoring of disease progression, and evaluation of care interventions and the effects of treatment as well as the early detection and prevention of endocrine emergencies.

In order to offer those people who have an endocrine disorder appropriate support and care that is patient-centred and responsive to individual needs, the nurse has to have a good understanding of endocrine anatomy and physiology along with the treatment of the various conditions.

References

Bevan, J. (2013). The endocrine system. In: *Macleod's Clinical Examination* (ed. G. Douglas, F. Nicol and C. Robertson), 77–96. Edinburgh: Elsevier.

Clare, C. (2017). The endocrine system. In: *Fundamentals of Anatomy and Physiology for Nursing and Healthcare Students*, 2e (ed. I. Peate and M. Nair), 479–512. Oxford: Wiley.

Dover, A.R. and Zammitt, N. (2018). The endocrine system. In: *Macleod's Clinical Examination*, 14e (ed. J.A. Innes, A.R. Dover and K. Fairhurst), 193–209. Edinburgh: Elsevier.

Jarvis, C. (2015). *Physical Examination and Health Assessment*, 7e. St Louis: Elsevier.

Marieb, E.N. and Hoehn, K. (2016). *Human Anatomy and Physiology*, 10e. San Francisco: Pearson Benjamin Cummings.

Nursing and Midwifery Council (2018). The Code. Professional Standards of Practice and Behaviour for Nurses, Midwives and Nursing Associates. https://www.nmc.org.uk/globalassets/sitedocuments/nmc-publications/nmc-code.pdf last accessed 8 May 2019.

Rhoads, J. and Wiggins Petersen, S. (2018). *Advanced Health Assessment and Diagnostic Reasoning*, 3e. Burlington: Jones and Bartlett.

Waugh, A. and Grant, A. (2018). *Ross and Wilson's Anatomy and Physiology in Health and Illness*, 12e. Edinburgh: Elsevier.

Williams, E., Chillag, S., and Rizvi, A. (2014). Thyroid bruit and the underlying 'inferno'. *American Journal of Medicine* 127 (6): 489–490.

de Wit, S.C., Stromberg, H.K., and Vreeland Dallred, C. (2017). *Medical Surgical Nursing: Concepts and Practice*, 3e. St Louis: Elsevier.

Chapter 19

Assessing the immune system

Aim

This chapter introduces the reader to the assessment of the immune system and the care required for those who experience problems related to this system.

Learning outcomes

By the end of the chapter the reader will be able to:

1. Provide a brief overview of the immune system and its functions
2. Discuss a number of conditions that might affect the immune system
3. Outline the various ways in which the nurse may undertake an assessment of the immune system
4. Describe care planning that is related to the immune system

Introduction

The immune system has a key role to play in the protection against various infections, but disorders of the immune system can lead to disease processes that can result in tissue injury and even death. Making a diagnosis that is related to an immune disorder or a suspected immune disorder will require the nurse to have an understanding of the immune system. Patient assessment is needed to determine if there is an immune disorder. The patient history is required and a detailed physical examination is needed to decide upon clinical tests so as to make a diagnosis and devise a care plan.

The immune system

The main purpose of the immune system is to defend the body from foreign invasion by disease-producing pathogens, for example bacteria and viruses.

There are many different organs and systems that work to ensure we are kept alive and healthy in an external environment that contains within it many threats to individual and community health. These include physical dangers, dangers related to poisonous chemicals and sharp objects, and those diseases producing micro-organisms known also as pathogens that can result in inflammation and infection. The immune system, working in collaboration with the lymphatic system, provides the defence against hazards to health and plays a major role in disease prevention.

Fundamentals of Assessment and Care Planning for Nurses, First Edition. Ian Peate.
© 2020 John Wiley & Sons Ltd. Published 2020 by John Wiley & Sons Ltd.

Throughout our lives, we are dependent upon the immune system to protect us from when we are born until we die. Nearly every disease, accident or disorder experienced is related to the immune system. The immune system is concerned with more than infections.

As the body is constantly exposed to a variety of foreign substances, infectious agents, and also abnormal cells, it is the immune system that is the key defender in providing protection. The immune system is an intricate system of cells, enzymes, and proteins offering protection and making us resistant or immune to infections that are caused by various micro-organisms. The immune system is a sophisticated system that has the capacity to do more than fight infection and offer protection from infectious diseases; its other functions include the removal and destruction of damaged or dead cells and the identification and destruction of malignant cells, helping to prevent them from development into tumours.

Blood cell development

The blood cells which form a chief part of the immune system are the white blood cells. All blood cells are descended from multipotent stem cells, which have the ability to change to different types of cells and in terms of the immune system they develop into two major branches of white blood cells. Figure 19.1 shows the development of white blood cells.

One branch will develop into the myeloid family of cells, these include the neutrophils and monocytes, whilst the other branch will develop into the lymphoid family of cells, made up of lymphocytes.

It can be seen that the myeloid family include the macrophages (consisting of monocytes and tissue macrophages) and granulocytes (consisting of neutrophils, eosinophils, and basophils). The lymphoid

345

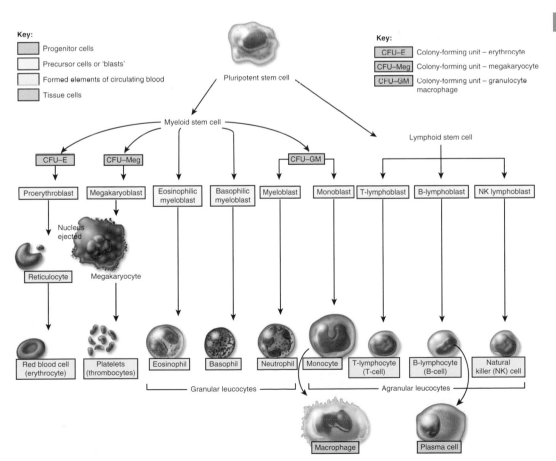

Figure 19.1 The development of white blood cells.

Table 19.1   A brief glossary of the blood cells (Vickers 2007).

B-lymphocytes	These lymphocytes arise in the bone marrow and differentiate into plasma cells, which produce immunoglobulins – also known as antibodies.
Bone marrow	The site in the body where most cells of the immune system are produced as immature (stem) cells.
Immunoglobulins	Immunoglobulins – known also as antibodies, they are highly specialised protein molecules whose job it is to connect with and hold on to foreign antigens so they cannot escape destruction by other cells of the immune system.
Monocytes	White blood cells are also phagocytes, found in the blood. However, they have the ability to migrate into tissues, where they are known as macrophages.
Plasma cells	These cells develop from B-lymphocytes and produce the immunoglobulins.
Platelets	Blood cells which have an important role to play in the clotting of blood.
Polymorphonuclear leucocytes	White blood cells also known as phagocytes, found in the blood.
Red blood cells	These cells carry oxygen from the lungs to the tissues.
Stem cells	Have the potential to differentiate and mature into the different cells of the immune system.
Thymus	An organ situated in the chest which instructs immature T-lymphocytes to become mature T-lymphocytes, which are then able to help fight infections.
T-effector lymphocytes	Known also as T-cytotoxic lymphocytes. These lymphocytes have the ability to produce chemicals that can kill foreign cells and micro-organisms, as well as assisting in the process of inflammation.
T-helper lymphocytes	Whilst in the thymus, these specialised lymphocytes develop the ability to help other lymphocytes to prepare for an immune response
T-lymphocytes	Whilst in the thymus, these specialised lymphocytes develop the ability to help other lymphocytes to prepare for an immune response
T-suppressor lymphocytes	These specialised lymphocytes can suppress the helper T-lymphocytes, helping to regulate the immune system by turning off the immune system response, so reducing the potential damaging effects of an overactive immune system.

branch of white blood provides T-lymphocytes and B-lymphocytes (many B-lymphocytes develop into plasma cells). Furthermore, the myeloid branch also provides the megakaryocytes (leading to platelets) and erythroid cells, which develop into erythrocytes (i.e. red blood cells).

All the white blood cells originate initially in the bone marrow as stem cells. However, as they mature through their various stages, they are found in different places around the body, including:

- The blood and lymph circulation
- The thymus
- The spleen
- The tonsils and other lymph nodes

They are also found in all the mucosal membranes, such as the lining of the mouth and the gastrointestinal tract.

Vickers (2007) provide a brief glossary of the blood cells (see Table 19.1).

The organs of the immune system

The prime organs of the immune system are all part of the lymphatic system. They consist of the:

- Thymus
- Spleen
- Lymph nodes
- Lymphoid tissues that are scattered throughout the gastrointestinal, respiratory, and urinary tracts.

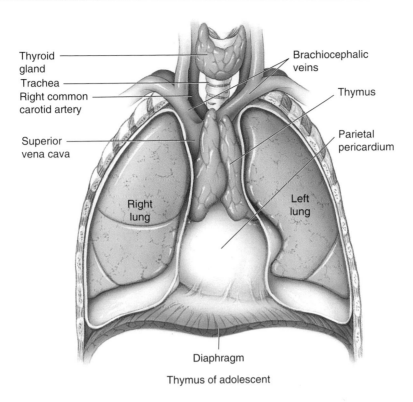

Thyroid gland

Trachea

Right common carotid artery

Superior vena cava

Brachiocephalic veins

Thymus

Parietal pericardium

Right lung

Left lung

Diaphragm

Thymus of adolescent

Figure 19.2   Location of the thymus within the body.

The thymus

The thymus is situated in the chest (see Figure 19.2), it shrinks (atrophies) with age. Within the thymus, blood stem cells mature and differentiate into various T-cell lymphocyte subclasses. They also acquire the ability to recognise and differentiate 'self' cells from 'non-self' cells.

'Self' cells are those which originate and belong to the individual with the thymus, whilst 'non-self' cells are cells which come from outside the individual. Even though the thymus starts to atrophy at puberty, T-cells will continue to develop in the thymus throughout an individual's life (Vickers 2017).

Review

The thymus and the thyroid are both endocrine glands. However, their functions differ. Make notes about these organs:

	Thyroid	Thymus
Location		
Function		

The lymphatic system

This is a specialised system of lymph vessels (similar to blood vessels) and lymph nodes. Lymphatic vessels contain a fluid called 'lymph', which drains into the organs of the lymph system from nearby organs. This lymph originates from plasma leaking from the blood capillaries.

Lymphocytes migrate from the blood system, passing through the walls of the smallest venous capillaries in the lymph node. Lymphocytes spend only a few minutes in the blood stream during each circuit of the body, but, in contrast, they spend several hours in the lymphoid system.

The lymphatic system can be considered as a parallel system to the blood circulatory system, but it does not have a pump as the heart does, pumping blood around the body. Instead lymph is agitated around the body by a combination of the smooth muscular walls of the lymph vessels and the flexing and relaxing of striated muscle as a person moves. The principal components of the lymphatic system are detailed in Figure 19.3, the system is made up of lymphatic vessels and lymphatic capillaries, as well as organs which are situated within their own capsule (encapsulated). These include:

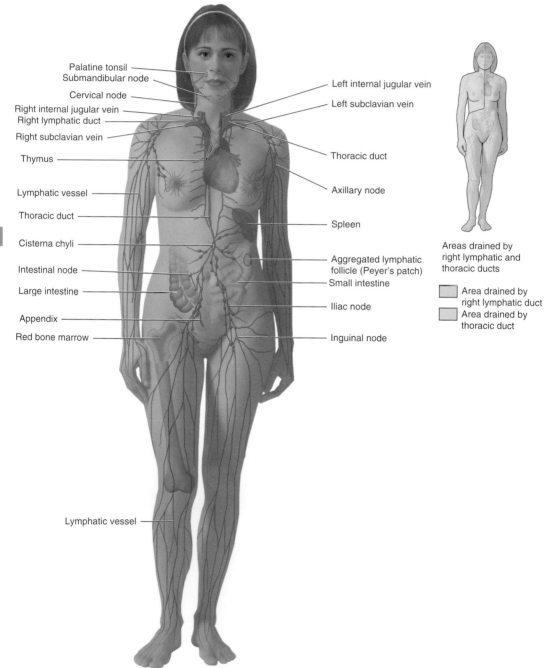

Figure 19.3   The lymphatic system.

- Spleen
- Tonsils
- Lymph nodes

The lymphatic system also includes unencapsulated lymphoid tissue in the gastrointestinal tract, the urogenital tract and the lungs.

The lymph vessels and capillaries form a network throughout the body, connecting the tissues of the body to the lymphoid organs, for example the spleen, and the lymph nodes.

Lymphatic capillaries have some anatomical similarities to blood capillaries in that their walls contain of a layer of endothelial cells. Lymphatic capillary walls, however, do not have a basement membrane, and this allows substances of relatively large molecular size, such as plasma proteins, to enter the lymphatic capillaries between the cells of the capillary walls.

The lymph eventually flows into two large lymph ducts. One is called the thoracic duct, receiving lymph from the:

- Lower limbs
- Digestive tract
- Left arm
- Left side of the thorax, head, and neck

The other large lymph vessel, the right lymphatic duct, receives lymph from the:

- Right arm
- Right side of the head, neck, and thorax

The two lymph ducts empty into the great veins in the neck, thus restoring fluid and proteins to the venous circulation.

349

Lymph nodes

Lymph enters the lymph nodes from the afferent lymphatic vessels, and from there it goes to the trabeculae. Afferent means 'leading towards', therefore, in the case of lymph nodes, afferent vessels are those vessels that lead towards the lymph node.

The lymph node is made up of a mesh of cells. Lymph at this stage contains antigens from infected cells and tissues. This lymph passes through this mesh in the lymph node and the antigens are trapped (see Figure 19.4).

Antigens entering the body at any point are quickly swept along the lymph vessels towards a lymphoid organ or lymph node.

Within the lymph node, B-cell lymphocytes are located in the primary lymphoid follicles as well as the secondary lymphoid follicles (containing the germinal centres). Inside these germinal centres the B-cells proliferate after encountering their specific antigen and its cooperating T-cell. The B-cells that are found at the centre of the secondary lymphoid follicles are actively dividing, whilst those at the periphery are antibody-forming.

Large numbers of phagocytic macrophages and plasma cells producing antibodies are located in the medulla of the gland. Macrophages and other antigen-presenting cells spend most of their lives migrating through the tissues until encountering antigens. These are then phagocytosed and carried to the nearest lymph node.

Macrophages in the lymph node also encounter trapped antigens within the meshwork of reticular cells, they phagocytose the dead cells and bacteria. The lymph which has destroyed the antigens in the lymph nodes leaves through the efferent lymphatic vessel.

Lymphoid tissue

As well as lymphatic vessels, the lymphatic system also contains lymphoid tissue. This consists of lymph glands, i.e. lymph nodes, which are approximately the size and shape of a broad bean, and lymphoid tissue, which is found in specific organs, particularly:

- Spleen
- Bone marrow
- Lungs

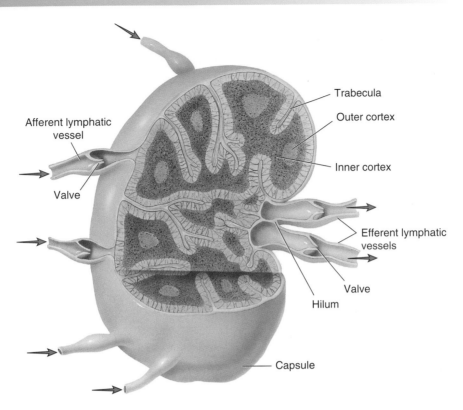

Afferent lymphatic
vessel

Valve

Trabecula

Outer cortex

Inner cortex

Efferent lymphatic
vessels

Valve

Hilum

Capsule

Figure 19.4 Structure of a lymph node.

- Liver
- Other lymphoid tissue.

The spleen

The spleen is located just behind the stomach and is about the size of a fist. It collects antigen from the blood for presentation to phagocytes and lymphocytes and also collects and disposes of dead red blood cells.

So far

- The lymphoid system allows lymphocytes to protect the tissues and vessels from infectious micro-organisms.
- It holds micro-organisms in antigen 'traps' in the lymph nodes and other lymphoid organs, bringing them into close proximity with other immune cells.
- This is a requirement for the cell-to-cell communication needed to recruit, direct, and regulate a coordinated immune response.
- Lymph glands are the major centres for lymphocyte proliferation and antibody production as well as for filtering the lymph.

Types of immunity

There are two types of immunity: the innate and the acquired.

Innate immunity

Innate immunity is acquired at birth. The foetus acquires some immunity via the placenta, this is called passive immunity and lasts for about three to six months; the main antibody which is able to cross the placenta is immunoglobulin (IgG). Although the time period for providing this passive immunity is limited, it is important at a time when the immune system is immature. After about six months, infants are more prone to respiratory and gastric infections, this is in part due to the loss of foetal antibodies before the B and T-lymphocytes are fully immunocompetent. A central role of the innate immune response is to prevent or restrict the entrance of micro-organisms into the body, so that tissue damage is limited. Inflammation is an example of an innate immune response (also called non-specific immunity).

Inflammation

When tissue damage occurs a number of proteins acting as the catalyst for the immune response are activated. This response is non-specific and attacks any and all foreign invaders attempting to rid the body of microbes, toxins, or other foreign matter aiming to prevent their spread to other tissues and preparing the site for tissue repair, restoring tissue homeostasis.

Take note

The most effective barrier against microbes is prevention. Preventing them from becoming pathogens, nurses and all health professionals must have insight and appropriate awareness and understanding of the effective measures needed to prevent cross-infection.

The responsibility of the cells of the immune system are to find and destroy any damaged cells and foreign tissues, and simultaneously recognise and preserve host cells. There are four phases related to the inflammatory response:

1. Redness
2. Swelling
3. Heat
4. Pain

When injury occurs almost immediately the damaged cells trigger a number of events to happen:

- Vasodilation
- Release of messenger molecules
- Initiation of complement
- Extravasation of vascular components
- Phagocytosis
- Pain

The mast cells that have been injured release histamine, causing arterioles to dilate and venules to constrict this promotes an increase in blood flow. The main mechanisms associated with vasodilation are: cells produce bradykinin (a vasodilator, also causes pain), damaged plasma membranes release arachidonic acid, a fatty acid, a precursor to prostaglandins. Prostaglandins (vasodilators) can increase pain. The histamine released from the degranulated mast cells enlarges pore size between the capillary cells, allowing proteins and other micromolecules to move into the interstitial spaces. Nitric oxide is released by the vascular epithelial cells, causing further vasodilation; the presence of macrophages release large quantities of nitric oxide.

Cells close to the injury release a series of chemical signals that radiate from the site of inflammation known as chemokines. The concentration of chemokines is greatest immediately surrounding the infection, these high levels of chemokines provide a signal for the attraction of phagocytic white blood cells including neutrophils. Figure 19.5 outlines the cells of the immune system.

As chemokine concentration increases as the phagocytes leave the capillary and enter the site of infection, macrophages arrive around 24 hours after. The phagocytes engulf and destroy the pathogens present recognising this as non-self-matter. The key molecule released is interleukin 1, attracting neutrophils and macrophages to the site of injury helping to clear away debris from the injured area.

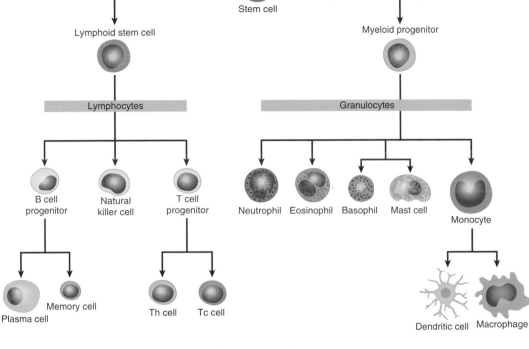

Figure 19.5   The cells of the immune system.

So far

Typical inflammatory response to tissue in injury is:

- Arterioles close to the injury site constrict briefly.
- This vasoconstriction is followed by vasodilation, increasing blood flow to the site of injury (redness and heat).
- Dilation of the arterioles at the injury site increases the pressure in the circulation.
- This increases the exudation of both plasma proteins and blood cells into the tissues in the area.
- Exudation causes oedema and swelling.
- Nerve endings in the area are stimulated, partly by pressure (pain).
- The clotting and kinin systems, as well as platelets, move into the area, blocking any tissue damage by starting the clotting process.
- White blood cells – phagocytes and lymphocytes – move into the area and start to destroy any infectious organisms in the vicinity of the trauma.
- The phagocytes and protein cells, with the substances produced, kill any bacteria or other micro-organisms in the vicinity, removing the debris resulting from the battle between the micro-organisms and the immune system – this includes exudate and dead cells (pus).
- All these parts of the immune and blood systems remain in the area until tissue regeneration occurs – this is known as resolution.

Table 19.2   The five types of antibodies.

Type of antibody	Purposes
IgA	Found in breast milk, mucous, saliva, and tears, inhibits antigens from crossing epithelial membranes and invading deeper tissue
IgD	Produced by B-cells and is found on their surface. Antigens bind to active B-cells here.
IgE	This is the least common antibody. Found bound to tissue cell membranes, specifically eosinophils
IgG	The most common and largest antibody. Attacks various pathogens, crosses the placenta to protect the foetus
IgM	This antibody is produced in large quantities, is the primary response and a potent activator of complement

Acquired immunity

Known also as specific immunity as it will only respond to known, specific organisms that the person has previously encountered (that have previously infected them), acquired immunity has a capability to remember when a particular immunological threat has been met and overcome, remembering how to defeat it and mobilise the immune system to deal with that threat (called immunological memory). The acquired immune system is based upon the lymphocytes that are closely associated to the lymphatic system.

The primary response (exposure for the first time) produces a slow and delayed rise in antibody levels. The delay is associated with activation of the T-lymphocyte system that stimulates B-lymphocyte separation.

Secondary response occurs on subsequent exposure to the same antigen and the response in this case is much faster; as the memory B-lymphocytes generated after the first infection divide and separate at a faster rate, antibody production occurs almost immediately. See Table 19.2 for the five types of antibody.

Natural and artificial acquired immunity

Immunity can be acquired naturally or artificially, and both forms can be active or passive (see Figure 19.6).

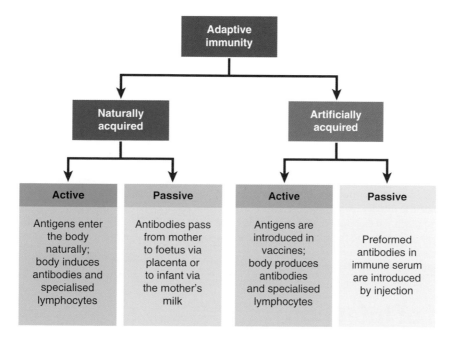

Figure 19.6   Types of acquired immunity.

When active immunity occurs, this means that the person has made a response to the antigen and this leads to the production of their own antibodies with activation of the lymphocytes. The memory cells offer long-lasting resistance.

Passive immunity occurs when the person has been given antibodies. This type of immunity is relatively short-acting as the antibodies will eventually break down.

Review

Go to this web site www.nhs.uk/conditions/vaccinations and make notes about the following vaccinations:

Vaccination	Notes
65 years The pneumococcal (PPV) vaccine	
65 years and over The flu vaccine	
70 years (and 78- and 79-year-olds as a catch-up) The shingles vaccine	

Infectious micro-organisms

Micro-organisms are microscopic cells living in the environment, on the skin, or inside bodies. They can cause infectious diseases, and they can do this as long as two conditions are met:

- They are able to grow and reproduce in the right conditions for that micro-organism
- They are in the right location for their growth and reproduction

These conditions are important as different micro-organisms have differing and sometimes exacting needs for their growth and reproduction. If environmental conditions are not right, then they will not flourish. However, once the conditions are right then the micro-organisms multiply at an astounding rate within the host's tissues. This leads to destruction or degeneration so that the host will become unwell and unable to function properly.

It is not the presence of micro-organisms that causes the problem, instead it is the fact that during their growth and reproduction (as well as part of the protection against the immune system) they produce waste products that are known as toxins, and it is these toxins that cause the problems. However, not all micro-organisms will pose problems for humans, for example humans need bacteria to help them break down food and digest it. These bacteria are known as commensal bacteria.

However, even commensal micro-organisms can become pathogenic if they find themselves in the wrong place. Those micro-organisms that live in the colon, for example, are beneficial but they may invade the urinary bladder, where they then become pathogenic micro-organisms as they are in the wrong place. An example of one of these is *Escherichia coli* (E. coli), which usually lives in the gut. If, however, it migrates to the bladder, then it can cause cystitis. When infections are triggered in this way, these are known as endogenous infections. All other infections are known as exogenous infections, coming from outside the body.

Spread of infection

The causative organisms of infectious disease in humans can be transmitted from the reservoir of infection by one of 10 ways (see Table 19.3).

Table 19.3 Routes of transmission.

Route of transmission	Mode and examples
Droplet spread	Microbial organisms are spread in mucous droplet nuclei that travel only short distances – less than 1 m from the reservoir to the host. From coughing and sneezing (as discussed below), but also by talking or laughing. Examples of disease spread by droplet transmission include: ● Influenza ● Pneumonia ● Pertussis (whooping cough)
Air currents (airborne transmission)	Airborne transmission refers to the spread of agents of infection by droplet nuclei in dust. Droplets may spread by more than 1 m from the reservoir to the host. An example of droplet transmission is what happens during sneezing and coughing. When a person coughs or sneezes, they expel a fine spray into the air around them. This is made up of many, many droplets of mucus that could contain infectious micro-organisms. Infectious micro-organisms that can be spread in this way include: ● Measles ● Tuberculosis (TB) ● Staphylococcal and streptococcal infections ● Certain fungal diseases – spread by the spores – such as histoplasmosis
Aerosol	Both domestic and industrial water supplies are potential sources of aerosol transmission. This has a similar action to that occurring with droplet transmission, except the reservoir is water, rather than another human. Examples of diseases that are spread by this method include: ● Legionnaire's disease ● Tuberculosis (TB)
Water	Pathogens are usually spread by water that has been contaminated with untreated, or poorly treated, sewage. The pathogenic organisms enter the host by contact with the mucosa, or by contact with broken skin. Examples of infections spread through water include: ● Leptospirosis – often picked up from rat urine whilst swimming in a river ● Schistosomiasis (commonly known as bilharzia) – caused by a fluke (similar to a worm), which is a parasite found in fresh water
Direct contact	Contact transmission is the spread of an infectious organism by direct or indirect contact, the direct transmission of an infectious organism by physical contact between its present host and a susceptible recipient host. Common forms of direct contact transmission are: ● Touching ● Kissing ● Sexual intercourse Many diseases that can be transmitted by direct contact include: ● Viral respiratory tract diseases (e.g. the common cold, influenza) ● Staphylococcal infections (e.g. septicaemia) ● Hepatitis A ● Measles ● Scarlet fever ● Sexually acquired infections (e.g. syphilis, gonorrhoea, genital herpes) ● Infectious mononucleosis (glandular fever) ● HIV Potential pathogens can also be transmitted by direct contact from animals (or animal products) to humans, e.g. rabies, anthrax. Indirect contact transmission occurs when the infectious micro-organism is transmitted from its present reservoir to a potential susceptible host by means of a non-living object.

(Continued)

Table 19.3   (Continued)

Route of transmission	Mode and examples
Soil	Soil is a potential reservoir for infectious micro-organisms. The route of entry from the soil into the body is usually by a skin lesion. Infection can occur: • When playing sport on a contaminated playing field • Whilst gardening on soil contaminated by the use of animal manure • Whilst farming on land that has been fertilised with animal manure. • Any fall on contaminated ground in which the skin becomes broken Examples of infectious diseases that can occur from soil include: • Tetanus • Gas gangrene
Inoculation	Inoculation can be accidental, for example by being bitten or scratched. Examples of infections caused this way include: • Cat scratch disease • Rabies Inoculation can occur following an injection as a result of needle stick injury or by someone injecting themselves with drugs. Examples of infections caused this way include: • HIV • Hepatitis B • Hepatitis C
Faceo-oral	This transmission of infectious micro-organisms can occur in several ways, including: • Hand-to-mouth – particularly in young children who may be exploring the anal area and then put their hands in their mouths • Sewage-contaminated food or water. • Certain sexual practices, in which there is oro-anal stimulation Examples of infectious diseases transmitted via this route, include: • Gastroenteritis • Enteric fevers
Vector	This is commonly held to be inoculation by the bite of a sucking arthropod (for example a 'tick') which is also a host, but there are other types of vector transmission. Vectors are animals that carry pathogens from one host to another. Arthropods are the most important group of disease vectors.
Contaminated intermediates	Caused by indirect contact transmission and occurs when the infectious micro-organism is transmitted from the initial reservoir to a potential susceptible host by means of a non-living object. These non-living objects, or inanimate intermediates, are called fomites. Examples include: • Clothes, bedding, and towels • Tissues and handkerchiefs • Drinking cups and eating utensils • Toys Other fomites can transmit infections such as: • Chickenpox • Staphylococci and streptococci infections • Tetanus

Source: Kannan (2016), Ward (2016).

So far

The immune system is a very complex system, with each of the various components interacting with others to provide protection needed to survive in this very perilous world. The immune system keeps us safe from infections and other potential harm that could occur.

Immunology is a dynamic subject, research and treatments (therapies) are continually bringing new knowledge to the fore.

The patient history

Undertaking an assessment of immunity requires the nurse to obtain the patient's history, undertake a physical examination, and assess blood results, specifically the white cell count with differentials. Assessment of immunity requires the nurse to adopt a structured approach and to listen carefully to the patient and their responses as this will help to structure the process. Silverman et al. (2014) considers the Calgary–Cambridge Observation Guide, which enables the nurse to follow a structured approach to the consultation, whilst at the same time being acutely aware of the need for effective communication and staying patient-focused throughout.

The following issues should be considered when undertaking a focused approach that can lead to a diagnosis:

- Recurrent infections
- Chronic conjunctivitis
- Chronic diarrhoea
- Arthritis-like symptoms
- Autoimmune diseases
- Allergies

Recurrent infections, chronic conjunctivitis, and chronic diarrhoea might indicate a possible assault on the immune system or may reveal an underactive, impaired-functioning immune system. Allergies, autoimmune disease, and arthritis symptoms are disease processes that can be related to autoimmunity. When the person's immune system response is altered and it does not recognise the body's cells as being part of the host, then these symptoms may occur.

Sore throat

Sore throat is a symptom as opposed to a diagnosis. This makes it important for the nurse to undertake a robust history and to perform a physical examination in order to establish a differential diagnosis and rule out any potentially more disturbing diagnoses. Sore throat, according to Kenealy (2014), occurs when an acute upper respiratory tract infection affects the mucosa of the throat.

Based on the findings in the health history and the patient's chief complaint the nurse then undertakes a physical examination. Problems affecting the throat can impact on a person's breathing and their ability to ingest food. The history provides an opportunity for the nurse to identify clues to potential risk factors for a number of disorders, including oral cancer (mouth, tongue, throat). See Table 19.4, a guide to history taking in relation to the chief complaint – sore throat.

The FeverPAIN clinical score can help to determine if a sore throat is more likely to be caused by bacteria. Higher scores will suggest more severe symptoms and likely bacterial cause. Each of the FeverPAIN criteria (Table 19.5) score 1 point (maximum score of 5).

A score of 0 or 1 is associated with a 13% to 18% likelihood of isolating streptococcus. A score of 2 or 3 is associated with a 34–40% likelihood of isolating streptococcus. A score of 4 or 5 is associated with a 62–65% likelihood of isolating streptococcus.

Obtaining the patient's past medical history requires the nurse to seek detailed information about any oral trauma or any surgery to the oral cavity. Ascertain if there is any history of upper respiratory tract infections and allergies. Past health conditions or surgery should be established along with dental history and any associated dental problems.

Table 19.4   A guide to history taking, chief complaint – sore throat

	To be determined/asked	To be considered
Onset	Ask if the onset was sudden or gradual	Bacterial infections usually occur suddenly and can relate to others in the household, school, university who are experiencing the same symptoms. Viral infections can be more gradual and can remain over time, they can be related to a post-bacterial infection
Duration	How long has the patient had the sore throat? How often do they experience sore throats?	There may be factors such as a dry humid environment or mouth breathing that are causing a sore throat – an itching feeling occurring in the morning
Severity	How severe, how bad is the sore throat, describe it	The severity of the sore throat can interfere with swallowing and when described as very sore is usually bacterial Virus-induced sore throats are usually less severe and are described as itching, scratchy
Associated signs and symptoms	Establish if there are any associated symptoms such as pyrexia, dysphagia, hoarseness	If there is pyrexia present this can indicate infection. An upper respiratory tract infection, allergy, smoking, inhalation of irritants, or overuse of the voice can be associated with hoarseness. Group A beta-haemolytic streptococcus (GABHS) is the most common cause of tonsillopharyngitis.
Exacerbating factors	Is the sore throat exacerbated by any environmental factors or any other changes?	Seasonal sore throats are often related to allergy. Exacerbating factors can also be allergy to pets or other allergens
Alleviating factors	Does anything alleviate the pain?	The use of over-the-counter gargles and pain relief can indicate there is inflammation related to infection
Medication history	History of current medications	Non-infectious sore throat may be caused by physical or chemical factors, for example snoring or smoking. Non-infectious sore throat may be medication-induced through the use of angiotensin-converting enzyme inhibitors, inhaled corticosteroids, or chemotherapy.

Source: Addey and Shephard (2012), Green (2015).

Cultural consideration

British South Asian patients report significantly higher rates of depressive symptoms following a recent cancer diagnosis, compared with White British Patients.

Source: Lord et al. (2013).

There are some diseases, such as cancers, that are familial (a genetic predisposition). Obtaining a family history can help focus the consultation further.

A description of current living arrangements (social history) is required. If the patient is exposed to multiple acute and chronic diseases within the family unit or living arrangements (for example, living in student halls of residence) this may be a significant issue, as working or living in crowded areas promotes transmission of disease. Use of tobacco and alcohol can increase the risk of oral cancers.

Oral piercings can be a risk factor for a number of oral conditions, including sore throat. Piercings can cause oedema of the tongue and this poses a threat to airway patency. They can also become infected and may bleed. The jewellery used can break off in the mouth and the patient may aspirate

Table 19.5 The FeverPAIN score.

Component	Score
Fever	
Purulence	
Attend rapidly (3 days or less)	
Severely **I**nflamed tonsils	
No cough or coryza	
Total	

Source: Little et al. (2014).

that dislodged piece, or a tooth can be chipped, which can also be aspirated. The person may have an allergic reaction to the piercing (metal or otherwise).

Sexual practices such as fellatio, cunnilingus, and oro-anal stimulation are activities that pose a risk of a number of infections that can manifest as sore throat.

6 Cs

When the subjective information has been gathered, history taking should be summarised and clarified with the patient (Green 2015). Clarifying with the patient can promote patient engagement and demonstrates the nurse's desire to work with the patient, involving them in their care. They may then feel better listened to and this has the potential to lead to enhanced concordance and patient satisfaction.

The details of the consultation are documented and reported using local policy and procedure and then the nurse progresses to the physical examination.

Take note

The consultation provides an ideal opportunity to offer health promotion and employ behaviour change methodologies, making every contact count.

So far

A structured comprehensive health history is required if the nurse is to go on and undertake a physical examination. The immune system is a complex system. Sore throat is a symptom and the skills required to gather secondary data around a sore throat are needed in order to make a diagnosis and to consider further diagnostic tests.

Physical examination

A number of oral diseases and disorders have manifestations in systems or other parts of the body other than the mouth or throat. Where appropriate a comprehensive review of body systems should be undertaken. Physical examination of the oral cavity requires the nurse to inspect and palpate.

Consent must always be gained prior to any physical examination and the nurse washes their hands prior to undertaking the procedure. Adhering to local infection prevention and control policy, the nurse should wear gloves when examining the mucous membranes. A full set of observations is required, including temperature, pulse, respiration rate, oxygen saturations, and blood pressure; this determines if the patient is systemically unwell and allows action to be taken should abnormalities be identified, such as immediate referral. Equipment required:

- Gauze
- Gloves
- Tongue depressor
- Light source (pen torch or otoscope)

Inspection

Saying hello to the patient and engaging in conversation with them can assist in assessing the clarity of the patient's voice. Note any abnormalities such as rough, wet, hoarse, or muffled voice which may be symptomatic of pathological causes (Wilson and Nicol 2013).

Take note

The nurse should not perform a physical examination if there is excessive drooling, stridor, or if the patient has a suspected airway occlusion or severe, acute difficulty in breathing. Any patient presenting in such a way must receive urgent medical attention and support. Assessing the throat, particularly if using a tongue depressor, can cause more distress and can exacerbate the problem.

When inspecting the mouth a good light source is essential. Observe the patient's lips first: the colour, oedema, any lesions and symmetry. If the patient has dentures or any dental appliances (for example a brace), ask them to remove these so there is a clear view of the mouth.

Using a bright light (a pen torch or an otoscope) with a tongue depressor, inspect the buccal mucosa and gums, noting colour, presence of ulcerations, lesions, or trauma. Ask the patient to protrude the tongue and observe for colour, lesions or masses. Asking the patient to raise the tongue to the roof of the mouth, inspect the underside for colour, lesions, and irritation. If the patient has teeth, note number and position. To inspect the roof of the mouth, ask the patient to tilt the head back, open the mouth, and shine the light on the roof of the mouth, noting colour and appearance. Observe the movement of the uvula using a tongue depressor to so this; it should rise symmetrically.

The posterior aspect of the throat is assessed using the tongue depressor to enhance visualisation, noting the size of the tonsils and any presence of exudate. There should be no lesions and the back of the throat should appear pink and moist.

Palpation

Explain to the patient that palpation of the head and neck will take place. Wash hands and don gloves, palpate the lips if appropriate and the tongue using gauze.

As lymph nodes are distributed throughout the body, examination, and evaluation often takes place as part of the regional examinations of the head and neck, breast and axillae, upper extremities, external genitalia, and/or lower extremities. It is best to use the pads of the index and middle fingers to note the size, shape, number, pliability, texture, mobility, and tenderness of nodes bilaterally.

Most lymph nodes lie too deep to be palpated for physical examination. Because lymph nodes are constantly interacting with extracellular fluid draining from nearby tissues, their examination can provide information about the presence and status of infections or malignancies in the area. Nodes draining the site of a soft tissue infection become enlarged and tender but usually remain soft, smooth, and mobile. Hard, non-tender, matted, or fixed nodes are more typical of a spreading malignancy. Diffuse lymphadenopathy can indicate systemic diseases, for example lymphomas, HIV, mononucleosis, or sarcoidosis. Finding a single abnormal node should support an examination of all nodes. The lymph nodes of the head and neck are shown in Figure 19.7.

Palpating the lymph nodes of the head and neck:

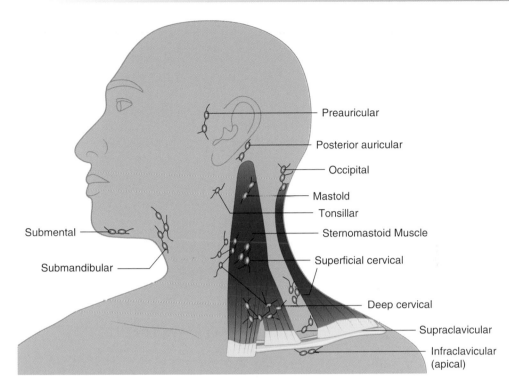

Figure 19.7 The lymph nodes of the head and neck.

1. Wash hands.
2. Ask the patient to slightly flex the head forward, and observe for noticeably visible node enlargement.
3. Palpate the head and neck nodes (see Figure 19.7) using both hands, one on each side, for each of the following steps. The nodes are not palpable in many cases.
4. Palpate the preauricular, posterior auricular, and mastoid nodes located in front of the ear, behind the ear and superficial to the mastoid process, respectively.
5. Palpate the occipital nodes posteriorly at the base of the skull.
6. Palpate the tonsillar nodes that are located at the angle of mandible, the submandibular nodes midway between the angle and tip, and the submental nodes a few centimetres from the tip.
7. Palpate the anterior and superficial cervical nodes in front of and overlying the sternomastoid muscle, respectively. Deep cervical nodes, beneath the sternomastoid muscle, are rarely palpable.
8. Palpate the posterior cervical nodes between the anterior edge of the trapezius and posterior edge of the sternomastoid.
9. Palpate the supraclavicular nodes deep within the angle formed by the sternomastoid muscle and clavicle. Some lung and abdominal cancers metastasise to these nodes and they may be noticed during the examination.
10. Palpate the infraclavicular nodes on the underside of the clavicle.
11. Wash hands.

Take note

When palpating the neck of an obese person there may be a need to palpate more deeply (gently) in order to assess lymph nodes. Take extra time to do this.

There may be a need to take a throat swab during the examination. If this is the case the nurse must adhere to local policy and procedure, explaining to the patient what it is they are doing and the rationale.

Take note

Patient referral should be instigated if the practitioner is concerned that the patient is systemically unwell or is at high risk of immunosuppression.

When the examination is complete, ensure that the patient is comfortable and dispose of used items in accordance with local policy and procedure and wash hands. Document and report findings.

The health history and the physical examination can lead the nurse to consider what other tests may be required in order to make a definitive diagnosis. When the diagnosis is made, care can be planned and provided using an individual patient-centred approach.

So far

Palpation and inspection are required in order to assess the oral cavity. The nurse must also assess the lymph nodes of the head and neck so as to confirm a diagnosis and to plan care working in partnership with the patient.

Maurice Samuda (Father)

Maurice has a history of Crohn's disease (an immune system disorder), he has been admitted to hospital with what he calls a 'flare up'. he was discharged three weeks ago after being diagnosed with a 'heart attack'. When the nurse is assessing Maurice's needs, he confides in her that things at home are tense and he has not been coping as well as he can, and the Crohn's has been agony and embarrassing. He tells the nurse that life is not so good, the nurse actively listens. Maurice has a sight hand tremor, he is sweating, and his breath smells of what the nurse thinks is alcohol.

As the assessment progresses and Maurice is more relaxed, the nurse asks, in a matter of fact way, as part of the assessment process, about alcohol consumption. The nurse asks if Maurice drinks alcohol (in a non-critical/judgemental way). Maurice says he does drink, and she asks him what he drinks and in an average week how much he drinks.

The quantity of alcohol that Maurice drank in an average week was calculated into units:

- One unit is 10 mL or 8 g of pure alcohol.

One unit is contained in one small glass of wine (76 mL), half a pint of beer or lager (250 mL), standard cider (218 mL), a standard alcopop (275 mL), or one standard measure of spirits (25 mL).

To avoid health risks caused by alcohol, the UK Chief Medical Officer's advice is not to drink more than 14 units a week on a regular basis. If a person regularly drinks as much as 14 units per week, it is best to advise them to spread drinking evenly over three or more days. Having several free drink days per week can help if a person wants to cut down the amount they drink. There is no safe level of drinking.

Maurice tells the nurse he drinks more now than he used to, around two to three bottles of wine a week. He enjoys whisky chasers when he has a few pints of lager a night (he confirmed this was around three to four pints a night) but he says he is now drinking cider more as its cheaper than lager and he drinks at home before going to the pub as its cheaper buying it from the supermarket. He reveals that he often has a quick 'snifter' in the morning before going into work and a drink before coming home 'to the bedlam that is there', 'I feel ashamed of that and I know I should be cutting down, but sometimes the hair of the dog helps me cope.' He tells the nurse, 'I get ratty as well with people for no reason, even if a mate says "take it easy" with the booze and I know they mean well.'

Calculate Maurice's average weekly alcoholic intake in units based on what he has shared with the nurse during the assessment.

CAGE (Ewing 1984) is an assessment tool that can be used to help determine if a patient's use of alcohol is a cause for concern

Description	Question
Concern by the person that there is a problem	Have you ever felt you should **c**ut down in your drinking?
Apparent to others that there is a problem.	Have you ever become **a**nnoyed by criticisms of your drinking?
Grave consequences	Have you ever felt **g**uilty about your drinking?
Evidence of dependence or tolerance	Have you ever had a morning **e**ye-opener to get rid of a hangover?

Two 'yes' responses would indicate there is possibility of alcoholism and this should be investigated further.

Undertake an assessment of Maurice's use of alcohol using CAGE and determine if it might be a cause for concern.

Another assessment tool, this tool is more sensitive than CAGE and is more complex to use, is the fast alcohol screening tool (FAST) (Hodgson et al. 2002). FAST is an alcohol harm assessment tool, consisting of a subset of questions from the full alcohol use disorders identification test (AUDIT). The FAST tool was developed for use in emergency departments. However, there are a number of health and social care settings where it can be used.

What local agencies (voluntary and statutory) might be of use to Maurice to help him manage his drinking?

Conclusion

Immunology is the study of the immune system and its effects on the body and on invading micro-organisms. However, the immune system does more than just protect the body from invasion by micro-organisms, and it is linked to many different organs and cells of the body. The immune system is an intricate system of cells, enzymes, and proteins, which together protect the body by making it resistant and immune to infection by micro-organisms.

Inflammation is the body's protective response against infection. The cells of the immune system travel to the site of injury or infection and cause inflammation. The four signs of inflammation include warmth, redness, swelling, and pain. Long-term inflammatory conditions include asthma, colitis, and Crohn's disease, arthritis, vasculitis, and nephritis. There are many different types of cells involved in the immune system, including lymphocytes, antibodies, and proteins secreted from B-cells, neutrophils, monocytes, eosinophils, and basophils. Infection is concerned with the invasion and multiplication of a pathogen within the body and inflammation is the protective response that the body makes against infection. Inflammation is a complex process that involves several types of immune cells, clotting proteins, and signalling molecules, all of which change over time.

Viral and bacterial infections, irritants and injuries, cause most sore throats and most get better in a few days without treatment. Sore throat is a common symptom. A structured approach to the consultation, history taking, and physical examination of those whose chief complaint is a sore throat will lead to an effective and efficient diagnosis and treatment plan.

References

Addey, D. and Shephard, A. (2012). Incidence, causes, severity and treatment of throat discomfort: a four-region online questionnaire survey. *BMC Ear, Nose and Throat Disorders* 12:19. https://doi.org/10.1186/1472-6815-12-9.

Ewing, J.A. (1984). Detecting alcoholism. The CAGE questionnaire. *Journal of the American Medical Association* 252 (14): 1905–1907.

Green, S. (2015). Assessment and management of acute sore throat. *Practice Nurse* 26 (10): 480–486.

Hodgson, R., Alwyn, T., John, B. et al. (2002). The fast alcohol screening tool. *Alcohol and Alcoholism* 37 (1): 61–66.

Kannan, I. (2016). *Essential of Microbiology for Nurses*. St Louis: Elsevier.

Kenealy, T. (2014). Sore throat. *BMJ Clinical Evidence* 2014: 1509.

Little, P., Stuart, B., Hobbs, F.D. et al. (2014). Antibiotic prescription strategies for acute sore throat: a prospective observational cohort study. *The Lancet: Infectious Disease* 14 (3): 213–219. https://doi.org/10.1016/S1473-3099(13)70294-9.

Lord, K., Kausher, I., Kumar, S. et al. (2013). Are depressive symptoms more common among British south Asian patients compared with British white patients with cancer? A cross-sectional survey. *BMJ Open* 3 (6): e002650.

Silverman, J., Kurtz, S., and Draper, J. (2014). *Skills for Communicating with Patients*, 3e. London: Radcliffe.

Vickers, P. (2007) Section 1: Anatomy and physiology of the immune system. In Immunology/Immunodeficiency's Antibody Defence. CD-ROM. Baxter, 3–51.

Vickers, P. (2017). The immune system. In: *Fundamentals of Anatomy and Physiology for Nursing and Healthcare Students*, 2e (ed. I. Peate and M. Nair), 513–550. Oxford: Wiley.

Ward, D. (2016). *Microbiology and Infection Prevention and Control for Nursing Students*. London: Learning Matters.

Wilson, J. and Nicol, F. (2013). The ear, nose and throat. In: *Macleod's Clinical Examination*, 13e (ed. G. Douglas, F. Nicol and C. Robertson), 297–314. Edinburgh: Elsevier.

Chapter 20

Assessing the skin

Aim

This chapter introduces the reader to the assessment of the skin and the care required for those who experience problems related to the skin.

Learning outcomes

By the end of the chapter the reader will be able to:

1. Provide a brief overview of the skin and its functions
2. Discuss a number of conditions that might affect the skin
3. Outline the various ways in which the nurse may undertake an assessment of the skin
4. Describe care planning that is related to the skin

Introduction

This chapter provides the reader with an overview of the anatomy and physiology of the skin, offering an understanding of the structures and functions of the skin and the related assessment. If the nurse understands the fundamental structures and functions of the skin, along with common assessment techniques, this can help the nurse to provide care for patients in an effective and patient-centred way.

The skin is a complex organ system that performs a variety of important activities. The skin acts as a protective barrier offering a defence against external organisms: it maintains temperature control (thermoregulation), assists in the sensing of our surroundings, removes waste products, and synthesises Vitamin D.

The skin

Shier et al. (2013) suggest that the skin is one of the more versatile organs of the body. The skin is often referred to as the integumentary system and is made up of the hair, nails, and skin, providing the body with an external cover, acting as a divider between the organs of the body and the external environment. The skin is the largest organ of the body and weighs 2.7–3.6 kg, with an average surface area of 1.9m² (Stephens 2018). It has many functions which are related to the structures that make up the layers of the skin. The skin has the ability to allow a person to experience pleasure, pain, and other stimuli from the external environment.

Fundamentals of Assessment and Care Planning for Nurses, First Edition. Ian Peate.
© 2020 John Wiley & Sons Ltd. Published 2020 by John Wiley & Sons Ltd.

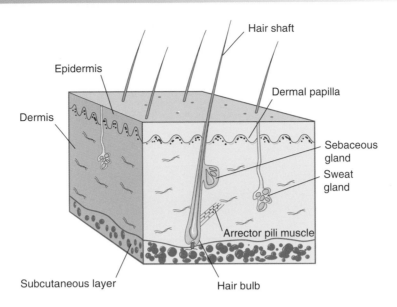

Figure 20.1   The components of the skin.

The skin accounts for around 15% of the total adult body weight and is composed of specialist cells and structures. The skin is continuous, with the mucous membranes that line the surface of the body. The skin and its derivatives, the hair, nails, sweat, and oil glands make up the integumentary system. The skin is composed of three layers:

- Epidermis
- Dermis
- Subcutaneous tissue

See Figure 20.1 for the components of the skin.

Throughout the body the skin's characteristics vary: the head for instance, contains more hair follicles than anywhere else, but the soles of the feet contain none. The thickness of the layers of the skin varies depending on where in the body this is located. The eyelids have the thinnest layer of the epidermis, this measures less than 0.1 mm. However, the palms of the hands and soles of the feet have the thickest epidermal layer, measuring approximately 1.5 mm. On the back the dermis is at its thickest – it is around 30–40 times as thick as the overlying epidermis (Jenkins et al. 2013). Skin type is another characteristic associated with the skin. The skin is constantly renewed. In relation to the other organs of the body, the skin has the ability to uncover a number of dysfunctions or pathologies.

The skin is composed of two distinct regions: the dermis and the epidermis. The subcutaneous facia (also known as the hypodermis) lies under the dermis. These masses of loose connective and adipose tissue attach to the skin and organs beneath; they are not part of the skin.

The epidermis

The superficial and thinnest aspect of the skin, the epidermis is the area of skin that can most commonly be seen. Whilst the skin covers the whole of the body, there are several regional distinctions, and these are associated with flexibility, distribution, and type of hair, density and types of gland, pigmentation, vascularity, innervations, and thickness (Jenkins et al. 2013).

The epidermis is composed of epithelium, called keratinised stratified squamous epithelium, containing four key cell types (see Figure 20.2):

- Keratinocytes
- Melanocytes
- Langerhans cells
- Merkel cells

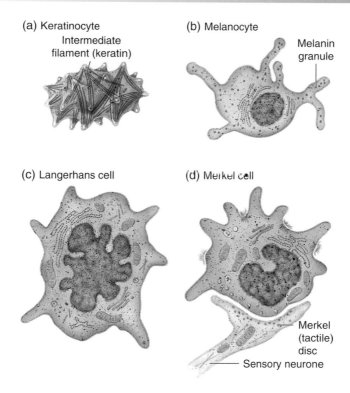

Figure 20.2 Types of cells in the epidermis.

Layers of the epidermis

Just as there are two distinct layers of skin – the dermis and epidermis – there are also a number of distinct layers of keratinocytes. Over time these layers are developed and form the epidermis. These layers are called strata and are only visible microscopically (see Figure 20.3). The superficial and deeper levels of the skin are:

- Stratum basale
- Stratum spinosum
- Stratum granulosum
- Stratum lucidum
- Stratum corneum

Table 20.1 discusses the microscopic layers.

The dermis

The dermis is the deepest aspect of the skin situated directly below the epidermis; it is composed mainly of dense connective tissue containing collagen and elastic fibres. Within the dermis are:

- Blood vessels
- Nerve
- Lymph vessels
- Smooth muscles
- Sweat glands
- Hair follicles
- Sebaceous glands

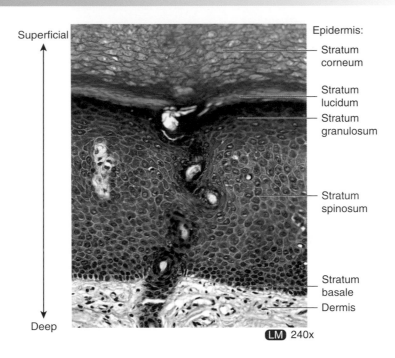

Superficial
Deep

Epidermis:
Stratum corneum
Stratum lucidum
Stratum granulosum
Stratum spinosum
Stratum basale
Dermis

LM 240x

Figure 20.3   Microscopic layers of the skin with various strata.

Table 20.1   The layers of the epidermis.

Layer	Location	Description
Stratum basale (sometimes called the basal cell layer)	The deepest layer	Cuboidal cells that are arranged as a single row; these divide and grow. The stratum basale also contains melanocytes.
Stratum spinosum	Above the stratum basale and below the stratum granulosum	These keratinocytes are tightly packed, flat, and have spine-like projections.
Stratum granulosum	Under the stratum corneum	Flattened cells arranged in approximately three to five layers. Protect the body from losing fluid and also protect from harm. Compact brittle cells as they lose their nucleus.
Stratum lucidum	When present, situated between the stratum corneum and the stratum granulosum	These cells are not present on the soles and palms. The cells have no nucleus and are tightly packed.
Stratum corneum	The most superficial of layers	Several layers of keratinised, dead epithelial cells. These cells are flattened and have no nucleus.

The elastic system associated with the dermis supports the components above, as well as allowing the skin to flex with movement and to return to its normal shape when at rest. The dermis can be divided into two layers:

- The papillary aspect
- The reticular aspect

The surface area of the dermis is much increased due to the projectile-like papillary layers; the papillary layers connect the dermis to the epidermis. The deeper aspect of the dermis is attached to the subcutaneous layer.

The accessory skin structures

The accessory structures are also known as the appendages. The following accessory structures of the skin will be outlined in this section of the chapter:

- Hair
- Skin glands
- Nails

The hair

Hair is found on most surfaces of the body apart from the palms, soles, and lips; the amount, its distribution, the colour and texture will vary depending on location, gender, age, and ethnic group. There are different types of hair, and the earliest type is distinctive at approximately the fifth month of foetal development. Known as lanugo, it is a very fine, downy, non-pigmented hair, covering the body of the foetus. Just prior to birth the lanugo of the eyelashes, eyebrows and scalp is shed and replaced by coarse hair, longer in length and heavily pigmented.

Hair colour is influenced by the melanocytes located in the hair bulb. Hair growth is determined by genetic and hormonal factors. Hairs are growths of dead keratin; each hair is a thread of keratin, formed from cells at the base of a single follicle (Timby 2016).

The key role of hair is to inhibit heat loss. The whole of the skin surface has hair follicles; each pore is an opening to a follicle located deep in the dermis on top of the subcutaneous layer. When heat leaves the body through the skin it becomes trapped in the air between the hairs. Each gland has attached to it a small smooth muscle called the arrector pili. These muscles contract becoming erect in response to cold, fear, and emotion. Contraction of the muscle can be seen on the skin in the form of 'goosebumps'.

Sebaceous glands accompany the hair follicles and sebum is exuded by these glands, lubricating the skin and at the same time ensuring that the skin and hair are waterproof as well as removing waste (e.g. old dead cells). Sebum is a slightly acidic substance and has antibacterial and antifungal properties. Sebaceous are foremost on the scalp, face, upper torso, and anogenital region. Figure 20.4 shows a pilosebaceous unit; this is made up of the follicle, the hair shaft, the sebaceous gland, and the arrector pili. The base of the onion-shaped bulb – the follicle – contains blood vessels, providing nourishment for the developing hair.

369

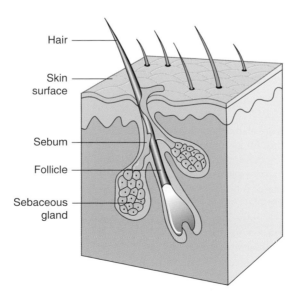

Figure 20.4   A pilosebaceous gland.

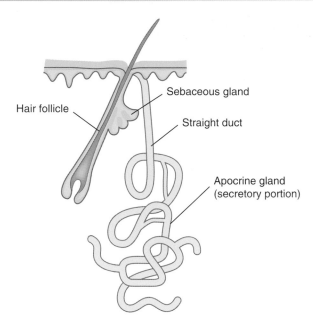

Figure 20.5   A sweat gland.

Skin glands

There are several glands located within the skin; these can be thought of as mini-organs of the skin which have a number of functions to carry out. The sweat glands are coiled tubes composed of epithelial tissue and open out to pores that are located on the skin surface (see Figure 20.5). All of the glands have separate nerve and blood supplies secreting a slightly acidic fluid made up of water and salts. There are two kinds of sweat gland: eccrine and apocrine.

Eccrine glands

Reaction to heat and fear and the production of secretions by the eccrine glands occur in response to activity of the sympathetic nervous system. These types of glands are located all over the body; there are, however, sites on the body where they are more numerous, for example the forehead, axillae, soles, and palms. The primary function of the eccrine glands is associated with thermoregulation. This is accomplished through the cooling effect of the evaporation of sweat on the surface of the skin.

Apocrine glands

The apocrine glands are also coiled; there are not as many as the eccrine glands and they are found in more localised sites, for example the pubic and axillary areas, the nipples and perineum. These glands are not fully active until the person reaches puberty; they are larger, deeper, and produce thicker secretions than the eccrine glands.

There are a number of modified types of apocrine glands (specialised types), for example those that are seen on the eyelids, the cerumen-producing glands of the external auditory canal, and the milk-producing glands of the breasts.

The apocrine glands first develop on the soles and palms, gradually appearing all over the body. It is understood that they secrete pheromones; released into the external environment, enabling communication through the sense of smell with other members of the species, provoking a number of reactions, including a sexual arousal reaction. A viscous material is excreted, resulting in body odour when activated by surface bacteria.

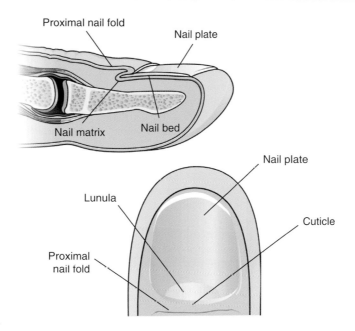

Figure 20.6   The nail.

Nails

The nails provide a protective covering for the ends of the fingers and the toes. Nails are tightly packed, dead, hard, keratinised epidermal cells that form a clean, solid covering over the digits (see Figure 20.6).

The horn-like structure of the nails is a result of the concentrated amount of keratin present; there are no nerve endings in nails. The majority of the nail body is pink, a result of the blood capillaries lying underneath. The white crescent present at the proximal ends of the nail, the lunula is formed by air mixed with keratin matrix. The cuticle (also called the eponychium) is stratum corneum extending over the proximal end of the nail body.

There are a number of factors that will influence the growth, for example the age of the individual, the time of year, the amount of exercise undertaken, as well as hereditary factors (Haneke 2006). The growth of nails can be delayed by trauma and inflammation; changes in the integrity of the nails can be caused by injury or infection. In some cases, evidence of systemic diseases can be identified by the condition of the nails, for example chronic cardiopulmonary disease or fungal infection (Timby 2016).

The functions of the skin

The nurse must have an understanding of the structure of the skin so as to understand the skin's various functions and to ensure that care provision is safe and effective.

Sensation

Receptor sites on the skin have the ability to sense change in the external environment with regard to temperature and pressure; these receptors situated throughout the skin are made up of a range of nerve endings. The messages picked up in the skin are then usually transferred to the brain.

Sensations that arise in the skin are known as cutaneous sensations; other sensations are those related to vibration, tickling, and irritations. There are some areas of the body that have more sensory receptors than others, such as the lips, genitalia, and tips of the fingers. The sensation of pain can signify actual or potential tissue injury.

Thermoregulation

The skin maintains homeostasis through thermoregulation, helping to keep the temperature of the body within narrow ranges, adapting and adjusting as the person engages in a number of different activities. Effective thermoregulation is essential for survival; temperature changes can influence alteration in the function of enzymes and this can impact on the chemical make-up of cells. The skin acts as a temperature regulator through a range of complex and integrated activities.

Changes to the size of blood vessels in the skin can help to regulate temperature. As body temperature rises, so the blood vessels dilate (vasodilation) this is a multifaceted bodily defence mechanism that strives to get hot blood from the deeper tissues beneath to the surface of the skin for cooling down: the surface of the skin is cooler, as heat radiates away from the body. As this occurs, the sweat glands secrete water onto the surface of the skin, evaporation occurs, and as a result of this, so too does cooling. The opposite occurs when the person is in a cold environment. The blood vessels constrict (vasoconstriction) and blood stays closer to the core of the body, preserving heat.

The hair plays an important part in thermoregulation. Pockets of air are trapped in the hair when the arrector pili are stimulated to contract, making the hairs stand up. The trapped air causes insulation, insulating the surrounding environment on the skin from the cooler atmosphere.

Protection

There are several ways the skin protects the body, for example the skin's ability to produce melanin, counteracting the harmful effects of ultraviolet light. Through its ability to intensify normal cell replacement when required and the ability to shed dead skin and causing the migration of cells, the skin maintains the integrity of the body. Wound healing is an example of how the skin provides protective mechanisms.

The skin protects the body from a build-up of poisonous substances as its eliminate waste products through its pores. The skin has the ability to help prevent body fluids from escaping, preventing dehydration and regulating the amount of fluid through the content and volume of sweat that is produced. As a waterproof barrier, the skin can also ensure that harmful fluids in the environment are prevented from entering the body.

Sebum contains bacterial chemicals that have the ability to destroy surface bacteria. When sweat is produced, the acidic pH has the potential to hamper the proliferation of bacteria. Phagocytic macrophages present in the dermis ingest and destroy viruses and bacteria that have penetrated the skin's surface.

Excretion and absorption

The skin has the ability to excrete substances from the body; sweat is composed of water, sodium, carbon dioxide, ammonia, and urea. Jenkins et al. (2013) notes that the body (despite its almost waterproof nature) can excrete approximately 400 mL of water daily; those leading a less active lifestyle will lose less, and a more active person will lose more.

The skin also has the ability to absorb substances from the environment. Materials are absorbed from the external environment into the body cells, and some of these substances when absorbed are toxic, for example heavy metals such as lead and mercury. There are some therapeutic and non-therapeutic medications that can be absorbed through the skin. A number of fat-soluble vitamins A, D, E and K, oxygen, and carbon dioxide are also absorbed.

Vitamin D synthesis

The skin is actively involved in the production and synthesis of vitamin D. For vitamin D to synthesise effectively, activation of a precursor molecule in the skin by ultraviolet rays in the sunlight (ultraviolet radiation) is needed. Enzymes that are present in the kidneys and liver alter the molecules, producing calcitriol. Calcitriol (a hormone) assists with the absorption of calcium found in food in the intestines into the blood.

A storage reservoir

The skin acts as a storage reservoir as 8–10% of total circulating blood flow is accommodated in the skin. The skin also stores fats as adipose tissue and water (Stephens 2018).

Psychological

The skin can be seen as sexually attractive and plays an important role as regards self-image (Gawkrodger 2013).

So far

The skin is an exceptional organ. It is also known as the integumentary system and is the largest organ in the body in weight and surface area. The skin has the ability to reveal how we are feeling and what emotional state we may be in: humans blush, sweat, and tremble.

This organ is the interface between the external and internal environments. The skin contributes to homeostasis and the physical changes noted can point to homeostatic imbalance. The skin is also composed of the accessory structures; the nails, hair, and a number of glands; these are called the appendages.

Assessing the skin

Skin assessment can occur using subjective and objective data, taking the form of a health care history and full physical assessment of a patient. Lawton (2016) notes that the principles of taking a comprehensive history apply. However, for patients presenting with a skin problem there are also specific questions which will need to be explored. The nurse needs to obtain a detailed history of the patient's skin condition, an overall assessment of the patient, an assessment of the patient's knowledge and understanding, and a systematic physical assessment.

There is no other organ in the body as easily inspected or palpated as the skin. The skin is also more easily exposed to injury, for example infection and trauma. There are a variety of diseases or injuries that can easily be observed on the surface of the skin, for example a skin rash, the presence of jaundice, or cyanosis.

Cultural considerations

There are important differences in presentation of dermatological disorders in dark skin as opposed to light skin. Nurses must be aware of the differences in dark-skin pigmentation as well as hair types, normal changes in dark skin and changes in colour and presentation related with dermatological conditions.

Source: Manning (2004).

The patient history

Assessing skin disorders is primarily undertaken thorough inspection. There are some dermatological conditions that have pathognomonic features (pathognomonic sign is a particular sign whose presence means that a specific disease is present beyond any doubt). However, obtaining a detailed health history is central to making a definitive diagnosis, obtaining the skin history can provide the nurse with important clues concerning the patient's chief complaint revealing local and systemic illness.

The most common dermatological chief complaints are pruritus, lesions (including lumps), and rash (Rhoads and Wiggins Petersen 2018; Tidman 2018). Changes in existing lesions and hair loss also feature as chief complaints.

Obtaining the history of the present illness requires the nurse to ask about lesion and rashes. Enquire about onset (initial appearance) and duration, are there single or multiple lesions, where is the lesion(s) located? Ask the patient to describe the size, shape, elevation, and colour. Is there any crusting, exudate, or pain? The nurse may ask, at this stage, to see the lesion(s)/rash. It is important to determine if there have been any changes in size, shape, elevation, and colour since onset. Determine if there are any associated symptoms pyrexia, pruritus, pain, headache, or any other systemic upset.

Take note

Exudate should be described and documented according to the colour and consistency of the fluid. Some common findings include:

- Serous (clear) or straw-coloured exudate: This is normal; however, it may indicate infection if not clear and watery.
- Fibrinous exudate: Cloudy and thin, and contains fibrin protein strands, this is normal.
- Serosanguinous exudate: Clear, pink, and watery, this is normal.
- Sanguineous exudate: Red, thin, and watery. This indicates trauma to blood vessels.
- Seropurulent exudate: Murky or yellow and thick and creamy in texture. Indicates active infection.
- Purulent exudate: Yellow/Grey/Green and thick in consistency. This indicates infection.
- Haemopurulent exudate: Dark, blood-stained, viscous, and sticky. The exudate contains neutrophils, dead/dying bacteria and inflammatory cells. This means an established infection is present. Consequent damage to dermal capillaries will lead to blood leakage.
- Haemorrhagic exudate: Red, thick, and usually infected, caused by trauma. Capillaries break down easily and spontaneous bleeding occurs. Haemorrhagic exudate is not to be confused with bloody exudate produced by excessive debridement.

Has there been any previous trauma to the skin, any malignancy, exposure to chemicals, irritants, has the patient eaten any new foods recently? What is the person's current medication regimen? These are known as precipitating factors.

The patient may tell you what it is that is aggravating the chief complaint. They may also inform you of factors that alleviate the complaint, this can be over-the-counter medications (creams or gels) or prescribed medications.

The past medical history is an important aspect of the health history for dermatological conditions just as it is for other conditions. Information gained at this stage can reveal recurrences or flare up of the condition any triggers or patterns (see Table 20.2).

The family and social history must also be given consideration. A number of skin disorders are familial or genetic. Explore family history with the patient gather data concerning parents, siblings, causes of deaths in the family and any chronic diseases or skin disorders. Gawkrodger (2013) comments that a family history is found in 10% of patients with malignant melanoma, psoriasis, and atopic eczema also have inherited traits. The social history provides information that will add to the data already amassed. What is the patient's occupation, jobs that result in prolonged sun exposure will increase cancer risk. Occupations that expose the employee to chemical contact, exposure to latex gloves and other chemicals may cause contact dermatitis, these are risk factors that should be noted and reported upon. Ask about hobbies and any chemicals that the person may have encountered. Does the patient smoke, ascertain what they smoke and how much (smoking can suppress the immune system and as such can inhibit the body's ability to repair cell damage)? Does the person drink alcohol? If so, how much and what is consumed? Use of amphetamines recreationally can cause skin-related problems such as dry, itchy skin. Ask about any foreign travel, consider tropical infections.

Table 20.2   The past medical history.

Surgery, past health	Any recent surgery? Surgery interrupts the natural defence of the skin providing conditions that can result in inflammation and infection. Immunodeficiency, endocrine dysfunction and thromboembolism can modify treatment of the skin
Skin, nail, hair conditions	Is there a history of skin cancer? Are there any nail, hair conditions. If so, what is the treatment?
Sunlight tolerance	Intolerance to sunlight puts the person at a higher risk of skin cancer. Is there any history of sunburn?
Allergy testing	Does the person have any allergy, has there been a test for allergies

Table 20.3 outlines questions to consider when asking a patient about a skin condition in relation to hair and nails.

Table 20.3   Questions to ask a patient in relation to hair and nails.

Hair	What recent changes in hair have occurred?
	Is there excessive hair loss, thinning, or baldness?
	Has the distribution of hair changed across the body?
	Has there been a recent change in hair products?
	Has the patient recently commenced a diet?
	Has there been an increase in hair growth (hirsutism), where?
Nails	What recent changes in the nails have occurred?
	Is there any splitting, breakage, or discolouration?
	Are there visible signs of infection?
	Have there been recent changes to the diet, dieting, or exposure to chemicals?

Source: Stephens (2018).

Take note

When detecting colour variation in dark skinned people refer to the table below.

Cyanosis	Inspect the person's conjunctiva, palms, soles, buccal mucosa and tongue. Look for a dark, dull colour
Erythema	Feel the area for warmth, take off gloves
Jaundice	Examine the sclera and hard palate. Look for a yellow colour
Pallor	Examine the sclera, buccal mucosa, tongue, lips, nail beds, palms, and soles. Look for any pale, ashen colour
Petechiae	Identify areas of lighter pigmentation, for example the abdomen, and examine these. Look for pinprick, tiny purplish red spots
Rashes	Palpate the area for changes in skin textures

Source: Adapted Clark (2010).

So far

The nurse is required to undertake a comprehensive, holistic health assessment of the person with a skin disorder. Collecting subjective data is the first stage. Amongst other things the nurse asks the person when it was that they first noticed the commencement of the skin disorder, how long they have had it, how often it occurs or recurs, what are the characteristics of the skin disorder, what route the disorder has taken, the severity of the skin disorder, any factors that precipitate or predispose the patient to the chief complaint. The nurse must also ascertain if there is a family history of the condition, if anything relieves the disorder (pharmacological and non-pharmacological), and if there are any related symptoms.

Physical examination

After the subjective data collecting phase has been completed, the nurse then moves the focus of the interview to undertaking a physical examination in order to gain a holistic understanding of the patient and their skin disorder.

Stephens (2018) suggests that examination of the skin is made up of a general assessment and a physical skin assessment. This can be part of a total assessment or a focused assessment for those people with a known or suspected problem.

The nurse should give consideration to the place in which the examination is to be undertaken as the patient may be requested to remove clothing, it is necessary to ensure an explanation is provided to why this is necessary. The area chosen for the examination will have bright natural light, it should be private and warm.

Curtains should be closed, dignity should be maintained, and as clothing will be removed a gown should be worn by the patient so as not to unnecessarily expose areas of the body that do not need revealing. Depending on where the skin disorder is, the patient may be assessed standing, sitting, or lying down. The nurse may be required to assist the patient into these positions and provide them with explanations and instructions. Personal protective equipment should be worn when assessing open lesions, infections, infestations, or when wounds or mucous membranes are oozing discharge, local policy and procedure must be followed. Some lesions may need measuring or photographing, others require close visualisation. Equipment required for the physical examination include:

- Gloves
- A good light source
- Magnifying glass
- A transparent ruler
- Measuring grids
- Tape measures
- Consent forms for photography

Inspection

Some elements of inspection may have been undertaken during the health interview. The skin conveys much information about the patient and this can often reflect their health status. Often the general appearance denotes the patient's self-caring abilities and the patient's mental and emotional state of mind.

One of the most essential aspects of a physical assessment is the opportunity to touch the patient and their skin. The nurse must always gain the patient's consent. The examination should take place in a clinical area with bright natural light. The patient may be embarrassed and uncomfortable on first meeting the nurse and the therapeutic nurse relationship comes to the fore, a chaperone must be provided.

The ability to touch the skin can tell the nurse much about the patient and their skin disorder. The nurse gathers information about the colour of the person's skin both in relation to ethnicity and the chief complaint, the texture and skin temperature, moisture, turgor, and presence of oedema. Other findings, for example scars, missing digits and limbs, and the presence of any open wounds, should be noted. The nurse assesses the distribution, character, and shape of lesions, the site and location as in Table 20.4.

When reporting on skin finding the nurse must be descriptive and specific about what is being observed. Notes should be taken of the size, shape, configuration, colour, texture, elevation, depression, and pedunculation (with or without a stalk). The nurse should be aware that secondary lesions may be superimposed on the primary lesions concealing identification hand magnification may be needed to help with identification. Figure 20.7 provides an overview of the terminology used with primary lesions and Figure 20.8 terminology used with secondary lesions.

Table 20.4   Character, distribution, and shape of lesions; questions to ask.

Character	Is there any redness, scaling, crusting, exudate? Are there excoriations, blisters, erosions, pustules, papules? Are the lesions all the same (monomorphic), for example a drug rash or variable (polymorphic) such as chickenpox?
Shape	Are the lesions small, large, ring-shaped, linear? Does it have a border, is it flat, fluid-filled, indurated?
Distribution	Is the disorder on the hands, feet, extremities of ears and nose, in areas exposed to light exposed or mostly confined to the trunk? Is the distribution localised or widespread. If widespread, is it symmetrical and is this central or peripheral? Is the disorder linear, regional (in a groin) or follows a dermatomal pattern such a shingles?

Source: Adapted Stephens (2018).

Table 20.5 offers a guide to examination.

Review

Describe and draw the following lesion configurations:

Lesion configuration	Description	Illustrate/draw
Discrete		
Annular		
Grouped		
Polycyclic		
Confluent		
Arciform		
Linear		
Reticular		

377

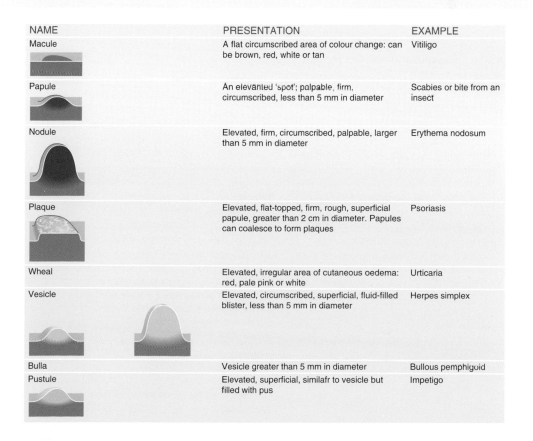

NAME	PRESENTATION	EXAMPLE
Macule	A flat circumscribed area of colour change: can be brown, red, white or tan	Vitiligo
Papule	An elevated 'spot'; palpable, firm, circumscribed, less than 5 mm in diameter	Scabies or bite from an insect
Nodule	Elevated, firm, circumscribed, palpable, larger than 5 mm in diameter	Erythema nodosum
Plaque	Elevated, flat-topped, firm, rough, superficial papule, greater than 2 cm in diameter. Papules can coalesce to form plaques	Psoriasis
Wheal	Elevated, irregular area of cutaneous oedema: red, pale pink or white	Urticaria
Vesicle	Elevated, circumscribed, superficial, fluid-filled blister, less than 5 mm in diameter	Herpes simplex
Bulla	Vesicle greater than 5 mm in diameter	Bullous pemphigoid
Pustule	Elevated, superficial, similafr to vesicle but filled with pus	Impetigo

Figure 20.7 Terminology used with primary lesions.

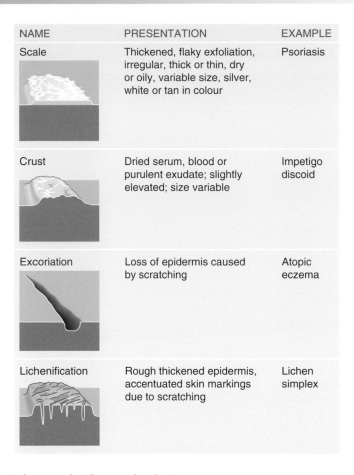

NAME	PRESENTATION	EXAMPLE
Scale	Thickened, flaky exfoliation, irregular, thick or thin, dry or oily, variable size, silver, white or tan in colour	Psoriasis
Crust	Dried serum, blood or purulent exudate; slightly elevated; size variable	Impetigo discoid
Excoriation	Loss of epidermis caused by scratching	Atopic eczema
Lichenification	Rough thickened epidermis, accentuated skin markings due to scratching	Lichen simplex

Figure 20.8   Terminology used with secondary lesions.

Table 20.5   A guide to skin examination.

Activity	Reasoning
Observe general skin colour	Abnormal findings can include regions of colour change; pallor, cyanosis, erythema
Identify morphology (the form or structure) of the lesion noting type of lesion, size, colour, shape, elevation arrangement and if needed use hand magnification, measure the lesion with the use of a transparent ruler if appropriate.	Identification and classification of a patient's skin lesion is an important step in making a diagnosis, it is the core of the dermatological diagnosis. Using the correct terminology to describe skin findings is essential for documenting findings and for communication with other clinicians. Differential diagnosis can be made when a critical assessment of the lesion is undertaken considering size and elevation, colour and arrangement.
Observe for any regional involvement and distribution	Where is the lesion found? Many skin conditions have a preference for a special area, for example in the folds of skin, head and neck, chest and back. Note: If the condition is localised, generalised, discrete, or confluent (does the lesion join up or run together, merge or form a patch).

Source: Adapted Rhoads and Wiggins Petersen (2018), Stephens (2018).

Review

A lesion refers to any single area of altered skin, it can be solitary or multiple. A rash is a widespread eruption of lesions. Dermatosis is a term that is used for a disease of the skin. Dermatological terminology can appear overwhelming at first, but adding to your dermatological vocabulary will help you better help those you offer care to.

Define the following terms:

Granuloma

Fungating

Excoriation

Exudate

Lichenification

Psoriasiform

Maceration

Vesicle

Bulla

Plaque

Sessile

After the skin has been examined the nurse should undertake an assessment of the hair and nails. Inspect the person's hair, explaining to the patient the rationale for this. Observe the colour, texture, and distribution. Note and record any scale and erythema of the scalp. Excessive hair in females is hirsutism and occurs in regions where males usually have hair:

- Beard
- Moustache
- Upper back
- Shoulders
- Sternum
- Axillae
- Pubis

Causes of hirsutism may be related to endocrinology disorders and may also be classed as idiopathic. Alopecia areata can be described an auto-immune disorder and can occur when a person has a medical condition and the hair falls out in round patches. It is a chronic inflammatory condition (British Association of Dermatologists 2012). Alopecia totalis refers to loss of scalp hair and alopecia universalis is where there is a total hair loss all over the body

Inspect the person's nails. Observe for consistency/texture, is there any separation of the plate from the nail bed? The nail surface should be smooth and consistent. Determine if there are any signs of fungal infection. The nail should be translucent in colour, changes in colour may indicate infection. Undertake and note the results of a capillary refill test

Visualisation provides the nurse with much information about the person's skin, it is the most used assessment technique. Palpation of the skin can also help to make a diagnosis. When using palpation, the nurse should use gloves wherever there is open skin. When testing skin turgor, the nurse must explain to the patient what the test is for and how it will be carried out. Gently pinch the patient's skin between the thumb and the forefinger and then release it; the skin should spring back into place. If the skin does not spring back into place, this may be an indication of dehydration.

When the examination is complete the nurse may be required to assist the patient to change from the gown into their clothes. Wash hands, report, and document findings as per local policy and procedure. A body map should be used to document findings. There are several ways in which the

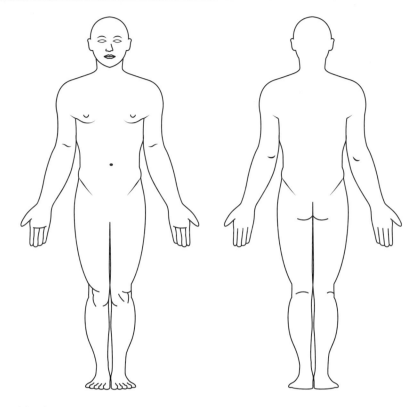

Figure 20.9   A body map.

nurse can make a correlation of patient reporting and clinical presentation of lesions. Computerised digital imaging systems and total body mapping photography can aid in lesion cataloguing, as this captures visual lesion characteristics and helps in objective monitoring of lesions (Skripnik Lucas et al. 2016). A basic line-drawn body map may also be effective (see Figure 20.9).

Findings based on the patient history and physical examination can assist the nurse in making a diagnosis and then formulate an individual plan of care for the patient. The findings can also assist in the ordering of further tests and investigations if a definitive diagnosis needs confirmation.

As the skin is the largest organ in the body and the one most commonly looked at by nurses, other healthcare professionals and other people, the impact of a skin disorder on a patient's life and their family can be significant. Emotional trauma can occur from the development of a number of skin conditions, Weller et al. (2015) suggest that these include psoriasis, atopic eczema, discoid eczema, alopecia areata and urticaria. The impact of emotional trauma can lead to stress, low self-esteem, social isolation, depression and in some cases suicide. Self-image and quality of life can be severely affected by a skin disorder as the scarring can be both physical and psychological, such as that witnessed in acne vulgaris in teenagers (Thomas 2005). It must also be remembered that psychological illnesses, for example depression, anxiety, and stress, have the potential to trigger or exacerbate a dermatological disorder. Stephens (2018) notes that within psychodermatology four groupings have been identified (see Table 20.6).

So far

Making a diagnosis in a patient with a skin disorder requires the nurse to predominantly inspect the skin. The physical examination and the recording of data must be undertaken in a systematic manner, the nurse must be specific and descriptive about skin findings (this also includes nails and hair).

Once secondary and primary data have been collected a diagnosis can usually be made. However, in order to make a definitive diagnosis there may be a need to order further tests and investigations.

Table 20.6   Psychodermatology.

Psychophysiological	Emotional stress causing inflammatory skin reactions
Primary psychiatric	Self-induced injury of the skin (iatrogenic).
Secondary psychiatric	Emotional consequences developing as a result of an existing skin disease such as anxiety, anger, and depression.
Cutaneous sensory disorders	Patients with no apparent dermatological skin or medical condition present with disagreeable skin sensations such as itching, soreness and pain and negative sensory symptoms such as numbness and hypoaesthesia

Source: Stephens (2018).

Winston Higgins (Uncle)

Mr Higgins is at the GP practice being seen by the practice nurse (the practice nurse is the GP surgery's specialist nurse – dermatology).

Winston's chief complaint concerns a 'mole' on his head. Mr Higgins explains to the nurse that he has had the 'spot' for a while now about 12 months, 'It started off itchy and red and then it got sore as I was picking at it and it started weeping.' 'I put some athlete's foot cream on it to see if that would help with the itching, but it didn't.' 'For sure,' Mr Higgins tells her, 'it is getting bigger now and uglier as it is changing shape.' 'It doesn't hurt, but it won't stop weeping, can you give me some cream for it?'

The nurse takes a patient history and examines Mr Higgins and the lesion, the nurse also uses the ABCDEE approach noting the following:

Asymmetry	The naevus (mole) was symmetrical, drawing a line through the mole the two halves did not match
Boarder	The boarders of a malignant lesion are uneven. The borders on Mr Higgins mole were uneven and appeared scallop-shaped as the nurse examines the mole with a hand-held magnifying glass.
Colour	The mole consisted of a variety of colours (shades of brown, black, red, and blue)
Diameter	The nurse measured the mole using a transparent ruler and it measured 8 mm across. A benign mole has a smaller diameter.
Elevation	The lesion, it was noted, was raised from the skin.
Evolving	A malignant mole will evolve over time in shape, elevation, colour. Mr Higgins had informed the nurse that there has been changes in size, shape, and colour over time

Source: Adapted Brown et al. (2017).

The nurse conducted a systemic examination and was alert for any other lesions.

Assessment can be undertaken by using the weighted 7-point check list, if the clinician has a concern, they need to make a referral (National Institute for Health and Care Excellence [NICE] 2017). All suspicious pigmented skin lesions that score 3 points or above must be referred urgently.

Assess Mr Higgins score using the 7-point check list

Score	Feature	Mr Higgins Score
Major features of the lesion (2 points)	Change in size Irregular shape Irregular colour	
Minor features of the lesion (1 point)	Largest diameter 7 mm or more Inflammation Oozing Change in sensation	
	Total	

A referral was made for Mr Higgins using the appropriate cancer care pathway. These are detailed by NICE (2017).

What other tests and investigations may be required related to Mr Higgins' condition?

Conclusion

This chapter has provided the reader with an overview of the anatomy and physiology of the skin. Being able to identify the various functions of the anatomical structures within the skin encourages the nurse to provide care that is based on the best available evidence. Understanding the various structures and functions of the skin, as well as developing and honing assessment techniques, allows the nurse to provide care for patients and to effectively intervene when a problem arises. A systemic and structured approach to skin history and physical examination when providing care to people with skin disorders is advocated.

The skin is an exceptional organ, and is also known as the integumentary system. There are a variety of diseases or injuries that can easily be observed on the surface of the skin, for example a skin rash, the presence of jaundice, or cyanosis. It is the largest organ in the body in weight and surface area. The skin has the ability to reveal how we feel and what emotional state we may be in: humans blush, sweat, and tremble. No other organ in the body is as easily looked over or palpated as the skin; the skin is also more easily exposed to injury, for example infection and trauma.

The role of the nurse in caring for those people with skin disorders requires the use of the nursing process and in particular a detailed assessment, diagnosis, planning, implementation of realistic patient care and regular evaluation.

References

British Association of Dermatologists (2012) British Association of Dermatologists' Guidelines for the Management of Alopecia Areata 2012. www.bad.org.uk/library-media%5Cdocuments%5CAlopecia_areata_guidelines_2012.pdf (accessed October 2018).

Brown, E.R.S., Fraser, S.J., Quaba, O. et al. (2017). Cutaneous melanoma: An update SIGN. *Journal of the Royal College of Physicians Edinburgh* 47: 214–217.

Clark, M. (2010). Skin assessment in dark pigmented skin: a challenge in pressure ulcer prevention. *Nursing Times* 106 (30): 16–17.

Gawkrodger, D. (2013). The skin, hair and nails. In: *Macleod's Clinical Examination* (ed. G. Douglas, F. Nicol and C. Robertson), 63–76. Edinburgh: Elsevier.

Haneke, E. (2006). Surgical anatomy of the nail apparatus. *Dermatology Clinic* 24 (3): 291–296.

Hogan-Quigley, B., Palm, L.M., and Bickley, L.S. *Bates' Nursing Guide to Physical Examination and History Taking*, 2e. Philadelphia: Lippincott.

Jenkins, G.W., Kemnitz, C.P., and Tortora, G.J. (2013). *Anatomy and Physiology: From Science to Life*, 3e. Hoboken: Wiley.

Lawton, S. (2016). Assessing the patent with a common dermatological problem. *Primary Health Care* 26 (10): 42–48.

Manning, J. (2004). The assessment of dark skin and dermatological disorders. *Nursing Times* 100 (22): 48–50.

National Institute for Health and Care Excellence (2017) Suspected cancer recognition and referral. www.nice.org.uk/guidance/ng12/resources/suspected-cancer-recognition-and-referral-pdf-1837268071621 (accessed October 2018).

Rhoads, J. and Wiggins Petersen, S. (2018). *Advanced Health Assessment and Diagnostic Reasoning*, 3e. Burlington: Jones and Bartlett.

Shier, D., Butler, J., and Lewis, R. (2013). *Hole's Anatomy and Physiology*, 13e. Boston: McGraw Hall.

Skripnik Lucas, A., Chung, E., Marchetti, M.A., and Marghoob, A.A. (2016). A guide for dermatology nurses to assist in the early detection of skin cancer. *Journal of Nursing Education and Practice* 6 (10): 71–79. https://doi.org/10.5430/jnep.v6n10p71.

Stephens, M. (2018). The person with a skin disorder. In: *Nursing Knowledge and Practice*, 2e (ed. I. Peate and K. Wild), 909–930. Oxford: Wiley.

Thomas, D.R. (2005). Psychological effects of acne. *Journal of Cutaneous Medicine and Surgery* 8 (suppl): 3–5.

Tidman, M.J. (2018). The skin, hair and nails. In: *Macleod's Clinical Examination*, 14e (ed. J.A. Innes, A.R. Dover and K. Fairhurst), 283–293. Edinburgh: Elsevier.

Timby, B.K. (2016). *Fundamental Nursing Skills and Concepts*, 11e. Philadelphia: Wolters Kluwer.

Weller, R., Hunter, H., and Mann, M. (2015). *Clinical Dermatology*, 5e. Oxford: Wiley.

Index

Page numbers in *italic* indicate figures, tables, and boxes.